NANDA International

NURSING DIAGNOSES:
DEFINITIONS & CLASSIFICATION
2009–2011

Book Committee

T. Heather Herdman, PhD, RN, *Chair*
Crystal Heath, MSN, RN
Margaret Lunney, PhD, RN, FAAN
Leann Scroggins, MN, RN, CCRN-A, APRN BC
Barbara Vassallo, EdD, RN, CS, ANPC

NANDA International
NURSING DIAGNOSES:
DEFINITIONS & CLASSIFICATION
2009–2011

Edited by

T. Heather Herdman, PhD, RN

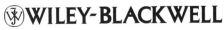

A John Wiley & Sons, Ltd., Publication

This edition first published 2009

Blackwell Publishing was acquired by John Wiley & Sons in February 2007. Blackwell's publishing programme has been merged with Wiley's global Scientific, Technical, and Medical business to form Wiley-Blackwell.

Registered office

John Wiley & Sons Ltd, The Atrium, Southern Gate, Chichester, West Sussex, PO19 8SQ, United Kingdom

Editorial offices

9600 Garsington Road, Oxford, OX4 2DQ, United Kingdom
2121 State Avenue, Ames, Iowa 50014-8300, USA

For details of our global editorial offices, for customer services and for information about how to apply for permission to reuse the copyright material in this book please see our website at www.wiley.com/wiley-blackwell.

The right of the author to be identified as the author of this work has been asserted in accordance with the Copyright, Designs and Patents Act 1988.

Wiley also publishes its books in a variety of electronic formats. Some content that appears in print may not be available in electronic books.

Designations used by companies to distinguish their products are often claimed as trademarks. All brand names and product names used in this book are trade names, service marks, trademarks or registered trademarks of their respective owners. The publisher is not associated with any product or vendor mentioned in this book. This publication is designed to provide accurate and authoritative information in regard to the subject matter covered. It is sold on the understanding that the publisher is not engaged in rendering professional services. If professional advice or other expert assistance is required, the services of a competent professional should be sought.

ISBN 978-1-4051-8718-3
ISSN 1943-0728

A catalogue record for this book is available from the British Library.

Set in 10 on 12 pt Palatino by SNP Best-set Typesetter Ltd., Hong Kong
Printed in the United States of America by Sheridan Books, Inc.

2 2009

Contents

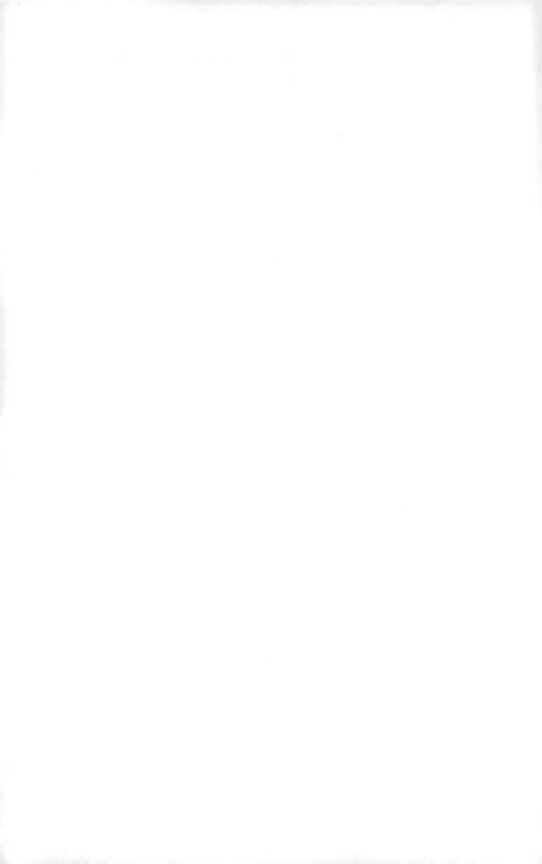

NANDA International Guidelines for Copyright Permission

The materials presented in this book are copyrighted and all copyright laws apply. Situations requiring approvals and/or copyright fees are listed below:

1. An author or publishing house requests use of the entire nursing diagnosis taxonomy in a textbook or other nursing manual to be sold.
2. An author or publishing house requests use of only the list of nursing diagnoses with no definitions or defining characteristics.
3. An author or company requests use of the nursing diagnosis taxonomy in an audiovisual material.
4. A software developer or computer-based patient record vendor requests use of the nursing diagnosis taxonomy in a program.
5. A nursing school, researcher, professional organization, or healthcare organization requests use of the nursing diagnosis taxonomy in a program.

Send all permission requests to:

Kris Kliemann
John Wiley & Sons Inc.
111 River Street
Hoboken
NJ 07030, USA

Tel: 001 201 748 6412
Email: kkliemann@wiley.com

Preface

The *2009–2011* edition marks a new look and feel for the *NANDA-I Nursing Diagnoses: Definitions & Classification* text. Perhaps the most obvious change is the physical size of the text. This change enables us to provide our readers with more content than we have previously been able to produce in the condensed "pocket size" publication. We are pleased to announce the addition of 21 new diagnoses, as well as 9 revised diagnoses. Six diagnoses have been retired from the taxonomy, but remain in an appendix within this edition to encourage users to consider revising and resubmitting those diagnoses. One diagnosis, *Disturbed Sleep Pattern*, was eliminated from the 2007–2008 edition of the *Definitions & Classification* text, and has been returned to this edition. I am especially excited to note that this edition of the *Definitions and Classification* text is the second in a row in which more than 20 new diagnoses have been added to the taxonomy. Although it is probable that all diagnoses are not used by all members, because of area of specialization, practice site, and/or cultural issues that make some diagnoses inappropriate, it is important to consider the breadth of nursing practice worldwide when accepting new diagnoses into the taxonomy.

You will notice that all of the nursing diagnosis codes are provided in parentheses following each diagnosis, along with the domain and class from the NANDA-I taxonomy of the diagnosis. We have also begun to include all submitted references for new and revised diagnoses, beginning with the previous cycle of diagnoses (2007–2008), rather than only including the three references identified by submitters as being the most critical. We believe that this will provide important information for all users, but particularly for those who may want to explore the diagnostic concept further in detail.

Other changes in this edition include the addition of a chapter by Dr Margaret Lunney on clinical judgment and assessment, and the role of each in the appropriate use of nursing diagnosis clinically. A new chapter by Leann Scroggins details the process for submission of a nursing diagnosis to NANDA-I's Diagnosis Development Committee (DDC) (originally published in the NANDA-I journal). Additional chapters provide insight on the use and applicability of nursing diagnoses within nursing education, nursing informatics, nursing research, and nursing administration. This information is offered as a brief introduction on the importance of nursing diagnoses to each of these critical areas within the nursing profession, particularly due to the increased interest being expressed by individuals in those areas who are beginning to see the need to look beyond the more obvious clinical applicability of the nursing diagnoses.

Another substantial change for the NANDA International organization is the decision to partner with Blackwell Publishing to publish and distribute the *NANDA-I Nursing Diagnoses: Definitions & Classification* worldwide. We are very excited to extend our partnership with Blackwell Publishers beyond production of our journal, *The International Journal of Nursing Terminologies and Classifications*, to include our two books: *NANDA-I Nursing Diagnoses: Definitions & Classification* and a new edition of *Critical thinking, nursing diagnoses, intervention and outcomes: Case studies and analyses*. We believe that NANDA-I will benefit greatly from the expertise provided by Blackwell Publishing, and specifically from the support in disseminating our work worldwide, and across multiple languages. We look forward to a successful partnership with Blackwell Publishing!

As a result of the increased awareness of the need for standardized nursing language to define the knowledge of nursing and to allow its presence to be captured and its effects measured through information systems, I want to encourage those of you who are not currently members of NANDA International to take the time now to join our organization. I would also ask you to encourage your colleagues – clinicians, students, administrators, educators, researchers or nurse informaticists – to join us as we continue the work of the organization. All our patients will benefit from the wisdom of the voices of nurses from a variety of practice areas and backgrounds. The Invitation to join NANDA International is found on page 428, and can be found at the NANDA-I website, www.nanda.org.

I was very encouraged during this cycle to see submissions from clinicians in practice and from nurses in several countries, including Brazil, Canada, Italy, Japan, Spain, and the USA. Without your dedication to standardized nursing language, there would be nothing to publish. We have increased the number of nursing diagnoses from 188 to 206 with this edition, but we still fall short in our efforts to describe the richness of nursing practice – the time is now, and your efforts in this regard can move us closer to the ability to describe nursing practice across site, patient population, and culture. I encourage you to review the chapter by Leann Scroggins, and commit to work on at least one diagnosis this year. Don't hesitate to contact the DDC to be assigned a mentor to guide you through this process (the committee chair can be reached through the NANDA-I website). Or, log on to www.nlinks.org and use the tools provided there to develop your concept analysis. We will be eagerly awaiting your contribution to our discipline – your submission to NANDA International's Diagnosis Development Committee.

This edition is the result of our first electronic voting on all new and revised diagnoses. This format enables members who may not be able to attend the biennial NANDA International conferences to contribute to the work of the organization through a thoughtful review and voting on proposed new and revised diagnoses. I want to thank Mary Hemminger, owner of Coherence Communications, LLC, for her work to enable us to launch this electronic format for diagnosis review. In the future, this process will enable us to review diagnoses as they move through the DDC cycle, rather than waiting until the end of the 2-year period as we have previously done. Approved new and revised diagnoses will then be made available to members on the NANDA-I website throughout the year.

I want to commend the members of the Board of Directors, all of the NANDA-I committee members, and committee chairs for their energy and enthusiasm for the work of the organization over the past 2 years. NANDA-I is a member-driven, volunteer organization that relies on the expertise of its members and end-users. The time commitment required of its Board members is substantial, as is that of its committee members and chairs. I have been honored to serve as president of this remarkable organization, and appreciate the opportunity to have represented its members in this manner.

Finally, I want to emphasize the critical role played by members of the Diagnosis Development Committee in the revision of several nursing diagnoses in this edition, in addition to their roles of mentoring submitters as required, and review of submitted new and revised diagnoses. These individuals play a key role in moving the work of this organization forward, and their efforts should not be underestimated. I wish especially to thank the co-chairs of the committee, Leann Scroggins and Dr Geralyn Meyers, for their dedication, organization, and commitment to continually improving the nursing diagnoses found within this text. Ms. Scroggins ends her second term as Chair of the DDC this year; I wish to acknowledge her dedication and commitment to the work of NANDA-I, and specifically to the DDC, for the past several years. Although members ultimately voted on a total of 21 new diagnoses during this cycle, it should be noted that the committee actually worked with many more diagnoses and their submitters; some of that work is still in progress and will continue into the next submission cycle. For this reason, I am dedicating this edition of the *Definitions and Classification* text to the members and co-chairs of the Diagnosis Development Committee, on behalf of the Board of Directors.

It is my hope that you find this edition of the *Definitions and Classification* text critical to your nursing practice – be that as a student, an educator, a clinician, an informaticist, an administrator, or a researcher. "Defining the knowledge of nursing" – clearly, this is the work of NANDA International.

T. Heather Herdman, PhD, RN
President, NANDA International

New Nursing Diagnoses, 2009–2011

Approved Diagnosis (New)	Submitter(s)
Ineffective **Activity** Planning	France Maltais BSc, MEd
Risk for **Bleeding**	Sheri Holmes, MSN, APRN BC
Readiness for Enhanced **Childbearing** Process	Yasuko Aoki, RN, RMW, Mitsuko Katayama, RN, RMW, PhD; Atsuko Kikuchi, RN, RMW; Minayo Kumazawa, RN, RMW, Med; Atsuko Koyama, RN, RMW; Masuko Saito, RN, RMW, DrMS; Toyo Yamazaki, RN, RMW; Mayumi Hamasaki, RN, RMW, MPH; Shigemi Kamitsuru, RN, PhD
Impaired **Comfort**	Mary Killeen PhD, RN; Kathy Kolcaba, PhD, RN
Risk for **Electrolyte** Imbalance	Jennifer Hafner, RN, BSN, PCCN, TNCC; Leah Mylrea Speltz BSN, RNC, ACCE, STABLE, ACLS, NNR; Kathy Weaver, RN
Risk for Disturbed **Maternal**/Fetal Dyad	Sheri Holmes, MSN, APRN BC
Dysfunctional Gastrointestinal **Motility**	Joan Klehr, RNC, MPH
Risk for Dysfunctional Gastrointestinal **Motility**	Joan Klehr, RNC, MPH
Neonatal Jaundice	David Wilson, MS, RNC
Ineffective Peripheral Tissue **Perfusion**	Jennifer Hafner, RN, BSN, PCCN, TNCC
Risk for Decreased Cardiac **Perfusion**	Jennifer Hafner, RN, BSN, PCCN, TNCC
Risk for Ineffective Cerebral Tissue **Perfusion**	Jennifer Hafner, RN, BSN, PCCN, TNCC
Risk for Ineffective Gastrointestinal Tissue **Perfusion**	Jennifer Hafner, RN, BSN, PCCN, TNCC

Approved Diagnosis (New)	Submitter(s)
Readiness for Enhanced **Relationship**	Yasuko Aoki, RN, RMW; Mitsuko Katayama, RN, RMW, PhD; Atsuko Kikuchi, RN, RMW; Minayo Kumazawa, RN, RMW, MEd; Atsuko Koyama, RN, RMW; Masuko Saito, RN, RMW, DrMS; Toyo Yamazaki, RN, RMW; Mayumi Hamasaki, RN, RMW, MPH; Shigemi Kamitsuru, RN, PhD
Risk for Impaired Renal **Perfusion**	Jennifer Hafner, RN, BSN, PCCN, TNCC
Impaired Individual **Resilience**	Angela Oldenburg, BA, RN, Shelly Eisbach, PhDc, MSN, RN; Melissa Lehan-Mackin, RN, BSN
Readiness for Enhanced **Resilience**	Angela Oldenburg, BA, RN; Shelly Eisbach, PhD, MSN, RN; Melissa Lehan-Mackin, RN, BSN
Risk for Compromised **Resilience**	Angela Oldenburg, BA, RN; Shelly Eisbach, PhDc, MSN, RN; Melissa Lehan-Mackin, RN, BSN
Self Neglect	Susanne Gibbons, C-GNP
Risk for **Shock**	Jennifer Hafner, RN, BSN, PCCN, TNCC
Risk for Vascular **Trauma**	Chistina Arreguy-Senna, Nurse, Master, PhD, Post-PhD; Emilia Campos de Carvalho, Nurse, Master, PhD

Revised Nursing Diagnoses, 2009–2011

Approved Diagnosis (Revised)	Submitter(s)
Risk Prone Health **Behavior**	DDC – minor editing
Defensive **Coping**	Céline Larouche
Risk for Imbalanced **Fluid** Volume	Louise Ritchie, MSc, BNur, RN; Geralyn Meyer, PhD, RN
Ineffective Self **Health** Management	Margaret Lunney, PhD, RN
Disturbed Personal **Identity**	Heidi Bjorge, RN, MNSc; Céline Larouche, Francine Fiset, BSN, MA, RN
Risk for Impaired **Liver** Function	DDC – minor editing
Chronic Low **Self** Esteem	Céline Larouche
Disturbed **Sleep** Pattern	DDC

Retired Nursing Diagnoses, 2009–2011

- Total Urinary **Incontinence**
- **Rape-Trauma** Syndrome: Compound Reaction
- **Rape-Trauma** Syndrome: Silent Reaction
- Effective **Therapeutic** Regimen Management
- Ineffective Community **Therapeutic** Regimen Management
- Disturbed **Thought** Process.*

These diagnoses can be found in Part 4, and the DDC encourages members and users of nursing diagnoses to work on these diagnoses and submit them for re-entry into the taxonomy.

* Work already in process on this diagnosis.

Introduction

This book is divided into five parts. Part 1 includes a chapter by Dr Margaret Lunney in which she discusses clinical judgment and assessment, and the role of each in the accurate clinical use of nursing diagnosis. A chapter by Leann Scroggins details the process for submission of a nursing diagnosis to NANDA-I's Diagnosis Development Committee (originally published in the NANDA-I journal). Additional chapters provide insight on the use and applicability of nursing diagnoses within nursing education, nursing informatics, nursing research, and nursing administration. This information is offered as a brief introduction on the importance of nursing diagnoses to each of these critical areas within the nursing profession, particularly because of the increased interest being expressed by individuals in those areas who are beginning to see the need to look beyond the more obvious clinical applicability of the nursing diagnoses.

Part 2 includes the traditional contents of the previous *NANDA International Nursing Diagnoses: Definitions & Classification* books – the diagnoses themselves, including definitions, defining characteristics, risk factors, and related factors, as appropriate. The diagnoses are listed alphabetically within Domain first, and then Class. This is new this year, and was done in response to requests from our non-English language users to facilitate ease of locating diagnoses within the book.

Taxonomy II splits the diagnoses into axes (see page 380 for a full explanation). Part 3 describes the structure of Taxonomy II and how it was developed. Figure 3.1 depicts *Taxonomy II Domains and Classes*; Table 3.1 shows *Taxonomy II: Domains, classes, and diagnoses*; and Table 2.2 shows the *NNN Taxonomy of nursing practice: Placement of nursing diagnoses*.

Part 4 contains those diagnoses that were noted in the 2007–2008 *Definitions & Classification* text to be slated for removal from the taxonomy, if work was not completed to bring them to a level of evidence ≥2.1. In some cases, these diagnoses are currently under revision; however, the work was not completed before the voting cycle for this edition of the text. The diagnoses are listed here in the hopes that members and/or end-users will wish to revise the diagnoses so that they can be returned to the taxonomy in our next edition.

Finally, Part 5 contains diagnosis submission guidelines, a process to appeal a decision of the Diagnosis Development Committee, and a glossary; a list of members of the NANDA International Board of Directors, Taxonomy and Diagnosis Development Committees; an invitation to join NANDA-I; and the index.

How to Use This Book

As noted above, the nursing diagnoses are listed alphabetically by Domain and then by Class. For example, *Ineffective Health Maintenance* is listed under Domain I (Health Promotion), Class 2 (Health Management). Similarly, *Disturbed Sleep Pattern* is listed under Domain 4 (Activity/Rest), Class 1 (Sleep/Rest).

We hope that the organization of *NANDA-I Nursing Diagnoses: Definitions & Classification 2009–2011* will make it efficient and effective to use. We welcome your feedback. If you have suggestions, please send them to us by email at president@nanda.org or by calling the office (USA) at +1 (920) 344 8670.

Part 1

An Introduction to Nursing Diagnoses: Accuracy, Application Across Setting, and Submission of Nursing Diagnoses to NANDA-I 2009–2011

Assessment, Clinical Judgment, and Nursing Diagnoses: How to Determine Accurate Diagnoses

Margaret Lunney, RN, PhD

Professor and Graduate Programs Coordinator
College of Staten Island, City University of New York
Department of Nursing
Chair, Research Committee
NANDA International

Assessment was identified as the first part of the nursing process. The nursing process is a theory of how nurses organize the care of individuals, families, and communities. The theory of nursing process has been broadly accepted by nurses since 1967 (Yura and Walsh, 1967). In the 1960s, it was thought that the nursing process was a four-part process of assessment, planning, implementation, and evaluation. But, soon after the first description of the nursing process, nurse leaders recognized that assessment data must be clustered and interpreted before nurses could plan, implement, or evaluate a plan to help patients.

The need to interpret data derives from the fact that short-term memory only holds 7 ± 2 bits of data (Newell and Simon, 1972). Thus nurses, like other human beings, continuously convert data into interpretations. For example, people interpret whether a person is female or male, based on over 20 bits of data, e.g., hair and dress styles, body language, facial structure, name, and voice. If a nurse decides to assist a patient to move from a bed to a chair, it is based on an interpretation of data showing that the patient wants or needs to be out of bed and needs assistance with moving from bed to chair. Some of the data that a nurse might use for this interpretation is that the patient is one day post-abdominal surgery, the patient has expressed pain, and the patient said that she or he felt "shaky." Nursing diagnoses are scientific interpretations of assessment data that are used to guide nurses' planning, implementation, and evaluation.

Only 6 years after Yura and Walsh's description of the nursing process in 1967, two nurses from St Louis, (USA), organized the first conference to identify the interpretations of data that represent the phenomena of concern to nurses. These nurses, Mary Ann Lavin and Kristine Gebbie, invited 100 nurses from the United States and Canada to participate in this event (Gebbie, 1998). This was the first conference on nursing diagnosis, out of which 80 nursing diagnoses were identified and defined. Since then, the list of approved diagnoses has been steadily grown and been refined through research-based submissions by nurses and the work of members of the nursing diagnosis association that sponsors this book, now known as NANDA International (NANDA-I).

Nurses are Diagnosticians

With use of the term "nursing diagnosis," it became apparent that nurses are diagnosticians. Before that time, the clinical judgment used in clinical practice to decide the focus of nursing care was invisible or not named. Today, in healthcare agencies where nurses do not use nursing diagnoses, or use them without a concern for accuracy, the invisibility of the nurse's role as a diagnostician may still exist. With the start of this formal classification of nursing diagnoses, however, it was broadly accepted that nurses are diagnosticians who use diagnostic reasoning in collaboration with patients to identify the best diagnoses to guide nursing interventions to achieve positive patient outcomes.

The diagnostic process in nursing differs from the diagnostic process in medicine in that, in situations when it is possible to do so, the person or persons who are the focus of nursing care should be intimately involved as partners with nurses in the assessment and diagnostic process. This is because the focus of nursing care is the person's achievement of well-being and self-actualization. People's experiences and responses to health problems and life processes have specific meanings to them and these meanings are identified with the help of nurses. It is also assumed that nurses do not make people healthy with their diagnoses and interventions; people make themselves healthy with their own behaviors. Thus, to achieve changes in behaviors that affect health, people and nurses together identify the most accurate diagnoses that have the potential to guide nursing care for achievement of positive health outcomes. Nursing interventions for diagnoses of human responses offer additional ways, besides treating medical problems, that the health of people can be promoted, protected, and restored.

The focus of nursing is the "health" of "human beings," two of the most complex scientific concerns: more complex, for example, than chemistry and astronomy. Health-related phenomena, such as sleep, comfort, or nutrition, are complex because they involve human experiences. We can never know for sure what other human beings are experiencing; yet the goal of nursing is to identify people's experiences or responses in order to support them. With human responses, there is also a tremendous overlap of cues to diagnoses and many contextual factors such as culture that can change the perspective of "what is the diagnosis?" Many studies have verified that interpretations of clinical cases have the potential to be less accurate than indicated by the data (Lunney, 2008).

With nursing diagnoses as the foundation of nursing care, nurses need to develop diagnostic competencies in order to become good diagnosticians. Diagnosticians are people who interpret data within their fields of expertise in order to provide needed services, e.g., an automobile mechanic must be able to diagnose why the car will not start in order to be able to fix it. A key element of data interpretations is that they are subject to error. A good diagnostician must be mindful that there are always risks to the accuracy of data interpretations. Becoming a nurse diagnostician, therefore, requires development of professional and personal skills and characteristics.

Two propositions are the basis for development of diagnostic competencies:

1. Diagnosis in nursing requires competencies in intellectual, interpersonal, and technical domains.
2. Diagnosis in nursing requires development of the personal strengths of tolerance for ambiguity and use of reflective practice.

Intellectual, Interpersonal and Technical Competencies

Intellectual Competencies

Intellectual competencies are discussed first because this is an invisible aspect of nursing that is very important for becoming a diagnostician. Intellectual skills include both knowledge of nursing diagnoses and the mental processes for use of knowledge. Nurses need to attain knowledge of diagnoses, their definitions and defining characteristics, especially those that are common to the populations with which they work, the interventions to treat the diagnoses, and the diagnostic processes that are used to interpret patient data. This knowledge is extensive and complex, so nurses should not be expected to memorize the available knowledge, but rather they need to know how to access the information that they need; the resources to obtain this knowledge should be available when needed.

Besides knowledge, thinking ability is the other important aspect of the intellectual domain. Even though, traditionally, thinking processes have not been emphasized in nursing, they are critical to use of nursing diagnoses. The cognitive skills of analyzing, logical reasoning, and applying standards are just three of the thinking processes that are needed for accurate diagnosis in nursing. These skills are developed, for example, through discussions of how data should be clustered to generate accurate diagnoses, the relation of data clusters to diagnoses, and comparisons of existing data to expected data based on research findings. Research findings in cognitive science and nursing show that adults at the same levels of education and experience vary greatly in thinking abilities (Lunney, 1992; Sternberg, 1997).

Research findings from cognitive science and other disciplines also show that thinking processes can be improved (Sternberg, 1997; Willingham, 2007). In nursing, research studies have shown that critical thinking abilities vary widely and that critical thinking can be improved with education and effort (Tanner, 2006). This is done through energy, focus, and support. To do this, students and nurses need to think about their thinking, referred to as metacognition (Pesut and Herman, 1992), by using the concepts of thinking that are relevant to nursing practice. A Delphi study of nurse experts in critical thinking (Scheffer and Rubenfeld, 2000) generated 7 cognitive skills and 10 habits of mind that were considered to be highly relevant to nursing practice (see list and definitions in Appendix). These 17 concepts of thinking should be used by nurses to think about their thinking. In any nursing situation, two or more cognitive skills are probably being used. The habits of mind support the cognitive skills. The combination of these critical thinking abilities that are needed for clinical situations are probably unique, so nurses need to cultivate all of these critical thinking processes and not just focus on a few of them.

Critical thinking abilities are essential to achieve accurate interpretations of patient data and appropriate selection of interventions and outcomes, so developing high-level thinking abilities is a high priority. To do this, nurses and nursing students can:

■ use thinking processes, rather than just receiving knowledge from others
■ when learning, think about the concepts, not just memorize knowledge
■ seek support from others, e.g., teachers, other nurses, patients, to validate thinking processes
■ develop confidence in ability to think.

Interpersonal Competencies

Nursing diagnoses are best used by nurses who have exquisite interpersonal communication skills. Such skills are needed so that patients will trust nurses enough to tell them about their responses to health problems and life processes. Trust is enhanced through a mature ability to communicate with others.

Nurses must assume that they do not know other people (Munhall, 1993). The only way other people can be known is through interpersonal processes, especially listening. Nurses who assume that they know patients without listening to them will not achieve diagnostic accuracy. The best use of nursing diagnoses is in partnership with patients and families. To work in partnership, nurses need to speak to people with respect and care, effectively listen, respect other people's opinions and views, and know how to validate perceptions with patients and families. Learning these skills is a challenge, so the interpersonal aspects of nursing need to be an integral part of learning to use nursing diagnoses.

Technical Competencies

Another baseline competency is the technical skill of conducting a nursing assessment. Obtaining valid and reliable data is the backbone of using nursing diagnoses, so nurses' development of their ability to conduct comprehensive and focused health histories and physical examinations is essential. This technical skill is learned in courses on the topic and using nursing textbooks on health assessment. For example, the diagnosis and treatment of pain requires sophisticated assessment knowledge, including ways to explore the types and locations of pain, factors that make the pain worse or better, etc. The same is true of many of the diagnostic concepts such as body image disturbance.

An assessment is a "nursing" assessment if it yields the data that are needed for nursing care. The assessment data that are generated by a biological systems review, which is done to yield medical diagnoses, are insufficient to yield the data needed for nursing diagnoses. Thus, other assessment frameworks such as the functional health patterns (Gordon, 2007) are being used in healthcare systems where the accuracy of nurses' diagnoses is considered important. The functional health pattern framework is used later in this chapter to demonstrate how to generate nursing diagnoses from assessment data.

Personal Strengths: Tolerance for Ambiguity and Reflective Practice

The personal strengths of tolerance for ambiguity and reflective practice need to be developed because decisions are so complex in nursing and the use of clinical judgment needs to be an ongoing learning process. Each decision that a nurse makes is relative to the context of the situation and to the specific nature of the individual, family or community with whom they are working. With experience, nurses become familiar with many types of contextual situations that can positively influence diagnostic abilities. Tolerance for ambiguity and reflective practice enable nurses to incorporate these contextual experiences to advance their professional development from novice to expert (Benner 1984; Benner et al., 1996).

Tolerance for Ambiguity

Tolerance for ambiguity is needed because there are numerous factors that influence clinical situations such as agency policies, the nurse's job description, and the availability of resources. Tolerance for ambiguity enables nurses to consider the broad range of influencing factors within the diagnostic process and be able to focus on the most accurate diagnoses for quality-based services to individuals, families and communities.

In addition, the human beings for whom nurses provide care are extremely complex and diverse, especially when the focus is the person's response or experience and not the illness itself. Thus, ambiguity is expected, so nurses need to adjust to the ambiguity. Nurse leaders and teachers can help by pointing out the ambiguity, treating it as a fact of life as a nurse, and being role models for tolerance for ambiguity.

Reflective Practice

Reflective practice is the ability to introspectively examine our own behaviors in relation to thinking, interpersonal events, and technical skills. This is a prerequisite to self-evaluation and, to accomplish it, to some extent we must expose ourselves, our frailties and our mistakes. There are good books and articles available that address the concept of reflection, (Johns 2007). Reflective practice supports continuous development or growth with the assumption that we benefit by thinking about our own behaviors and our own thinking.

Assessment and Nursing Diagnosis

Nursing assessments at all levels of analysis (individuals, families and communities), consist of subjective data from the person or persons and objective data from diagnostic tests and other sources. Assessments of individuals consists of a health history (subjective data) and a physical examination (objective data) (Weber and Kelly, 2007). Assessments of families consist of obtaining specific information from the family (subjective data) and observing family interactions (objective data) (Wright and Leahey, 2005). Assessments of communities consist of obtaining information from key informants within the community (subjective data) and statistical data (objective data) (Anderson and McFarland, 2006).

There are two types of assessments that are done to generate accurate nursing diagnoses: comprehensive and focused. Comprehensive assessments cover all aspects of a nursing assessment framework such as the 11 functional health patterns to determine the health status of the individual, family, or community. Comprehensive assessments of individuals are done, for example, when admitting a patient to a hospital or to home care services. Focused assessments focus on a particular issue or concern, such as pain, sleep, or respiratory status. Focused assessments are done when specific symptoms need to be explored further, e.g., a person says "I am having difficulty with breathing," or something generates increased risk of a particular problem, e.g., when a person needs the medication of coumadin, there is increased risk of bleeding.

The goals for a nursing assessment are that:

- it focuses on the data needed to identify human responses and experiences
- it is conducted in partnership with the individual, family or community, wherever possible
- the findings are based on research and other evidence.

Assessment Framework

For nursing, assessment frameworks need to be broad enough to yield data to guide nursing care for health promotion, health protection (primary, secondary, and tertiary prevention), and health restoration. "Health promotion is directed toward increasing the level of well-being or self actualization of a given individual or group. Health promotion focuses on efforts to approach or move toward a positive balanced state of high level health and well being" (Pender et al., 2006, p. 37). An example of a health promotion diagnosis is *Readiness for Enhanced Sleep*. Health protection is a process of helping people to reduce risks to health and protect themselves from existing risk states (Pender et al., 2006). An example of a health protection diagnosis is *Risk for Infection*. Health restoration, also referred to as illness management, is a process of helping people to manage health problems. The actual nursing diagnoses such as *Pain, Anxiety, Fear*, and *Ineffective Self Health Management* are examples of diagnoses in the realm of health restoration.

A nursing assessment framework that is widely used to generate accurate nursing diagnoses is the functional health pattern framework (Gordon, 2007). This framework includes 11 patterns of individuals (see Assessment Tool, Appendix A), families, or communities.

Diagnostic Reasoning Associated with Nursing Assessment

Principles should include:

- Diagnostic hypotheses are considered throughout the assessment process and are used along with the formal assessment guide to generate the data needed for diagnoses.

- In a comprehensive assessment, diagnoses are not finalized until completion of the assessment. Assessment of each pattern informs the nurse and patient about the diagnostic hypotheses.
- When possible, the individual, family or community is involved from start to finish with the assessment and diagnostic processes.

Recognizing the Existence of Cues

Nurses *mentally recognize* cues early in the diagnostic process and continue to integrate cue recognition throughout the process. Cues are units of data, (e.g., a person's rate of breathing), which a nurse collects during intentional or unintentional assessment. Intentional assessment involves deliberate collection of data as a foundation for nursing actions. Unintentional assessment involves noticing cues that are important without planning to do so. In clinical situations, nurses notice cues to diagnoses by thinking about what they see, hear, smell, touch, and taste. Information pertaining to the health-care consumer is *thought about* in relation to the *nurse's knowledge* of the health state or life situation of the consumer. Nurses attend to information based on established ideas of what should occur in various situations. A nurse may not notice a person's rate of breathing, for example, unless it looks unusual in the context of a health problem (e.g., the individual is one day post-abdominal surgery), or other aspects of the clinical situation (e.g., the individual has just completed vigorous exercise). A nurse's recognition of a unit of data as a cue with special meaning is dependent on *knowledge stored in memory*. Knowledge bases in memory are used for comparison of current data with expected data.

Mentally Generating Possible Diagnoses

The meaning that nurses assign to cues noticed early in the diagnostic process can be understood only if there are possible and plausible explanations for the cues within the context of the situation. This is an *active thinking process* whereby the nurse explores knowledge in memory for possible explanations of data. Often, there are many possible diagnoses or explanations that may be considered. Sometimes, there is only one plausible meaning for cues noticed early in the diagnostic process, for example, if a woman who is newly admitted to a hospital unit for a surgical procedure is rapidly asking the nurse many questions, and exhibits a fast rate of breathing, the cues are not specific enough to consider only one possible diagnosis. The nurse in this instance would consider a number of possible explanations for this set of cues such as fear, anxiety, ineffective breathing pattern, and others. A nurse diagnostician avoids deciding on a diagnosis prematurely: before there are sufficient data to support a diagnostic judgment. Flexibility of thinking enables nurses to make a broad search of the mind for possible diagnoses. Logical reasoning in collaboration with the patient enables nurses to derive the most accurate diagnosis when the data are sufficient to do so.

Comparing Cues to Possible Diagnoses

Cues are analyzed in relation to possible diagnoses through a *mental process of evaluation*. Evaluation involves a process of mental matching wherein the existing cues are matched with the expected cues for the diagnoses being considered. Information about the expected cues for diagnoses is found in this book and current literature on specific phenomena such as pain, coping, and fluid volume. During the evaluation of cues and related diagnoses, nurses may decide that there is not enough evidence to make a diagnostic decision *or* that there is enough evidence for one likely diagnosis. If a nurse decides that there are not enough data to make a diagnosis, the next step involves a focused search for additional cues. If a nurse decides that there is enough supporting evidence, a diagnosis is made and then validated.

Conducting a Focused Data Collection

To confirm or rule out diagnoses that are under consideration, additional cues may be collected by focusing questions to obtain data for one or more diagnoses. With the preoperative patient mentioned above, for example, the nurse might ask the patient how she feels about the surgical procedure. The answer to a broad question such as this can yield data to support many possible diagnoses in the psychosocial realm. If the patient mentions fear of death or fear of the unknown in relation to the surgery, the nurse can begin to confirm *Fear* as the diagnosis and eliminate some of the other possibilities such as anxiety. When the nurse conducts a medical history and physical examination, biological reasons for the fast rate of breathing can also be confirmed or ruled out. A focused data collection concludes when the nurse synthesizes available data and selects one or more of the diagnoses being considered, rules out all of the diagnoses being considered, or revises the diagnoses being considered to incorporate new ones. If a diagnosis under consideration is supported through focused data collection, the next step is to validate the diagnosis. If all of the diagnoses are ruled out or not confirmed, new diagnoses are considered or the nurse concludes that there is no diagnosis. If new diagnoses are considered, a focused data collection continues until the revised set of diagnoses are confirmed or ruled out through supporting evidence (cues).

Validating Diagnoses

As human behavior is complex and nurses cannot truly "know" what other people are experiencing (Munhall, 1993), it is important for nurses' thinking and technical processes to be accompanied by collaborative processes with consumers and other providers. In most instances, nurses should decide on diagnoses with healthcare consumers; a nurse may say, "From the information you have just given me, it seems that you are experiencing *Fear* associated with surgery. Is that correct?" Based on the patient's response, the nurse validates or rejects the diagnosis. In cases when patients are unable to collaborate with nurses because they are too sick, developmentally unable, or mentally incompetent, nurses can validate diagnoses with family members or other providers; a nurse may say, "From the information you have given me about your son, it seems that he is having difficulty coping with the stress of the illness. Is that correct?" To validate with another provider, a nurse may say: "From my physical examination, I concluded that Mary's airway clearance is impaired. Do you agree?" Validation of diagnoses with others helps to ensure the accuracy of diagnoses as the bases for subsequent stages of the nursing process. To save the time, energy, and costs associated with interventions for diagnoses, diagnoses should be validated as highly accurate.

Case Study Example

The following case study was developed by Maria Cruz, RN, who was a bachelor's degree student at the College of Staten Island when she wrote this case study. The Functional Health Patterns Assessment tool in the Appendix on p. 18 was used and the nurses' use of NOC and NIC, explained in the following section, is also included.

CW is a 30-year-old man who currently works in the marketing department for a major credit card company in Manhattan. He attends a university part-time in the evenings to complete his Masters degree in Business Administration.

CW believes that he is in good general health, and being healthy is very important to him. The last time he was "sick" was last fall when he had a head cold. CW maintains his health status by trying to eat healthily, exercising at a gym, and maintaining good personal hygiene. He limits his intake of alcohol to social occasions and said he smokes "once in a blue moon."

He has psoriasis, a skin condition that he developed as a child. Currently, he has a large patch on his left shin that is dry, scaly, and very itchy. He stated that the last time he saw the dermatologist was 2 years ago and he really should see him more often. He "put it off" because he knows that the condition is chronic. CW is taking two medications on a regular basis: Propecia, a steroid cream that he occasionally uses for the psoriasis, and minoxidil for his thinning hair. He uses the cream whenever the psoriasis "acts up," which temporarily relieves itching. He expressed the possibility and desire to better manage flare-ups of the psoriasis.

CW has a family history of mental illness and becoming overweight. Both his grandmothers were diagnosed with depression, and they are on many medications. His father is very heavy now, but when he was younger he was fit and healthy. He fears that the same may happen to him.

CW expressed concern about maintaining his health status, but he has not had a physical check-up in over 2 years. He stated that if he feels well he sees no reason to go to a physician. As psoriasis is a chronic condition, he sometimes feels that the lesions will occur no matter what he does. According to him, the cream is messy and stains everything, which is a barrier to using the cream. With regard to self-efficacy, CW is capable of using the cream, but has not committed to doing so. The fact that the cream is messy and stains creates a negative activity-related affect for CW.

CW tries to eat balanced meals but finds it difficult sometimes due to his hectic work and school schedule. He eats low-fat, low-sugar, and low-sodium foods that are good sources of protein and dairy. A typical day's meals include vegetables and fruits and he has a "weakness" for sweets and desserts. He has a good appetite and in order to maintain his weight he has been going to Weight Watchers for the past year. He reached his goal weight for his height and needs to "stick to a plan" to stay there. He sometimes has difficulties making healthy choices at the supermarket because there are too many things to choose from, but he loves to cook and try new things. He bites his nails when he feels stressed.

CW's pattern of urine elimination is within normal limits, voiding light yellow urine about five times a day. He has no trouble moving his bowels, although he does have small hemorrhoids, which bother him from time to time.

CW has a daily routine of walking to the bus stop, which is about three blocks away, to go to work. He sits at a desk most of the day, but goes to the gym three times a week for a cardiovascular workout. He also enjoys taking his dog on walks. Three nights a week he attends college classes. He loves going out to dinner with friends and family, going to the movies, or watching movies at home. He is a frequent traveler to local destinations such as Atlantic City, and he also likes going abroad.

During the week CW usually gets about 8 hours of sleep each night and, on the weekend, he sleeps longer. CW uses a sound machine that makes "white noise" to help him fall asleep. He started using this when he first moved to the city from upstate because all the night sounds in the city made it difficult for him to fall asleep. Even though he now lives in a quiet area, he says he can't sleep without the soothing sounds that the machine makes. Because of his schedule, CW does not find too much time to rest during the day, but he takes a nap on the bus while commuting.

CW's senses are within normal limits. He has 20/20 vision and his hearing is normal. He denies any problems with his sense of taste, touch, or smell; he denies pain.

CW has a positive self-perception and moderate self-esteem. He describes himself as an extrovert, spontaneous, family-oriented person with an intimate social circle of friends and colleagues. His strengths include his determination and his "all or nothing" attitude. He is ambitious, although he feels he is also simple and modest. Sometimes "I spread myself too thin," trying to accomplish too many things at one time. This may add to his feelings of being easily distracted and having trouble focusing at work. His physical self is also somewhat positive. He is happy about his general appearance, height, and symmetrical body. He feels that he has too much body hair and not enough hair on his head, and tries to hide the patches of psoriasis, e.g., he wears jeans, not shorts.

At work, CW assumes a leadership role when he leads his marketing team. As a student he deals with responsibilities of going to class and doing assignments. He is proud of being a homeowner. He describes his relationships as loving, peaceful, supportive, open, and non-conflicting. He is the youngest of three children, and he has a close relationship with his mother and sisters. Overall he is happy and satisfied with these aspects of his life, although he wishes he were closer to his dad. He gets a lot of support from family, friends, and his partner.

CW states that he has no concerns about sexuality. He practices safe sex and is currently in a committed relationship.

Currently, CW has a long list of stressors. He has to balance the stress of both school and work, and is in the process of selling his house and buying a new one before the end of the summer. He stated that, like any relationship, he feels stressed about helping his partner with goals such as getting US citizenship and passing the driver's license test. He feels that the daily routine of keeping up with the responsibilities of owning a house, going to work, and school add to his stress level, which he rates as moderate. In dealing with stress, he has one bad habit – biting his nails. On the positive side he tries to get things done so work does not "pile up" and he takes frequent vacations. Surprisingly, although he has all these stressors, he feels that he thrives on them, not that they hold him back or have a negative impact on his health.

CW's cultural and family traditions promote a balance between hard work and rest. He is not very religious and he is unsure how religion plays a role in his health. At this point in life, he feels that his goals are being met and he is satisfied with his health status.

Analysis of Health Data: Nursing Diagnoses

There were several NANDA-I diagnoses that the nurse considered. These included: *Impaired Skin Integrity*, *Ineffective Health Maintenance*, *Deficient Knowledge*, *Disturbed Body Image*, *Powerlessness*, *Readiness for Enhanced Coping*, and *Readiness for Enhanced Self Health Management*. *Impaired Skin Integrity* is not the best diagnosis to guide nursing care because the problem of psoriasis mostly requires medical interventions. *Ineffective Health Maintenance* was rejected because CW generally has a healthy lifestyle. Although *Deficient Knowledge* was considered as a diagnosis, it is more appropriate as a contributing factor to his management of the therapeutic regimen for his psoriasis and there is not very much that the nurse can teach him that he does not already know. There are not enough data to support the diagnoses of *Disturbed Body Image* and *Powerlessness* and, as CW perceives that he has no health problems, a health promotion diagnosis is more appropriate. Even though CW admits to having a lot of stress, he includes many stress management techniques in his daily routines, so there is less data support for *Readiness for Enhanced Coping* than *Readiness for Enhanced Self Health Management (RESHM)*. The diagnosis of *RESHM*, defined as "a pattern of regulating and integrating into daily living a program for treatment of illness and its sequelae that is sufficient for meeting health-related goals and can be strengthened" is the one that CW and I decided to address.

Defining characteristics for RESHM are that CW expressed a desire to want to change how he manages his skin condition and an awareness that perhaps flare-ups can be reduced. His sporadic pattern of treatment may not be the most effective, and maybe there are newer easier treatments for him to consider. In addition CW already maintains his health in a number of ways, which reduces his risk for the condition to worsen.

Interpersonal influences that can have an impact on CW's behavior are his partner, his family, and his dermatologist (Pender et al., 2006). Perhaps his family and significant other could support and encourage him to use the cream daily by reminding him and reinforcing positive outcomes. One situational influence in this case is that, as CW has not been to his physician in a long time, he may not be aware of other possible options available, which may be even more effective than his current treatment.

Nursing Outcomes Classification

Based on our discussion, we decided to use the Nursing Outcomes Classification (NOC) outcome *Health-Promoting Behavior* (1602), defined as "personal actions to sustain or increase wellness" (Moorhead et al., 2004, p. 307). The outcome scale is: 1 = never demonstrated, 2 = rarely demonstrated, 3 = sometimes demonstrated, 4 = often demonstrated, and 5 = consistently demonstrated. His score on the overall outcome is 3 and his goal is 5. For indicator 160207, "performs healthy behaviors routinely," CW is at level 3 and his goal is 5. For indicator 160213, "obtains recommended health screenings," CW is at 2 and his goal is 5.

Nursing Interventions Classification

In order to treat the diagnosis and achieve the desired outcome, we chose the Nursing Interventions Classification (NIC) intervention of *Patient Contracting* (4420), defined as "negotiating an agreement with an individual that reinforces a specific behavior change" (Dochterman and Bulechek, 2004, p. 538). The activities for this intervention that will be used are: help CW to identify the health practice that he wishes to change, i.e., better management of his skin condition, and identify the goals of care. For CW, one goal is to see his dermatologist on a regular basis and to find a way to treat his skin condition that he is more likely to routinely use. During our discussion, we learned that there are some barriers for CW to carry out his current plan, and perhaps developing a regimen with these barriers in mind will help to improve management. It is important for the nurse to assist CW in developing a plan to meet the goals, and facilitate a written contract with all agreed-upon elements. Another activity is to assist CW in developing a flow chart, through use of a journal to record his skin condition and daily use of the cream. Perhaps this would help show him if continued use would have a better effect than sporadic use. Finally, we coordinated opportunities to review the contract and goals. This gives CW and me a chance to see his progress and whether or not his plan is working.

References

Anderson, E.T. & McFarlane, J.A. (2006). *Community as partner: Theory and practice in nursing*, 4th edn. Philadelphia: Lippincott.

Benner, P. (1984). *From novice to expert: Excellence and power in clinical nursing practice*. Menlo Park, CA: Addison Wesley.

Benner, P., Tanner, C.A., & Chesla, C.A. (1996). *Expertise in clinical practice: Caring, clinical judgment, and ethics*. New York: Springer.

Dochterman, J.M. & Bulechek, G. (eds) (2004). *Nursing interventions classification* (NIC). St Louis, MO: Mosby.

Gebbie, K. (1998). Utilization of a classification of nursing diagnosis. *Nursing Diagnoses* **9**(2 suppl): 17–26.

Gordon, M. (2007). *Manual of nursing diagnosis*, 11th edn. Boston: Jones & Bartlett.

Johns, J. (2007). Toward easing suffering through reflection. *Holistic Nursing* **25**: 204–10.

Lunney, M. (1992). Divergent productive thinking factors and accuracy of nursing diagnoses. *Research in Nursing & Health* **15**: 303–11.

Lunney, M. (2008). The critical need to address accuracy of nurses' diagnoses. *OJIN: Online Journal of Issues in Nursing*. American Nurses Association. Available at: www.

nursingworld.org/MainMenuCategories/ANAmarketplace/ANAperiodicals/
OJ%20IN/tableofcontents/vol31998/vol3no21998/AccuracyofNursesDiagnoses.aspx
(accessed June 7 2008).

Moorhead, S., Johnson, M., & Maas, M. (eds) (2004). *Nursing outcomes classification* (NOC).
St Louis, MO: MOSBY.

Munhall, P.L. (1993). "Unknowing": Toward another pattern of knowing in nursing.
Nursing Outlook **41**: 125–8.

Newell, A. & Simon, H. (1972). *Human problem solving*. Englewood Cliffs, NJ: Prentice
Hall.

Pender, N.J., Murdaugh, C.L., & Parsons, M.A. (2006). *Health promotion in nursing practice*,
5th edn. Upper Saddle River, NJ: Prentice Hall.

Pesut, D.J. & Herman, J.A. (1992). Metacognitive skills in diagnostic reasoning: Making
the implicit explicit. *Nursing Diagnosis* **3**: 148–54.

Scheffer, B.K., & Rubenfeld, M.G. (2000). A consensus statement on critical thinking.
Journal of Nursing Education **39**: 352–9.

Sternberg, R.J. (1997). *Thinking styles*. New York: Cambridge University Press.

Tanner, C.A. (2006). Thinking like a nurse: a research-based model of clinical judgment
in nursing. *Journal of Nursing Education* **45**: 204–11.

Weber, J. & Kelly, J. (2007). *Health assessment in nursing*. Philadelphia, PA: Lippincott/
Williams & Wilkins.

Willingham, D.T. (2007). Critical thinking: Why is it so hard to teach? *American Educator*
31(2): 8–19.

Wright, L.M. & Leahey, M. (2005). *Nurses and families: A guide to family assessment and
interventions*, 4th edn. Philadelphia: FA Davis.

Yura, H. & Walsh, M. (1967). *The nursing process*. Norwalk, CT: Appleton–Century–
Crofts.

Appendix: Functional Health Pattern Assessment Framework

Directions

1. The categories on the left provide guidance to the type of information that is included in the pattern description. The pattern of the client should be described on the right. The description as written should be understandable by others, for example,
   Correct: no history of related physical and psychological problems
   Incorrect: none
2. Use interviewing techniques as described in the literature, e.g., include silence and statements, not just questions.
3. As all of the data represent subjective data, quotation marks should not be used. Every sentence should represent the words of the individual and family, *or* their words are paraphrased.
4. As the subject of every sentence is "I" or "we," the subject should not be repeated throughout. The person's responses can be written as incomplete sentences, e.g., attend church every day at 9am (the subject is assumed to be "I" or "we").
5. When people have long stories to tell in relation to an assessment category, the data can be shortened by paraphrasing, but be careful to retain the essence of their descriptions.
6. As much as possible, record your data in the form of cues, not inferences. Cues are units of sensory data. Inferences are the subjective meanings that persons apply to cues.
7. Avoid interjecting diagnoses into the database, e.g., *anxious* (a nursing diagnosis) about her relationship with her family. This statement should only be in the database if it is said by the patient.
8. Consider the assessment categories of this form as incomplete for any particular client. *Follow through on cues that are raised in the assessment.* For example, if Mary states she smokes one pack of cigarettes per day, identify whether she knows the dangers of smoking, how she feels about smoking, what is her motivation to quit, does smoking affect other aspects of her life, and, does she have other risk factors for heart and lung disease?

Date: _____ Nurse: _____

Client: _____ Age: _____ Sex: _____ Occupation: _____
Physician(s): _____ Pharmacist: _____
Reason for Contact: _____

Health Perception–Health Management Pattern

Meaning of health	
Description of health status	
Health promotion: food and fluids, exercise, lifestyle and habits, stress management	
Health protection: screening programs, visits to primary healthcare professionals, diet, exercise, stress management, rest, economic factors	
Self examination of: breast and/or testicles, blood pressure, other	
Knowledge of self-examination	
Medical history, hospitalizations and surgery; family medical history	
Behaviors to manage health problems: diet, exercise, medications, treatments	
Names, dosage, and frequency of prescription and nonprescription drugs	
Risk factors related to health, e.g., family history, lifestyle and/or habits, poverty	
Relevant PE (physical examination) data: Complete	

Nutrition–Metabolic pattern

Usual number of meals and snacks	
Types and amounts of foods and fluids	
24-hour recall or 3-day history	
Shopping and cooking habits	
Satisfaction with weight	
Influences on food choices, e.g., religious, ethnic, cultural, economic	
Perceptions of metabolic needs	
Related factors, e.g., activity, illness, stress	

Ingestion factors: appetite, discomfort, taste and smell, teeth, oral mucosa, nausea or vomiting, dietary restrictions, food allergies	
History of related physical and/or psychological problems	
Relevant PE data: general survey, skin, hair, nails, abdomen	

Elimination Pattern

Usual voiding pattern: frequency, amount, color, odor, discomfort, nocturia, control, any changes	
Usual defecation pattern: regularity, color, amount, consistency, discomfort, control, any changes	
Health/cultural beliefs	
Level of self-care: toileting, hygiene	
Aids for excretion, e.g., medications, enemas	
Actions to prevent cystitis	
History of related physical and/or psychological problems	
Relevant PE data: abdomen, genitals, prostate	

Activity–Exercise Pattern

Typical activities of daily living (ADLs)	
Exercise: type, frequency, duration, intensity	
Leisure activities	
Beliefs about exercise	
Ability for self-care: dressing (upper and lower), bathing, feeding, toileting independent, dependent, or assistance needed	
Use of equipment, e.g., cane or walker	
Related factors, e.g., self-concept	
History of related physical and/or psychological problems	
Relevant PE data: respiratory, cardiovascular, musculoskeletal, neurological	

Sleep–Rest Pattern

Usual sleep habits: number of hours, time of sleep and awakening, bedtime rituals, sleep environment, rested after sleep	
Cultural beliefs	
Use of sleep aids, e.g., drugs, relaxation tapes	
Scheduled rest and relaxation	
Symptoms of sleep pattern disturbance	
Related factors, e.g., pain	
History of related physical and/or psychological problems	
Relevant PE data: general survey	

Cognitive–Perceptual Pattern

Description of special senses: vision, hearing, taste, touch, smell	
Aids to senses, e.g., glasses, hearing aid	
Recent changes in senses	
Perception of comfort/pain	
Cultural beliefs regarding pain	
Aids to relieve discomfort	
Educational level	
Decision-making ability	
History of related physical, developmental, or psychological problems	
Relevant PE data: general survey, neurological	

Self-Perception–Self-Concept Pattern

Social self: occupation, family situation, social groups	
Personal identity: description of self, strengths and weaknesses	
Physical self: any concerns about body, likes/dislikes	
Self-esteem: feelings about self	
Threats to self-concept, e.g., illness, changes in roles, history of related physical and/or psychological problems	
Relevant PE data: general survey	

Role-Relationship Pattern

Description of roles with family, friends, co-workers	
Role satisfaction/dissatisfaction	
Effect of health status	
Importance of family	
Family structure and support	
Family decision-making processes	
Family problems and/or concerns	
Child rearing patterns	
Relationships with others	
Significant relationships	
History of related physical and/or psychological problems	
Relevant PE data: general survey	

Sexuality–Reproductive Pattern

Sexual concerns or problems	
Description of sexual behavior, e.g., safe sex practices	
Knowledge related to sexuality and reproduction	
Impact of health status	
Menstrual and reproductive history	
History of related physical and/or psychological problems	
Relevant PE data: general survey, genitals, breasts, rectal	

Coping–Stress Tolerance Pattern

Nature of current stressors	
Perceived level of stress	
Description of overall and specific responses to stress	
Usual stress management strategies and their effectiveness	
Life changes and losses	
Coping strategies usually used	
Perceived control over events	
Knowledge and use of stress management techniques	

Relationship of stress management to family dynamics	
History of related physical and/or psychological problems	
Relevant PE data: general survey	

Value-Belief Pattern

Cultural/ethnic background	
Economic status, health behaviors that relate to cultural/ethnic group	
Goals in life	
What is important to client and family	
Importance of religion/spirituality	
Impact of health problems on spirituality	
Relevant PE data: general survey	

Analysis of Data, Nursing Diagnoses, Outcomes, and Interventions

- Record the key points of your discussion with individual and family regarding *strengths* and *weaknesses*.
- Analyze *each* of the patterns *and* the relationships between and among the patterns. Incorporate PE data (normal and abnormal) into your decision-making.
- State the highest priority nursing diagnosis according to the individual/family. Do you agree? If not, why not? Consider health promotion, risk states and problem diagnoses.
- Record appropriate and realistic outcomes that were decided on with the patient. Explain what type of intervention(s) a nurse can use (stay within the domain of nursing) *to support* this person in achieving the outcomes.

Nursing Diagnosis in Education

Martha Craft-Rosenberg, PhD, RN, FAAN and
Kelly Smith, MSN, RN

The use of nursing diagnoses is central to nursing education. The assessment and diagnosis of individuals, families, and communities teach students hypothetical reasoning and critical thinking. Further, those who come to nurses for assistance expect the achievement of improved health outcomes for which nurses are increasingly held accountable. Outcomes and the selection of interventions rest on accurate and valid nursing diagnoses.

Teaching nursing students to use nursing diagnoses begins with assessment and history-taking. As students assess and collect data (information) about individuals, families, and communities, they are identifying the "signs and symptoms" or defining characteristics of the nursing diagnosis concepts. The factors or variables influencing diagnoses are integrated with the history, charts, and other evidence. These variables provide the context, the "related factors," that are combined with the defining characteristics to make nursing diagnoses. When possible, nurses treat related factors with interventions to prevent or reduce their impact. When it is not possible for nurses to treat a related factor, they treat the defining characteristics with selected nursing interventions.

Assessment and Identifying Defining Characteristics

The defining characteristics are those characteristics in individuals, families, and communities that are observable and verifiable. They serve as cues or inferences that cluster as manifestations of an actual illness or wellness health state, or nursing diagnosis. Suppose, for example, that an individual (Sarah) states to a nursing student that she is "sick to my stomach" and asks for an emesis basin. The nursing student further observes that Sarah is swallowing a great deal and gagging. These defining characteristics are suggestive of the nursing diagnosis *Nausea*.

History and Identifying Related Factors

The related factors provide the context for the defining characteristics. Related factors are factors that appear to show some type of patterned relationship with the nursing diagnosis. These factors may be described as antecedent to, associated with, related to, contributing to, or abetting the diagnosis. They are identified as characteristics or history of individuals, families, and communities. In the case of Sarah, she may tell us that she is taking large doses of aspirin on the advice of her physician, and that she takes the aspirin on an empty stomach. In this case students can establish an outcome of "freedom from nausea" and use the NIC nursing intervention of *"Nausea Management"* (Dochterman and Bulechek, 2004), especially the activity of "Reduce or eliminate personal factors that precipitate or increase the nausea (taking aspirin on an empty stomach)."

Selecting the Nursing Diagnosis Label

The nursing diagnosis label is selected based on two characteristics. First, the definition of the diagnosis label should convey a combination of the defining characteristics and related factors. Second, the diagnosis selected is the term with defining characteristics and related factors that fits the data that students collect on assessment and history-taking. In this case the definition of *Nausea* is "A subjective unpleasant, wave-like sensation in the back of the throat, epigastrium, or abdomen that may lead to the urge or need to vomit" (p. 353). In the example, Sarah stated that she is "sick to my stomach" and exhibited other defining characteristics. Her history provided an antecedent of nausea – the ingestion of large doses of aspirin on an empty stomach.

Risk Diagnoses

Nurses have always been responsible for identifying individuals, families, and communities at risk and protecting them from this risk. A risk diagnosis "describes human responses to health conditions/life processes that may develop in a vulnerable individual, family, or community. It is supported by risk factors that contribute to increased vulnerability" (p. 419). For example, the diagnosis of *Risk for Impaired Skin Integrity* includes both internal and external factors that influence vulnerability. The interventions that a nurse selects to reach the outcomes are based on these influencing factors.

Health-Promotion Diagnoses

A health-promotion diagnosis is a clinical judgment of a person's, family's, or community's motivation and desire to increase well-being and actualize human health potential as expressed by a readiness to enhance specific health behaviors such as nutrition and exercise. Health-promotion diagnoses can be used in any health state and do not require current levels of wellness. This readiness is supported by defining characteristics. Interventions are selected in concert with the individual/family/community to best ensure the ability to reach the stated outcomes.

Wellness Diagnoses

A wellness diagnosis describes human responses to levels of wellness in an individual, family, or community that have a readiness for enhancement. This readiness is supported by defining characteristics. As with all diagnoses, nurse-sensitive (sensitive to nursing interventions) outcomes are identified and nursing interventions are selected that provide a high likelihood of reaching the outcomes.

Prioritizing Diagnoses

Prioritizing diagnoses is one type of critical thinking that most nursing educators expect from students. Faculty members often request a list of nursing diagnoses from students. Students compile this list while they are reading the history of individuals, families, and communities. After assessment, the students need to make decisions about prioritizing diagnoses. Priorities are established based on the needs of individuals, families, and communities. When nursing students are assigned to clinical experience for a short period of time, faculty members may ask them to choose nursing diagnoses that they can address during this time frame.

Linking Nursing Diagnoses to Outcomes and Interventions

Accurate and valid nursing diagnoses determine the nurse-sensitive outcomes. These outcomes guide the selection of interventions that are likely to produce the desired treatment effects. Again, interventions will treat either related factors (or risk factors) or defining characteristics. Faculty members and their students can use the linkage book (Johnson et al., 2006) or the linkages to nursing diagnoses provided in the back of the NIC (Dochterman and Bulechek, 2004) and NOC (Moorhead et al., 2004) books. These linkages with nursing diagnoses provide clear examples for linking diagnoses, interventions, and outcomes. Some faculty members, however, may require their students to identify outcomes and select nursing interventions independently in order to apply critical thinking skills. Faculty members using nursing diagnoses will detect an increase in critical and analytical thinking from students, which will have a clear focus on prioritized individual, family, and community needs. Faculty members who are new to this process will learn with their students initially, but both will be amazed at the speed with which this "natural" process is applied.

References

Dochterman, J.M. & Bulechek, G. (eds) (2004). *Nursing interventions classification* (NIC). St Louis, MO: Mosby.

Johnson, J., Bulechek, G., Butcher, H., et al. (2006). *NANDA, NOC, and NIC Linkages: Nursing diagnoses, outcomes, & interventions*, 2nd edn. St Louis, MO: Mosby.

The Value of Nursing Diagnoses in Electronic Health Records

Jane Brokel, PhD, RN and Crystal Heath, MSN, RN

In 2004, the healthcare industry accounted for $1.9 trillion dollars, 16% of the US gross domestic product (Doeksen, 2006). MECON (1995) and the Healthcare Financial Management Association, in 1995, reported that nursing labor costs accounted for more than 50% of the total healthcare labor costs. As a result, in the mid-1990s hospital corporations reduced labor costs by reducing nursing personnel (Wunderlich et al., 1996; DeMoro, 2000). Consequently, the prospective payment system was driving the reductions in inpatient admissions and lengths of stay although hospitals experienced increasing complexity of care for inpatients. In addition, the prospective payment system was moving care from the hospital settings to other ambulatory settings such as home care. These changes have implications for nursing labor resource requirements (Kovner et al., 2000). Yet no specific nursing data were ever used to guide the decisions on where reduction of personnel should occur.

Previous studies had found that nursing diagnoses associated with each patient explained a portion of length of hospital stay, length of stay on the intensive care unit (ICU), and total hospital charges (Welton and Halloran, 1999). Nursing diagnoses also explained a portion of the number of home health nursing visits (Marek, 1996). Titler and team (2006) studied the movement of patients with hip fractures from the hospital. Her team found that the documented nursing interventions provided during hospital care predicted whether the patients were discharged home or to another intermediate nursing facility setting. In view of the fact that nursing interventions and costs are a significant source of hospital expenditure, there is still very little quantitative analysis on nurses' contributions to overall patient outcomes. Now, nurse staffing levels are under continual review with even legislative debates to determine ratios of nurses to patients. Using standardized nursing languages within clinical information systems can provide nurses and others with the information that demonstrates contributions of nursing care (Titler et al., 2006). These complex studies compile the data from multiple healthcare information systems and even paper systems, which have a wide variation in documentation methods.

Nursing services are not always identified as revenue generating for a hospital because nursing services historically have been included as overhead in the room and board (Hendricks and Baume, 1997). As the care provided by nurses has not been collected and analyzed, the effect on outcomes and the benefits of nursing assessments, interventions, and coordination of care for the patient and hospital are not quantified. To provide the quantifiable information required to effectively evaluate the value of nursing, standardized nursing terminologies must be uniformly included in the electronic health record (EHR) so the data are systematically collected and analyzed (Lavin et al., 2004).

As nursing personnel are the main source of hospital expenditure, the ability to extract standard nursing terms from the EHR will provide answers for the management of healthcare costs. Nursing data are more important than ever in today's environment in order to improve patient safety and manage health care efficiently and cost-effectively (Jerant et al., 2001). Cost-effectiveness analysis is dependent on an ingredients method (Levin and McEwan, 2001). Basically, every intervention uses ingredients that have a value or costs. If the ingredients can be *identified* and their costs ascertained, the total cost of the intervention and the cost per unit of effectiveness, benefit, or utility can be calculated (Levin and McEwan, 2001). Terminologies such as NANDA International's nursing diagnoses, NIC interventions, NOC outcomes and indicators, when used together, provide the best opportunity to answer questions about the safety, efficiency, and cost-effectiveness of nursing practice for patient populations. Several frameworks have been proposed to use the terminologies together in EHRs, such as VIPS Models (Ehnforss et al., 1998), OPT Model (Pesut and Herman, 1999), NNN Taxonomy of Nursing Practice (McCloskey and Bulechek, 2004), and the KPO Model (von Krogh et al., 2005).

Nursing documentation in current practice primarily consists of lengthy, paper-based, narrative notes. This approach has significant variations in terms of describing nursing findings and actions, and therefore disadvantages anyone's ability to analyze care. Narrative notes are ambiguous, and contain redundancies and various nuances within the text. In addition, as these notes are usually handwritten, they are frequently illegible, misinterpreted, and generally available to only one person at a time. As a result of these issues, narrative notes are difficult to enter into a computerized system where they can be retrieved for daily evaluation of patient care or analyzed for research and decision support (Bates et al., 2003).

The inclusion of NANDA-I nursing diagnoses in conjunction with the Nursing Intervention Classification (McCloskey and Bulechek, 2004) and the Nursing Outcome Classification (Moorhead et al., 2004) in the EHR provides a comprehensive means for capturing the unique contribution of nursing in a consistent and quantifiable format. This consistency can provide the following benefits:

- Facilitate communication efforts of the healthcare team. These nursing terms, along with uniform medication and medical terms, will provide continuity of care within nursing units and across nursing settings (Figoski and Downey, 2006).

- A language that links nursing concepts for the nursing process within the EHR and facilitates the eventual data exchange of nursing process concepts.
- A means of describing the knowledge and skills essential to nursing practice (Lunney, 2006).
- A common method to allow nurse executives and administrators to collect and analyze nursing-specific data that will provide evidence of the effects and contributions that nursing care provides, as well as the ability to cost out nursing services to third party payers (Jerant et al., 2001). A common means to capture data on patient outcomes that will assist design and build new knowledge to support evidence-based practice (Lavin et al., 2004).
- A mechanism to facilitate health ministry and legislative debate with policy development (Lavin et al., 2004).
- A common language in the education process to teach clinical decision-making to nursing students (Garcia et al., 2006; Gloskey et al., 2006; Gordon, 2006; Johnson, 2006).
- Information to advance the science of nursing care.
- In order for the EHR to truly reflect the total care provided by healthcare professionals, it must include nursing data to reflect the nursing process (von Krogh et al., 2005).

Standardized nursing terminologies such as NANDA-I, NIC, and NOC provide the means of collecting nursing data that are systematically analyzed within and across healthcare organizations. Furthermore, these data are essential to provide the foundation for any cost/benefit analysis for nursing practice.

References

Bates, D.W., Ebell, M., Gotlieb, E., Zapp, J., & Mullins, H.C. (2003). A proposal for electronic medical records in U.S. primary care. *Journal of the American Medical Informatics Association* **10**(1): 1–10.

DeMoro, D. (2000). Engineering a crisis. How hospitals created a shortage of nurses. *Revolution* **1**(2): 16–23.

Doeksen, G.A. (2006). The changing face of economic development: Health care as an economic engine. Paper presented at the EcoMod International Conference on Regional and Urban Modeling, Brussels, Belgium.

Ehnfors, M., Ehrenberg, A., & Thorell-Ekstand, I. (1998). *VIPS Boken. The VIPS book.* Stockholm: Vordforbunder.

Figoski, M. & Downey, J. (2006). Perspectives in continuity of care. Facility charging and nursing intervention classification (NIC): The new dynamic duo. *Nursing Economics* **24**: 102–11.

Garcia, T., Hansche, J., & Lobert, J.H. (2006). A user's guide to operationalizing NANDA, NIC, and NOC in a nursing curriculum. *International Journal of Nursing Terminologies & Classifications* (17), 33–4.

Gloskey, D., Kravutske, M.E., & Zugcic, M. (2006). Do you need to educate RNs on how to document using the nursing outcome classification? *International Journal of Nursing Terminologies & Classifications* (17): 34–5.

Gordon, M. (2006). Tips on teaching nursing diagnosis. *International Journal of Nursing Terminologies & Classifications* (17): 35.

Hendricks, J. & Baume, P. (1997). The pricing of nursing care. *Journal of Advanced Nursing* **25**: 454–62.

Jerant, A.F., Azari, R., & Nesbitt, T.S. (2001). Reducing the cost of frequent hospital admissions for congestive heart failure. A randomized trial of a home telecare intervention. *Medical Care* **39**: 1234–45.

Johnson, M. (2006). Linking NANDA, NOC and NIC. *International Journal of Nursing Terminologies & Classifications* **17**: 39–40.

Kovner, C.T., Jones, C.B., & Gergen, P.J. (2000). Nursing staffing in acute care hospitals, 1990, 1996. *Policy, Politics, & Nursing Practice* **1**: 194–204.

Lavin, M.A., Avant, K., Craft-Rosenberg, M., Herdman, T.H., & Gebbie, K. (2004). Contexts for the study of the economic influence of nursing diagnoses on patient outcomes. *International Journal of Nursing Terminologies and Classifications* **15**: 39–47.

Levin, H.M. & McEwan, P.J. (2001). *Cost-effectiveness analysis*, 2nd edn. Thousand Oaks, CA: Sage.

Lunney, M. (2006). Staff development. Helping nurses use NANDA, NOC, and NIC: Novice to expert. *Journal of Nursing Administration* **36**: 118–25.

Marek, K.D. (1996). Nursing diagnoses and home care nursing utilization. *Public Health Nurse* **13**: 195–200.

McCloskey, J. & Bulechek, G. (2004). *Nursing interventions classification*, 4th edn. St Louis, MO: Mosby.

MECON and Healthcare Financial Management Association. (1995). *From increasing revenues to controlling costs: Benchmark data for strategic planning* [Supplement]. Westchester, IL: MECON.

Moorhead, S., Johnson, M., & Maas, M. (2004). *Nursing outcomes classification* (NOC). St Louis, MO: Mosby.

Pesut, D.J. & Herman, J. (1999). Clinical reasoning. In: *The art & science of critical and creative thinking*. Detroit, MI: Delmar.

Titler, M., Dochterman, J., Xie, X., et al. (2006). Nursing interventions and other factors associated with discharge disposition in older patients after hip fractures. *Nursing Research* **55**: 231–42.

von Krogh, G., Dale, C., & Naden, D. (2005). A framework for integrating NANDA, NIC, and NOC terminology in electronic patient records. *Journal of Nursing Scholarship* **37**: 275–81.

Welton, J.M. & Halloran, E.J. (1999). A comparison of nursing and medical diagnoses in predicting hospital outcomes. Transforming health care through informatics: Cornerstone for a new information management paradigm. *Proceedings from AMIA 1999 Annual Symposium*, pp. 171–5. Bethesda, MD: AMIA.

Wunderlich, G., Sloan, F., & Davis, C. (eds) (1996). *Nursing staff in hospitals and nursing homes: Is it adequate?* Washington, DC: National Academy Press.

Nursing Diagnosis and Research

Margaret Lunney, PhD, RN

Since 1973, the diagnoses approved for the NANDA-I *Taxonomy of Nursing Diagnoses* were developed and submitted by nurses using a variety of research methods. Each diagnosis is research based, with some diagnoses having stronger research evidence than others. Over the last four decades, the research methods have become more sophisticated and the Diagnosis Development Committee has required more stringent evidence as the basis for approving new diagnoses.

To remain evidence based, however, the NANDA-I Taxonomy needs ongoing research support (Whitley, 1999). Some of the types of studies needed are concept analyses, content validation, construct and criterion-related validation, consensus validation, studies of accuracy of nurses' diagnoses, and implementation studies. The references cited can be used as resources for these research methods.

Concept Analyses

Concept development and analyses have been and continue to be an important aspect of the development and approval of new diagnoses (Avant, 1990). Concept identification and formulation are the first step in developing a new diagnosis and refining previously accepted diagnoses. Each nursing diagnosis is a concept that needs to be developed using systematic methods (Walker and Avant, 2005). A classic study, for example, was Whitley's (1992) concept analysis of *fear*. At the 2006 NNN Alliance conference, a concept analysis was reported to develop a new wellness health promotion diagnosis: *Supportive Family Role Performance* (Lamont, 2006). Melo Ade, Campos de Carvalho, & Rotter Pelà (2007) used content analyses to recommend changes in the diagnoses of sexual dysfunction and ineffective sexuality patterns.

Content Validation

Content validation studies are often foundational for refining approved diagnoses and developing new diagnoses. In these studies, there are two possible groups of subjects – nurses who work with patients who experience the specific diagnoses or patients who currently are experiencing the diagnosis (Fehring, 1986). A problem with nurses as subjects, however, especially if it is a new diagnosis, is that they are being asked to state from memory the relevance of defining characteristics. Clinical validation studies, in which patients are assessed for defining characteristics at the time that they experience the specific human response, provide better data for content validation studies.

For decades, the data from clinical validation studies have served as support for nursing diagnoses, (Zeitoun, de Barros, Michel & de Bettencourt, 2007; Bartek et al.; 1999; Carlson-Catalano et al., 1998; and Kim et al., 1984). The challenges of conducting clinical studies are significant but worthwhile because data are from actual patients who are currently experiencing the human response of interest to the researcher. Methodological considerations for such studies were described by Carlson-Catalano and Lunney (1995), Grant et al. (1990), and Maas et al. (1990). Sparks and Lien-Gieschen (1994) provided revised guidelines for scoring and interpreting defining characteristics as highly or moderately relevant for making a diagnosis. These scoring revisions are important to avoid development of long lists of defining characteristics. Some of the currently approved diagnoses have long lists of defining characteristics that could be reduced if clinical studies were done using the aforementioned guidelines.

Construct and Criterion-Related Validity

"Knowledge development of diagnoses in the NANDA-I Taxonomy means that a series of studies needs to be done for each individual diagnosis as well as groups of diagnoses", (Parker and Lunney, 1998, p. 146). The various types of studies needed to establish construct and criterion-related validity are reliability, epidemiological, outcome, causal analysis, and generalizability studies (Parker and Lunney, 1998). Reliability studies can establish the stability and coherence of diagnoses. Epidemiological studies of the incidence and prevalence of specific diagnoses in settings and populations can show the importance and co-occurrence of diagnoses, e.g., in retrospective analyses of 123,241 sequential admissions to a university hospital, Welton and Halloran (2005) demonstrated that nursing diagnoses were good predictors of hospital outcomes, adding 30–146% of explanatory power to diagnosis-related groups (DRGs) and all payer-refined DRGs. Epidemiological studies can also be done to show the relationships among diagnoses, interventions, and outcomes. Outcome, or effectiveness, studies can illustrate the prognoses of diagnoses and the best interventions to help people who are experiencing specific diagnoses. Effectiveness studies are being done by a research team in Iowa, e.g., Shever, Titler, Dochterman, Fei & Picone (2007). A study be Müller-Staub, Needham, Odenbreit, Lavin & van Achterberg (2007) showed that there was improved documentation of patient outcomes after teaching nurses to use nursing diagnoses and interventions. A symposia of three examples of effectiveness studies was presented at the 2006 NNN Alliance conference (Dochterman, 2006). Causal analysis studies, using experimental designs, can show the relation of diagnoses to theories and the importance of using standardized diagnoses to achieve high-quality nursing care. Generalizability studies can show the importance of nursing diagnoses across institutions and medical diagnoses or *International Classification of Diseases*, 9th edn (ICD-9 – Mortality Statistics Branch 1987, National Center for Health Statistics, Centers for Disease Control and Prevention) categories. A good resource for conducting validity and reliability studies is a book on measurement (e.g., Waltz et al., 2005).

Consensus Validation

Consensus validation techniques are being used to establish the connections of NANDA, NIC, and NOC with specific populations for the purposes of developing standards of practice and identifying the specific terms to be included in electronic health records (Westmoreland et al., 2000; Carlson, 2006a, 2006b; Minthorn, 2006). Westmoreland et al.'s study validated that their clinical practice guidelines delineated the right services and knowledge related to these services (p. 19). Carlson (2006a) recommends participatory action research methods for practicing nurses to identify the specific NANDA, NIC, and NOC terms that apply to patients served by their agency or unit. This process is being used in a variety of settings and can be adopted by nurses in any setting and locality. In the near future, the Research Committee will be promoting this process as a standardized method to establish standards of practice and to select terms for EHRs.

Studies of Accuracy of Nurses' Diagnoses

Studies of accuracy of nurses' diagnoses and factors that influence accuracy are needed because previous studies established that accuracy varies widely (Lunney, 2008). The accuracy of nurses' diagnoses is important because this is the foundation for choices of interventions and outcomes. Examples are a clinical study by Lunney, Karlik, Kiss and Murphy (1997) and a mail survey by Hasegawa, Ogasawara, and Katz (2007). Crossetti and Saurin (2006) presented a study related to accuracy at the 2006 NNN Alliance conference.

Implementation Studies

The importance of using nursing diagnoses in clinical practice is that the quality of nursing care is expected to improve (Lunney, 2008). Yet, there are insufficient data at the present time to convince others that this is so. Two recent studies demonstrated the positive effects of implementing standardized nursing languages (Müller-Staub, 2007; Thoroddsen & Enfors, 2007), but many more such studies are needed.

Summary

Nursing diagnosis studies are sorely needed to maintain and enhance the evidence-base of the NANDA-I Taxonomy. The Research Committee is eager to provide assistance to anyone considering undertaking a study. Contact margell@si.rr.com or Lunney@mail.csi.cuny. edu.

References

Avant, K.C. (1990). The art and science in nursing diagnosis development. *Nursing Diagnosis* **1**(2): 51–6.

Bartek, J.K., Lindeman, M., & Hawks, J.H. (1999). Clinical validation of characteristics of the alcoholic family. *Nursing Diagnosis: Journal of Nursing Language and Classification* **10**: 158–68.

Carlson, J.M. (2006a). Consensus validation process: A standardized research method to identify and link their relevant NANDA, NIC and NOC terms for local populations [Abstract]. *International Journal of Nursing Terminologies and Classifications* **17**(1): 23–4.

Carlson, J.M. (2006b). Professional nursing latent tuberculosis infection standards of practice development using NANDA, NIC and NOC [Abstract]. *International Journal of Nursing Terminologies and Classifications* **17**(1): 62.

Carlson-Catalano, J. & Lunney, M. (1995). Quantitative methods for clinical validation of nursing diagnoses. *Clinical Nurse Specialist: Journal of Advanced Nursing Practice* **9**: 306–11.

Carlson-Catalano, J., Lunney, M., Paradiso, C., et al. (1998). Clinical validation of ineffective breathing pattern, ineffective airway clearance and impaired gas exchange. *IMAGE: Journal of Nursing Scholarship* **30**: 243–8.

Crossetti, M.G.O. & Saurin, G. (2006). Critical thinking and nursing diagnosis accuracy in a university hospital [Abstract]. *International Journal of Nursing Terminologies and Classifications* **17**(1): 29–30.

Dochterman, J. (2006). Effectiveness research: Three examples [Abstracts]. *International Journal of Nursing Terminologies and Classifications* **17**(1): 85–7.

Fehring, R.J. (1986). Validating diagnostic labels: Standardized methodology. In Hurley, E. (ed.), *Classification of nursing diagnoses: Proceedings of the sixth conference*, pp. 183–90. St Louis, MO: NANDA.

Grant, J.S., Kinney, M., & Guzzetta, C.E. (1990). Using magnitude estimation scaling to examine the validity of nursing diagnoses. *Nursing Diagnosis,* **1**(2): 64–9.

Hasegawa, T., Ogaswara, C., Tachibana, S., et al. (2006). Validity of written case studies as a tool to measure nurses. Ability for making nursing diagnoses. *International Journal of Nursing Terminologies and Classifications* **17**(1): 36–7.

Hasegawa, T., Ogasawara, C., & Katz, E.C. (2007). Measuring diagnostic competency and the analysis of factors influencing competency using written case studies. *International Journal of Nursing Terminologies and Classifications,* **18**: 93–102.

Kim, M.J., Amoroso-Seritella, R., Gulanick, M., et al. (1984). Clinical validation of cardiovascular nursing diagnoses. In: Kim, M.J., McFarland, G.K., & McLane, A.M. (eds), *Classification of nursing diagnoses: Proceedings of the fifth national conference*, pp. 128–138. St Louis: Mosby.

Lamont, S.C. (2006). Supportive role performance: Development of a new wellness diagnosis [Abstract]. *International Journal of Nursing Terminologies and Classifications* **17**(1): 40–1.

Lunney, M., Karlik, B.A., Kiss, M., & Murphy, P. (1997). Accuracy of nurses' diagnoses of psychosocial responses. *Nursing Diagnosis,* **8**: 157–66.

Lunney, M. (2001). *Critical thinking and nursing diagnosis: Case studies and analyses.* Philadelphia: NANDA.

Lunney, M. (2008). Critical need to address accuracy of nurses' diagnoses. *OJIN: Online Journal of Issues in Nursing, Retrieved on February 21, 2008 from http://www. nursingworld.org/MainMenuCategories/ANAmarketplace/ANAperiodicals/OJIN/Tableof Contents/Vol31998/VolNo21998/accuracyofnursesdiagnoses.aspx*

Maas, M.L., Hardy, M.A., & Craft, M. (1990). Methodologic considerations in nursing diagnosis research. *Nursing Diagnosis* **1**(1): 24–30.

Melo Ade, S. Campos de Carvalho, E., & Rotter Pelà, N.T. (2007). Proposed revisions for the nursing diagnoses sexual dysfunction and ineffective sexuality patters. *International Journal of Nursing Terminologies and Classifications* **18**: 150–5.

Minthorn, C. (2006). Meeting Magnet criteria with studies of NANDA, NIC and NOC. [abstract] *International Journal of Nursing Terminologies and Classifications* **17**: 46.

Mortality Statistics Branch, National Center for Health Statistics, Centers for Disease Control and Prevention (1987). *International classification of diseases*, 9th revision (ICD). Hyattsville, MD. Available at: ftp://ftp.cdc.gov/pub/Health_Statistics/NCHS/ Publications/ICD-9/ucod.txt (accessed June 7, 2008).

Müller-Staub, M., Needham, I., Odenbreit, M., Lavin, M.A., & van Achterberg, T. (2007). Improved quality of nursing documentation: Results of a nursing diagnoses, interventions and outcomes implementation study. *International Journal of Nursing Terminologies and Classifications* **18**: 5–17.

Parker, L. & Lunney, M. (1998). Moving beyond content validation of nursing diagnoses. *International Journal of Nursing Terminologies and Classifications* **9**(suppl 2): 144–50.

Shever, L.L., Titler, M., Dochterman, J., Fei, Q., & Picone, D.M. (2007). Patterns of nursing intervention use across 6 days of acute care hospitalization for three older patient populations. *International Journal of Nursing Terminologies and Classifications* **18**: 18–29.

Sparks, S.M. & Lien-Gieschen, T. (1994). Modification of the diagnostic content validity model. *Nursing Diagnoses* **5**(1): 31–5.

Thoroddsen, A. & Ehnfors, M. (2007). Putting policy into practice: Pre-and posttests of implementing standardized languages for nursing documentation. *Journal of Clinical Nursing* **16**: 1826–38.

Walker, L.O. & Avant, K.C. (2005). *Strategies for theory construction in nursing*, 4th edn. Norwalk, CT: Appleton & Lange.

Waltz, C.F., Strickland, O.L., & Lenz, E.R. (2005). *Measurement in nursing and health sciences research*, 3rd edn. New York: Springer.

Welton, J.M. & Halloran, E.J. (2005). Nursing diagnoses, diagnosis-related groups, and hospital outcomes. *Journal of Nursing Administration* **35**: 541–9.

Westmoreland, D., Wesorick, B., Hanson, D., & Wyngarden, K. (2000). Consensus validation of clinical practice model practice guidelines. *Journal of Nursing Care Quality* **14**(4): 16–27.

Whitley, G.G. (1992). Concept analysis of fear. *Nursing Diagnoses* **3**(4): 155–61.

Whitley, G.G. (1999). Processes and methodologies for research validation of nursing diagnoses. *Nursing Diagnoses* **10**(1): 5–14.

Zeitoun, S.S., de Barros, A.L., Michel, J.L., & de Bettencourt, A.R. (2007). Clinical validation of the signs and symptoms and the nature of the respiratory nursing diagnoses in patients under invasive mechanical ventilation. *Journal of Clinical Nursing* **16**: 1417–26.

Nursing Diagnosis in Administration

Dickon Weir-Hughes, EdD, RN, FRSH

Since the advent of the nursing diagnosis movement in the 1970s, some of the finest nurse scholars have been attracted to support the work. Many of these activists have been clinically focused academics, researchers, and educationalists, and some have also been expert clinicians. It is notable, however, that chief nurses/nurse directors, administrators, or managers have generally been less active in this important area of nursing development. This is intriguing because nursing diagnosis is so fundamental to the provision of high quality nursing care, and the benefits are so numerous, that it would seem obvious that even the busiest nurse leader would make its development and implementation a priority. In an era when both cost containment and evidence-based practice are key objectives for nurse leaders, classifying, clarifying, and documenting the phenomena that are of professional concern to nurses are essential.

Why Implement Nursing Diagnosis in a Clinical Environment?

The implementation of nursing diagnosis brings a number of benefits to patient care: improved and more consistent care planning; improved nurse-to-nurse, nurse-to-physician, and nurse-to-patient communication; and better recognition of phenomena that nurses find challenging to assess and describe, such as psychological, spiritual, and sexual issues. From an organizational point of view, nursing diagnosis helps to improve clinical governance and risk management, and clearly demonstrates a commitment to bring together nursing theory, education, and clinical practice – in other words, evidence-based nursing. Importantly, it also enables nurse leaders and researchers to evaluate nursing practice across an organization in a consistent and thought-provoking way.

A number of studies, including those by Halloran and Kiley (1987), published in a range of peer-reviewed journals between 1985 and 1987 examine the whole notion of the use of diagnostic-related groups (DRGs) and related systems that attach payment to procedures or medical conditions rather than actual patient dependency. Halloran and Kiley examined 1288 adult medical and surgical patients in an urban teaching hospital in the US. The complexity of medical treatment was measured by use of the DRG relative cost weight. The nursing indicator was derived from a set of nursing diagnoses. The study findings concluded that DRG cost weight is a poor predicator of dependency (and therefore costs of care) and that the nursing-dependency index, based on a series of 61 nursing diagnoses, added significantly to the DRG weight in explaining length of stay and other issues. Given that the nursing resource is one of the most significant areas of expenditure for any healthcare organization and that organizations frequently rely on the number of nurses that it has available to take in more work, this is a significant finding. The Halloran and Kiley study, and one by Frank and Lave (1985), indicate that, to be cost-efficient in relation to length of stay, it is essential to include a nursing-dependency factor based on nursing diagnoses in forward planning. It is sobering that, 20 years later, nurse leaders still have not taken forward the use of nursing diagnosis in ways recommended by these seminal pieces of work.

Evidence-based Practice: Integrating Theory and Practice

The nursing research and outcomes opportunities that emerge as a result of using nursing diagnosis are phenomenal and unparalleled. Almost 150 years ago Florence Nightingale (1863) commented on the paucity of comparative outcomes data on nursing interventions. "In an attempt to arrive at the truth, I have applied everywhere for information, but in scarcely an instance have I been able to obtain hospital records fit for any purpose of comparison. They would show the subscribers how their money was being spent, what good was really being done with it. They would enable us, besides, to ascertain the influence of the hospital upon the course of operations and diseases passing through its wards; and the truth thus ascertained would enable us to save life and suffering and to improve the management of the sick" (pp. 175–6).

Although major strides have been made in some places, it is concerning that 150 years later many nursing organizations, whether in hospitals or community settings, are still failing to evaluate their practice in a consistent manner. Nursing diagnosis data collected from clinical areas allow nurses to evaluate their individual clinical practice and explicitly integrate theory and practice. As well, the data allow nurse leaders and researchers to evaluate, audit, and establish practice priorities organizationally through conducting prevalence studies. This information can then help to define the content of inservice education and even university-based educational offerings.

Nursing in the Era of Electronic Patient Records

The essence of nursing is the therapeutic professional relationship between nurse and patient. Although information systems may appear to be cold and literal, there is no reason why an electronic patient records system should do anything but enhance the clinical role of the nurse by saving time and improving documentation. Within some such systems, however, there is a tendency to see nursing reduced to an automated list of tasks generated by standardized care pathways. This reductionist approach to professional nursing is neither clinically safe nor commercially savvy because it ignores the needs of individual patients. Assessing, meeting, and evaluating such individual needs are key to safe patient care, and providing the levels of patient satisfaction omnipresent in the ever more consumer-driven health sector in which nurses practice.

It is well recognized that the implementation of any healthcare information system provides the opportunity to review and improve clinical practice. Unfortunately, it is also recognized that some system implementations have had extremely negative consequences on nursing practice and, therefore, patient care. These consequences are manifested in a variety of ways. From a clinical point of view, poorly planned and under-professionally led systems reduce nursing to a care pathway-generated list of tasks that ignores the needs of individuals, and which serves only as a retrograde step to developing patient-focused care. This sort of implementation has been found to give rise to unsafe, unthinking nursing practice, which creates a major clinical governance issue.

From a leadership perspective, systems that radically change nursing practice overnight create enormous problems for clinical staff, who have to get used not only to a new IT system but also to numerous new concepts in documenting and planning care, such as using standard nursing language. However, when well managed and professionally led, there are numerous benefits to bringing together nursing diagnosis and an electronic patient record (EPR). Systems that support nursing diagnosis functionality enable nurses to plan care using gold standard, evidence-based nursing. This is key to the reputation of the system vendor and essential for the credibility and legal status of healthcare organizations. From a research and audit perspective, using an EPR based on nursing diagnoses means that comparative data about nursing diagnoses, prevalence, incidence, and linkages to interventions and outcomes can be retrieved quickly and easily. This information can be used to inform an organization's nursing strategy, workforce design, and curriculum planning, and to define in-service education priorities.

Leading the Implementation of Nursing Diagnosis in Clinical Practice

The key nursing diagnosis challenge for nurse leaders is its implementation into everyday clinical practice. Implementation is variable throughout the developed world and even within health systems.

However, successful implementation requires expert, high level nursing leadership, ideally at a board or organizational "top team" level. A range of leadership skills is required for successful implementation, with high levels of technical ability, influencing skills, delegation, strategic thinking, networking, and following through. It is vital that nurse leaders thoroughly understand the use and development of nursing diagnosis and can inspire, harness enthusiasm, manage dissent, and answer questions from clinicians with an in-depth understanding of the challenges. As stakeholders in the future of nursing, it is vital to engage nurses at all levels in this important developmental work.

The amount of attention paid to nursing diagnosis in undergraduate nursing programs varies quite significantly worldwide. In terms of inservice education and implementation support, nurses typically need preparation and/or updating in critical thinking and the use of nursing diagnosis and associated assessment tools. Typically, this teaching can be covered in an intensive 1- or 2-day program with follow-up support in clinical areas from mentors who have this knowledge. Nurses also need paper-based manuals of nursing diagnoses. In many environments, nursing diagnosis is used within EPRs and therefore IT training will be required. It is important to understand that teaching nursing diagnosis and critical thinking should be nurse led, not IT led, so the focus will be on nursing. Suggested ways of engaging stakeholders and raising awareness include having nursing diagnosis in all regular teaching programs, encouraging attendance at international nursing diagnosis conferences, organizing Grand Rounds where cases are presented using nursing diagnosis, and starting focused journal clubs.

Conclusion

Using nursing diagnosis is key to the future of evidence-based, professionally led nursing care. Thus, it needs to be a priority for all nurse leaders in administration and management in order to make nursing practice visible, which is vital to the future of our profession and to enabling us to more effectively meet the needs of patients.

References

Frank, R. & Lave, J. (1985). The psychiatric DRGs: Are they different? *Medical Care* **23**: 1148–55.
Halloran, E. & Kiley, M. (1987). Nursing dependency, diagnosis-related groups, and length of stay. *Health Care Financing Review* **8**(3): 27–36.
Nightingale, F. (1863). *Notes on hospitals.* London: Longman, Roberts, Green.

The Process for Development of an Approved NANDA-I Nursing Diagnosis

Leann M. Scroggins, MS, RN, CRRN-A, APRN BC

Clinical Nurse Specialist
Mayo Clinic, Rochester, MN
Chair, Diagnosis Development Committee
NANDA International

This article is designed to assist in the development of a nursing diagnosis that will meet the inclusion criteria for acceptance into the NANDA classification system. It is recommended that the submitter follow the steps below to move through the process. If at any point there are questions, please contact the Chair of the Diagnosis Development Committee for assistance and guidance: info@nanda.org.

An additional resource that will facilitate completion of the process include:

■ NANDA-I website: www.nanda.org/html/nursing_diagnosis_devmt.html.

Reviewing the following information will provide a good basis on which to begin this important work.

To be accepted for publication and inclusion in NANDA-I Taxonomy II, a nursing diagnosis submission must minimally have a label, definition defining characteristics or risk factors, related factors (if an actual diagnosis), supported by references and examples of appropriate interventions and outcomes. The official definition of a nursing diagnosis is "a clinical judgment about individual, family, or community responses to actual or potential health problems/life processes. A nursing diagnosis provides the basis for selection of nursing interventions to achieve outcomes for which the nurse is accountable" (NANDA-I, 2007–2008, p. 332).

Taxonomy II is a multiaxial structure. The seven axes of the taxonomy are dimensions of the human response. To create a diagnosis, it is essential to consider all seven axes (Figure 1.1).

Axis 1: The Diagnostic Concept

The diagnostic concept is the principal component of the diagnosis. The diagnostic concept may consist of one or more nouns. When more than one noun is used (e.g., activity tolerance), each noun contributes a unique meaning to the concept, as if the two were a single noun. The meaning of the combined term is, however, different from the nouns

Figure 1.1 *The NANDA-I model of a nursing diagnosis*

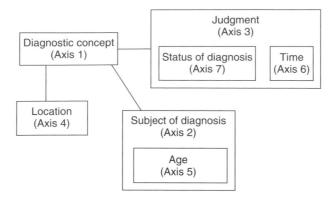

stated separately. Frequently an adjective (e.g., spiritual) may be used with a noun (e.g., distress) to denote the diagnostic concept (e.g., *Spiritual Distress*).

In some cases, the diagnostic concept and the diagnosis are the same (e.g., *Pain*). This occurs when the nursing diagnosis is stated at the most clinically useful level and the separation of the diagnostic concept adds no meaningful level of abstraction. The following are examples of diagnostic concepts. For a complete listing refer to *NANDA-I Nursing Diagnoses: Definitions & Classification 2009–2011*, pp. 382–384.

Examples of diagnostic concepts in Taxonomy II:

- *Activity intolerance*
- *Airway clearance*
- *Mobility*
- *Hope*
- *Pain*
- *Parenting*
- *Grieving.*

Axis 2: Subject of the Diagnosis

The subject of the diagnosis refers to the individual or individuals for whom the nursing diagnosis is determined. NANDA-I has identified the following subjects for whom nursing diagnoses may be determined:

- Individual
- Family (e.g. Interrupted Family Processes)
- Group (currently no Group diagnoses have been identified)
- Community (e.g. Ineffective Community Coping)

Axis 3: Judgment

A judgment is a descriptor or modifier (Table 1.1) that limits or specifies meaning to the diagnostic concept. The following are examples of descriptors or modifiers. For a complete listing of descriptors and modifiers, refer to p. 384–385 of *NANDA-I Nursing Diagnoses: Definitions & Classification 2009–2011*.

Some diagnoses, depending on the level of specificity, do not require a modifier or descriptor. Examples of such diagnoses include "*Nausea*" and "*Fatigue*".

Table 1.1 *Judgment*

Descriptor/Modifier	Definition
Compromised	Damaged, made vulnerable
Decreased	Lessened (in size, amount, or degree)
Delayed	Late, slow, or postponed
Disturbed	Agitated, interrupted, interfered with
Impaired	Damaged, weakened
Readiness for	In a suitable state for an activity or situation

Axis 4: Location

Location describes the parts/regions of the body and or their related functions – all tissues, organs, anatomical sites or structures. Following are examples of locations. For a complete listing refer to p. 385 of *NANDA-I Nursing Diagnoses: Definitions & Classification 2009–2011*.

- Cerebral
- Kinesthetic
- Oral
- Renal
- Tactile.

Location does not pertain to all diagnoses.

Axis 5: Age

Age refers to the age of the person who is the subject of the diagnosis. Specific ages identified by NANDA-I are shown in Table 1.2.

Table 1.2 *Specific Age of Diagnostic Subjects*

Fetus	School-age child
Neonate	Adolescent
Infant	Adult
Toddler	
Preschool child	Older adult

Axis 6: Time

Time describes the duration of the diagnostic concept. The time parameters identified by NANDA-I include:

- Acute
- Chronic
- Intermittent
- Continuous.

Axis 7: Status of the Diagnosis

Status refers to the actuality or potentiality of the diagnosis or the categorization of the diagnosis. NANDA-I has identified the following:

- Actual: existing in fact or reality, existing at the present time. A diagnosis is considered "Actual" unless otherwise specified. An actual diagnosis describes human responses to health conditions/life processes that exist in an individual, family, or community. It is supported by defining characteristics (manifestations, signs and symptoms) that cluster in patterns of related cues or inferences. An example of an actual diagnosis is *"Nausea"*.
- Health Promotion: behavior motivated by the desire to increase well-being and actualize human health potential (Pender, Murduagh, & Parsons, 2006).

  Health promotion diagnoses are clinical judgments of a person's, family's, or community's motivation and desire to increase well-being, actualize human health potential, and enhance specific health behaviors such as nutrition and exercise. Health-promotion diagnoses can be used in any health state and do not require current levels of wellness. This readiness is supported by defining characteristics.

  An example of an existing health-promotion diagnosis is, *"Readiness for Enhanced Hope."* Each label of a health-promotion diagnosis begins with the phrase "Readiness for Enhanced."

- Risk: vulnerability, especially as a result of exposure to factors that increase the chance of injury or loss. A Risk diagnosis describes human responses to health conditions/life processes that may develop in a vulnerable individual, family, or community. It is supported by risk factors that contribute to increased vulnerability. An example of a risk diagnosis is, *"Risk for impaired skin integrity."* Each label of a risk diagnosis begins with the phrase "Risk for."
- Wellness: the quality or state of being healthy. A Wellness diagnosis describes human responses to levels of wellness in an individual, family, or community that have a readiness for enhancement. This readiness is supported by defining characteristics. An example of a wellness diagnosis is, *"Readiness for enhanced family coping."* Each label of a wellness diagnosis begins with the phrase "Readiness for Enhanced."

To begin developing the nursing diagnosis consider the following:

1. Is this concept a human response? (Axis 1) If yes, then proceed.
2. Is this concept consistent with the definition of a nursing diagnosis?

   "A nursing diagnosis is a clinical judgment about individual, family, or community responses to actual or potential health problems/life processes. A nursing diagnosis provides the basis for selection of nursing interventions to achieve outcomes for which the nurse is accountable." (NANDA-I, 2009–2011, p. 419)

   If yes, then proceed.
3. Who is the subject of this concept? (Axis 2)
   _____ Individual patient/client
   _____ Family
   _____ Group
   _____ Community
4. Is this concept already included in NANDA-I?
   Review the related existing diagnoses currently in the NANDA-I taxonomy.
   Is the concept currently represented? If there is a similar diagnosis, it may be appropriate to revise the existing diagnosis rather than creating a new diagnosis. If this concept is not included as a current NANDA-I diagnosis, then it is appropriate to proceed with the development of a new diagnosis.
5. Is a descriptor or a modifier required to accurately identify this concept? (Axis 3) If yes, select the appropriate descriptor/modifier (see overleaf):

Descriptor/Modifier	Definition
☐ Anticipatory	Realize beforehand, foresee
☐ Compromised	Damaged, made vulnerable
☐ Decreased	Lessened (in size, amount, or degree)
☐ Defensive	Used or intended to defend or protect
☐ Deficient	Insufficient, inadequate
☐ Delayed	Late, slow, or postponed
☐ Disabled	Limited, handicapped
☐ Disorganized	Not properly arranged or controlled
☐ Disproportionate	Too large or too small in comparison with norm
☐ Disturbed	Agitated, interrupted, interfered with
☐ Dysfunctional	Not operating normally
☐ Effective	Producing the intended or desired effect
☐ Enhanced	Improved in quality, value, or extent
☐ Excessive	Greater than necessary or desirable
☐ Imbalanced	Out of proportion or balance
☐ Impaired	Damaged, weakened
☐ Ineffective	Not producing the intended or desired effect
☐ Interrupted	Having its continuity broken
☐ Low	Below the norm
☐ Organized	Properly arranged or controlled
☐ Perceived	Observed through the senses
☐ Readiness for	In a suitable state for an activity or situation
☐ Situational	Related to a particular circumstance

Is a descriptor/modifier, other than those identified above required for this concept?

If yes, identify and define the descriptor or modifier which best describes this concept:

Descriptor/Modifier: _____

Definition: _____

6. Is Location (Axis 4) relevant for the diagnostic concept? Examples of current diagnoses requiring location to be specified are, "Impaired skin integrity" and "Risk for peripheral neurovascular dysfunction."

If yes, identify the location: _____

7. Should Age (Axis 5) be specified in this diagnostic concept? An example of a current diagnosis requiring age to be specified is, "Adult failure to thrive."

If age should be identified in your diagnostic concept, please identify the appropriate age term: _____

8. Is the Axis 6, Time required to describe this diagnostic concept? If yes, select the appropriate term:
   - ☐ Acute
   - ☐ Chronic
   - ☐ Intermittent
   - ☐ Continuous
9. Select the appropriate Status (Axis 7) for this diagnostic concept:
   - ☐ Actual diagnosis: existing in fact or reality, existing at the present time. A diagnosis is considered "Actual" unless otherwise specified.
   - ☐ Health-promotion diagnosis: behavior motivated by the desire to increase well-being and actualize human health potential (Pender, Murduagh, & Parsons, 2006)
   - ☐ Risk diagnosis: vulnerability, especially as a result of exposure to factors that increase the chance of injury or loss
   - ☐ Wellness diagnosis: the quality or state of being healthy
   - ☐ Syndrome: a cluster or group of signs and symptoms that almost always occur together. Together, these clusters represent a distinct clinical picture (McCourt, 1991, p. 79)

It is now appropriate to begin creating the new diagnosis. Taxonomy II is a multiaxial structure. The seven axes of the taxonomy are dimensions of the human response. To create a diagnosis, it is essential to consider all seven axes (see Figure 1.1).

Congratulations! Many steps have been completed in developing this diagnosis and the diagnostic label may now be identified. Verify that the appropriate axes have been incorporated into your proposed label:

- Diagnostic concept
- Subject of the diagnosis
- Judgment about the diagnosis (descriptor/modifier)
- Location
- Age
- Time
- Status of the diagnosis

State the proposed label here: _____

Label and Definition

The next step in creating this diagnosis is to define the label that has been selected.

Go to the literature, focusing on literature published in the last 5 years. Most of the literature should be nursing but you may find supporting literature in related fields such as the psychosocial sciences.

It is best to have research-based literature but, if such literature does not exist, non-research-based literature may be referenced. The literature must support both the label and the definition. References addressing nursing interventions are not appropriate as supporting references for the label and definition.

The definition must provide a clear, precise description of the label without using the language of the label. The definition gives meaning and helps differentiate this diagnosis from other similar diagnoses. Create the definition here:

_____

_____

_____

Identify the references used to support the label and definition:

_____

_____

Defining Characteristics versus Risk Factors

If this diagnosis is an actual, health-promotion, or wellness diagnosis, identify the Defining characteristics for the diagnosis.

If this diagnosis is a risk diagnosis, identify the Risk factors for the diagnosis. Select which of the following are appropriate for this diagnosis:

☐ Defining characteristics
Defining characteristics are observable cues/inferences that cluster as manifestations of an actual, health promotion or wellness diagnosis.
☐ Risk factors
Risk factors are environmental factors and physiological, psychological, genetic, or chemical elements that increase the vulnerability of an individual, family, or community to an unhealthful event. Risk factors are identified for Risk diagnoses.

Defining characteristics or risk factors must be supported by literature. Like the literature supporting the label and definition of this diagnosis, literature supporting each defining characteristic or risk factor should also focus on literature published in the last 5 years. Again, most of the literature should be nursing but supporting literature in related fields such as the psychosocial sciences may also be used.

It is best to have research-based literature but, if such literature does not exist, non-research-based literature may be referenced. The literature must support the defining characteristics or risk factors. References addressing nursing interventions for the proposed diagnosis are not appropriate as supporting references for defining characteristics or risk factors.

Table 1.3 *Defining Characteristics with References*

Defining characteristics	Supporting reference (no. from list below)
Defining characteristic #1	Reference #___
Defining characteristic #2	Reference #___
Defining characteristic #3	Reference #___

References:

1.
2.
3.
4.

Table 1.4 *Risk Factors*

Risk factors	Supporting reference (no. from list below)
Risk Factor #1	Reference #___
Risk Factor #2	Reference #___
Risk Factor #3	Reference #___

References:

1.
2.
3.
4.

If this diagnosis is an *Actual, Wellness,* or *Health Promotion* diagnosis, list the defining characteristics in Table 1.3. Following this list of defining characteristics, list and number the references supporting the defining characteristics. Indicate the number of the supporting reference with each defining characteristic.

If the diagnosis is a *Risk* diagnosis, list the risk factors in Table 1.4. Following the list of risk factors, list and number the references supporting the risk factors. Indicate the number of the supporting reference with each risk factor.

Taxonomy Rules

The following are some "taxonomy rules" that apply to attributes of nursing diagnoses, both defining characteristics and risk factors. Check each of these rules to make certain the attributes for the proposed diagnosis are stated correctly.

- The attributes of a nursing diagnosis may not contain the following stop-words (i.e., "and," "&," "or," ":," ";," "/," "( )," "e.g.").
- The attributes of a nursing diagnosis may not contain quotes.
- The number of attributes should be limited to those that actually drive the decision of whether or not the diagnosis exists.

Congratulations! A label, definition and either defining characteristics or risk factors all supported by literature have been developed! If the diagnosis is a *wellness*, *health promotion* or *risk* diagnosis, each of the steps necessary to submit your proposal to NANDA-I for inclusion into Taxonomy II has been completed. Please refer to the "Protocol for Submission of Diagnoses" in one of the following references for assistance in the submission process:

- *Nursing Diagnoses: Definitions & Classification* 2009–2011
- NANDA-I website: www.nanda.org/html/nursing_diagnosis_devmt.html.

Related Factors

If the diagnosis is an *actual* diagnosis, there is still more work to do. . . .

Identify Related Factors

Related Factors show a patterned relationship with the nursing diagnosis. Such factors may be described as antecedent to, associated with, related to, contributing to, or abetting. Only actual nursing diagnoses have related factors. Related factors must be supported by literature.

Similar to the literature supporting the label, definition, and defining characteristic or risk factors, the literature supporting related factors should also be published in the last 5 years. Again, most of the literature should be nursing but you may find supporting literature in related fields such as the psychosocial sciences.

It is best to have research-based literature but, if such literature does not exist, non-research-based literature may be referenced. The literature must support the related factors. References addressing nursing interventions for the proposed diagnosis are not appropriate as supporting references for the related factors.

Please list the *Related Factors* in Table 1.5 and link the related factor to the supporting reference by identifying the number of the reference(s).

Table 1.5 *Related Factors*

Related factors	*Supporting reference (no. from list below)*
Related Factor #1	Reference #____
Related Factor #2	Reference #____
Related Factor #3	Reference #____

References:

1.
2.
3.
4.

Indicate the number of the supporting reference with each related factor.

The following "taxonomy rules" apply to related factors. Check each of these rules to make certain that the related factors are stated correctly. (follow by the two bullet points).

■ The related factors of a nursing diagnosis may not contain the following stop-words (i.e., "and," "&," "or," ":," ";," "/," "( )," "e.g.").
■ The related factors of a nursing diagnosis may not contain quotes.

Congratulations! A label, definition, defining characteristics and related factors all supported by literature have been created!

All the steps necessary to submit the proposal to NANDA-I for inclusion into Taxonomy II have been completed. Please refer to the "Protocol for Submission of Diagnoses" in one of the following references for assistance in the submission process:

■ *Nursing Diagnoses: Definitions & Classification 2009–2011*
■ NANDA-I website: www.nanda.org/html/nursing_diagnosis_devmt.html.

References

NANDA International (2007). *Nursing diagnoses: Definitions & classification*, 2007–2008. Philadelphia: NANDA-I. Available at: www.nanda.org/html/nursing_diagnosis_devmt.html (accessed May 23, 2008).

Pender, N.J., Murduagh, C., & Parsons, M.A. (2006). *Health promotion in nursing practice*, 5th edn. Upper Saddle River, NJ: Pearson/Prentice-Hall.

McCourt, A.E. (1991). Syndromes in nursing: a continuing concern. In: Carrol-Johnson, R.M. (ed.), *Classification of nursing diagnoses: Proceedings of the ninth Conference of North American Nursing Diagnosis Association*, pp. 79–82. Philadelphia: JB Lippincott.

Part 2
NANDA-I Nursing Diagnoses 2009–2011

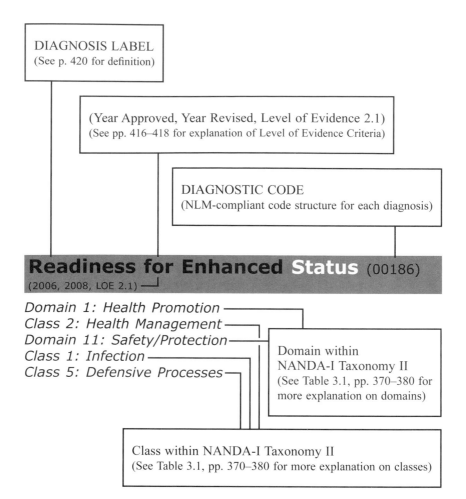

DIAGNOSIS LABEL
(See p. 420 for definition)

(Year Approved, Year Revised, Level of Evidence 2.1)
(See pp. 416–418 for explanation of Level of Evidence Criteria)

DIAGNOSTIC CODE
(NLM-compliant code structure for each diagnosis)

Readiness for Enhanced Status (00186)
(2006, 2008, LOE 2.1)

Domain 1: Health Promotion
Class 2: Health Management
Domain 11: Safety/Protection
Class 1: Infection
Class 5: Defensive Processes

Domain within
NANDA-I Taxonomy II
(See Table 3.1, pp. 370–380 for
more explanation on domains)

Class within NANDA-I Taxonomy II
(See Table 3.1, pp. 370–380 for more explanation on classes)

Domain – "a sphere of activity, study or interest" (Roget, 1980, p. 287)

Class – "a subdivision of a larger group; a division of persons or things by quality, rank, or grade" (Roget, 1980, p. 157)

Diagnosis Label – Provides a name for a diagnosis. It is a concise term or phrase that represents a pattern of related cues. It may include modifiers.

Diagnostic Code – 32-bit integer or 5-digit code that is assigned to a nursing diagnosis; compliant with the National Library of Medicine (NLM) recommendations concerning healthcare terminology codes.

Roget's II: The new thesaurus (1980). Boston: Houghton Mifflin.

Domain 1
Health Promotion

Ineffective Health Maintenance (00099)
(1982)

Domain 1: Health Promotion
Class 2: Health Management

Definition Inability to identify, manage, and/or seek out help to maintain health

Defining Characteristics

- Demonstrated lack of adaptive behaviors to environmental changes
- Demonstrated lack of knowledge about basic health practices
- Lack of expressed interest in improving health behaviors
- History of lack of health-seeking behavior
- Inability to take responsibility for meeting basic health practices
- Impairment of personal support systems

Related Factors

- Cognitive impairment
- Complicated grieving
- Deficient communication skills
- Diminished fine motor skills
- Diminished gross motor skills
- Inability to make appropriate judgments
- Ineffective family coping
- Ineffective individual coping
- Insufficient resources (e.g., equipment, finances)
- Lack of fine motor skills
- Lack of gross motor skills
- Perceptual impairment
- Spiritual distress
- Unachieved developmental tasks

Ineffective Self Health Management
(00078)
(1994, 2008, LOE 2.1)

Domain 1: Health Promotion
Class 2: Health Management

Definition Pattern of regulating and integrating into daily living a therapeutic regime for treatment of illness and its sequelae that is unsatisfactory for meeting specific health goals

Defining Characteristics

- Failure to include treatment regimens in daily living
- Failure to take action to reduce risk factors
- Makes choices in daily living ineffective for meeting health goals
- Verbalizes desire to manage the illness
- Verbalizes difficulty with prescribed regimens

Related Factors

- Complexity of healthcare system
- Complexity of therapeutic regimen
- Decisional conflicts
- Economic difficulties
- Excessive demands made (e.g., individual, family)
- Family conflict
- Family patterns of healthcare
- Inadequate number of cues to action
- Knowledge deficit
- Regimen
- Perceived barriers
- Powerlessness
- Perceived seriousness
- Perceived susceptibility
- Perceived benefits
- Social support deficit

References

Banister N.A., Jastrow, S.T., Hodges, V., Loop, R., & Gillham, M.B. (2004). Diabetes self-management training program in a community clinic improves patient outcomes at modest cost. *J Am Dietetic Assoc* **104**: 807–10.

Benavides-Vaello S., Garcia, A.A., Brown, S.A., et al (2004). Using focus group to plan and evaluate diabetes self-management interventions for Mexican Americans. *Diabetes Educ* **30**: 238–56.

Bodenheimer, T., Lorig, K., Holman, H., et al (2002). Patient self-management of chronic disease in primary care. *JAMA* **288**: 2469.

Brown, C.M. & Segal, R. (1996). Ethnic differences in temporal orientation and its implications for hypertension management. *J Health Soc Behav* **37**: 350.

Bythe, F.M., March, L.M., Nicholas, M.K., & Counsins, M.J. (2005). Self-management of chronic pain: a population-based study. *Pain* **113**: 285–92.

Chinn, M.H. et al (2000). Developing a conceptual framework for understanding illness and attitudes in older, urban African Americans with diabetes. *Diabetes Educ* **26**: 439.

Cousins, S.O. (2000). My heart can't take it: older women's beliefs about exercise benefits and risks. *J Gerontol B Psychol Sci Soc Sci* **55B**: 283.

Curtin, R.B., Sitter, D.C.B., Schatell, D., et al (2004). Self-management, knowledge, and functioning and well being of patients on hemodialysis, *Neph Nurs J* **31**: 378–86.

Deakin, T., McShane, C.E., Cade, J.E., & Willams, R.D. (2005). Group-based training for self management strategies in people with type 2 diabetes mellitus. *Cochrane Database Sys Rev* **18**(2): CD003417.

DeWalt, D.A., Pignone, M., Malone, R., et al (2004). Development and pilot testing of a disease management program for low literacy patients with heart failure. *Patient Educ Couns* **55**: 78–86.

DiLorio, C., Shafer, P.O., Letz, R., Henry, T.R., Schomer, D.I., & Yeager, K. (2004). Project EASE: a study to test a psychosocial model of epilepsy medication management. *Epilepsy Behav* **5**: 926–36.

Funnell, M.M. & Anderson, R.M. (2004). Empowerment and self-management of diabetes. *Clin Diabetes* **22**: 123–7.

Gallant, M.H., Beaulieu, M.C., & Carnevale, F.A. (2002). Partnership: an analysis of the concept within the nurse–client relationship. *J Adv Nurs* **40**(2): 149.

Georges, C.A., Bolton, L.B., & Bennett, C. (2004). Functional health literacy: an issue in African–American and other ethnic and racial communities, *J Natl Black Nurses Assoc* **15**(1): 1–4.

Goldberg, H.I., Lessier, D.S., Mertens, K., Eytan, T.A., & Cheadle, A.D. (2004). Self management support in a web-based medical record: A pilot randomized controlled trial. *J Comm J Qual Saf* **30**: 629–35, 589.

Goodwin, J.S., Black, S.A., & Satish, S. (1999). Aging versus disease: the opinions of older black, Hispanic, and non-Hispanic white Americans about the causes and treatment of common medical conditions. *J Am Geriatr Soc* **47**: 973.

Gray, J.A. (2004). Self-management in chronic illness. *Lancet* **364**: 1467–8.

Grey, M., Knafl, K., & McCorkle R. (2006). A framework for the study of self- and family management of chronic conditions. *Nurs Outlook* **54**: 278–86.

Griffiths, R., Johnson, M., Piper, M., et al (2004). A nursing intervention for the quality use of medicines by elderly community clients. *Int J Nurs Pract* **10**: 166.

Haidet, P., Kroll, T., & Sharf, B. (2006). The complexity of patient participation: lessons learned from patients' illness narratives. *Patient Educ Couns.*, **62**(3): 323–9. Epub 2006 Aug 2. Last accessed June 23, 2008.

Harmon, M., Castro, F., & Coe, K. (1996). Acculturation and cervical cancer: Knowledge, beliefs, and behaviors of Hispanic women. *Women's Health*, **24**(3): 37.

Harvey, I.S. (2006). Self management of a chronic illness: an exploratory study on the role of spirituality among older African American women. *J Women Aging* **18**(3): 75–88.

Hibbard, J.H. (2004). Moving toward a more patient-centered health care delivery system. *Health Affairs (Millwood)*, Suppl Web Exclusives: CAR 133–5. Last accessed June 24, 2008.

Huang, C.L., Wu, S.C., Jeng, C.Y., et al (2004). The efficacy of a home-based nursing program in diabetic control of elderly people with diabetes mellitus living alone. *Publ Health Nurse* **21**(1): 49.

Kastermans, M.C. & Bakker, R.H. (1999). Managing the impact of health problems on daily living. In: Ranz, M.J. & Lemone, P. (eds), *Classification of nursing diagnoses: Proceedings of the thirteenth conference.* Glendale. CA: CINAHL Information Systems.

Kennedy, M.S. (2005). Education benefits women with IBS: nurses teach self management techniques. *Am J Nurs* **105**(1): 22.

Kennedy, A.P., Nelson, E., Reeves, D., et al (2004). A randomized controlled trial to assess the effectiveness and cost of a patient oriented self–management approach to chronic inflammatory bowel disease. *Gut*, **53**: 1639–45.

Koch, T., Jenkin, P., & Kralik, D. (2004). Chronic illness self-management: locating the "self". *J Adv Nurs.*, **48**(5): 484–92.

Domain 1

Krein, S., Heisler, M., Piette, J., Makki, F., & Kerr, E. (2005). The effect of chronic pain on diabetes patients' self-management. *Diabetes Care,* **28**(1): 65–70.

McMurray, S.D., Johnson, G., Davis, S., et al (2002). Diabetes education and care management significantly improve patient outcomes in a dialysis unit. *Am J Kidney Dis* **40**: 566.

Marabini, A., Brugnami, G., Curradi, F., et al (2002). Short term effectiveness of an asthma educational program: results of a randomized controlled trial. *Respir Med* **96**: 933.

Midwest Bioethics Center (2001). Healthcare narratives from diverse communities – a self-assessment tool for health-care providers. *Bio-ethics Forum* **17**(3–4): SS1.

Millard, L., Hallett, C., & Luker, K. (2006). Nurse–patient interaction and decision making in care: patient involvement in community nursing. *J Adv Nurs* **55**: 142–50.

Mohammadi, E., Abedi, H.A., Gofranipour, F., et al (2002). Partnership caring: a theory of high blood pressure control in Iranian hypertensives, *Int J Nurs Pract* **8**: 324.

Munir, F., Leka, S., & Griffiths, A. (2005). Dealing with self-management of chronic illness at work: predictors for self-disclosure. *Soc Sci Med* **60**: 1397–407.

Neafsey, P.J., Strickler, Z., Shellman, J., et al (2002). An interactive technology approach to educate older adults about drug interactions arising from over-the-counter self medication practices. *Public Health Nurs* **19**: 255.

Newman, S., Steed, L., & Mulligan, K. (2004). Self management interventions for chronic illness. *Lancet* **364**: 1523–37.

Nguyen, H.Q., Carrieri-Kohlman, V., Rankin, S.H., Slaughter, R., & Stulberg, M. (2005). Is Internet-based support for dyspnea self-management in patients with chronic obstructive pulmonary disease possible? Results of a pilot study. *Heart Lung* **34**(1): 51–62.

Opler, L.A., Ramirez, P.M., Dominguez, L.M., et al (2004). Rethinking medication prescribing practices in an inner-city Hispanic mental health clinic. *J Psychiatr Pract* **10**: 134–40.

Ogedegbe, G., Mancuso, C.A., & Allegrante, J.P. (2004). Expectations of blood pressure management in hypertensive African–American patients: a qualitative study. *J Natl Med Assoc* **96**: 442–9.

Patterson, B.L., Russell, C., & Thorne, S. (2003). Critical analysis of everyday self care decision making in chronic illness. *J Adv Nurs* **35**: 335–41.

Pearson, J., Mensing, C., & Anderson, R. (2004). Medicare reimbursement and diabetes self-management training: national survey results. *Diabetes Educ* **30**: 914, 916, 918.

Robbins, B., Rausch, K.J., Garcia, R.I., et al (2004). Multicultural medication adherence: a comparative study. *J Gerontol Nurs* **30**(7): 25–32.

Rogers, A., Kennedy, A., Nelson, E., et al (2005). Uncovering the limits of patient centeredness: implementing a self management trail for chronic illness, *Qual Health Res* **15**: 224–39.

Stevens, S. & Sin, J. (2005). Implementing a self-management model of relapse prevention for psychosis into routine clinical practice. *J Psych Ment Health Nurs* **12**: 495.

Thackeray, R., Merrill, R.M., & Neiger, B.L. (2004). Disparities in diabetes management practice between racial and ethnic groups in the United States. *Diabetes Educ* **30**: 665–75.

Thorne, S.E. & Paterson, B.L. (2000). Two decades of insider research: what we know and don't know about chronic illness experience. *Annu Rev Nurs Res* **18**: 3.

Warsi, A., Wang, P.S., LaValley, M.P., et al (2004). Self management education programs in chronic disease. *Arch Intern Med* **164**: 1641–9.

Watts, T., Merrell, J., Murphy, F., et al (2004). Breast health information needs of women from minority ethnic groups. *J Adv Nurs* **47**: 526–35.

Wen, L.K., Shepard, M.D., & Parchman, M.L. (2004). Family support, diet, and exercise among older Mexican Americans with type 2 diabetes. *Diabetes Educ* **30**: 980–93.

Whittemore, R., Melkus, G.D., & Grey, M. (2005). Metabolic control, self management and psychosocial adjustment in women with type 2 diabetes. *J Clin Nurs* **14**: 195–204.

Impaired Home Maintenance (00098)

(1980)

Domain 1: Health Promotion
Class 2: Health Management

Definition Inability to independently maintain a safe growth-promoting immediate environment

Defining Characteristics

Objective

- Disorderly surroundings
- Inappropriate household temperature
- Insufficient clothes
- Insufficient linen
- Lack of clothes
- Lack of linen
- Lack of necessary equipment
- Offensive odors
- Overtaxed family members
- Presence of vermin
- Repeated unhygienic disorders
- Repeated unhygienic infections
- Unavailable cooking equipment
- Unclean surroundings

Subjective

- Household members describe financial crises
- Household members describe outstanding debts
- Household members express difficulty in maintaining their home in a comfortable fashion
- Household members request assistance with home maintenance

Related Factors

- Deficient knowledge
- Disease
- Inadequate support systems
- Injury
- Impaired functioning
- Insufficient family organization
- Insufficient family planning
- Insufficient finances
- Lack of role modeling
- Unfamiliarity with neighborhood resources

Readiness for Enhanced Immunization Status (00186)

(2006, LOE 2.1)

Domain 1: Health Promotion
Class 2: Health Management
Domain 11: Safety/Protection
Class 1: Infection
Class 5: Defensive Processes

Definition A pattern of conforming to local, national, and/or international standards of immunization to prevent infectious disease(s) that is sufficient to protect a person, family, or community and can be strengthened

Defining Characteristics

- Expresses desire to enhance behavior to prevent infectious disease
- Expresses desire to enhance identification of possible problems associated with immunizations
- Expresses desire to enhance identification of providers of immunizations
- Expresses desire to enhance immunization status
- Expresses desire to enhance knowledge of immunization standards
- Expresses desire to enhance record-keeping of immunizations

References

Bundt, T.S. & Hu, H.M. (2004). National examination of compliance predictors and the immunization status of children: Precursor to a developmental model for health systems. *Military Medicine* **169**: 740–5.

Centers for Disease Control (1997). Recommended childhood immunization schedule. United States 1997. *Mortality and Morbidity Weekly Report* **46**(2): 35–40.

Centers for Disease Control. (2002). Recommended adult immunization schedule: United States, 2002–2003. *Mortality and Morbidity Weekly Report* **51**: 904–8.

Das, J & Das, S. (2003). Trust, learning and vaccination: A case study of a North Indian village. *Social Science & Medicine* **57**(1), 97–112.

Davis, T.C., Frederickson, D.D., Kennen, E.M., et al. (2004). Childhood vaccine risk/benefit communication among public health clinics: A time motion study. *Public Health Nursing* **21**: 228–36.

Hull, S., Hagdrup, N., Hart, B., et al. (2002). Boosting uptake of influenza immunization: A randomised controlled trial of telephone appointing in general practice. *British Journal of General Practice* **52**: 712.

Lambert, J. (1995). Every child by two. A program of the American Nurses Foundation. *American Nurse* **27**(8): 12.

Lopreiato, J.O. & Ottolini, M.C. (1996). Assessment of immunization compliance among children in the Department of Defense health care system. *Pediatrics* **97**: 308–11.

McMurray, R., Cheater, F.M., Weighall, A., Nelson, C., Schweiger, M., & Mukherjee, S. (2004). Managing controversy through consultation: A qualitative study of communication and trust around MMR vaccination decisions. *British Journal of General Practice* **54**: 520–5.

Mell, L.K., Ogren, D.S., Davis, R.L., et al. (2005). Compliance with national immunization guidelines for children younger than 2 years, 1996–1999. *Pediatrics* **115**: 461–7.

Scarborough, M.L. & Landis, S.E. (1997). A pilot study for the development of a hospital-based immunization program. *Clinical Nurse Specialist* **11**(2): 70–5.

Shui, I., Kennedy, A., Wooten, K., Schwartz, B., & Gust, D. (2005). Factors influencing African–American mothers' concerns about immunization safety: A summary of focus group findings. *Journal of the National Medical Association* **97**: 657–66.

Taylor, J.A., Darden, P.M., Slora, E., Hasemeier, C.M., Asmussen, L., & Wasserman, R. (1997). The influence of provider behavior, parental characteristics, and a public policy initiative on the immunization status of children followed by private pediatricians: A study from Pediatric Research in Office Settings. *Pediatrics* **99**: 209–15.

Wood, D., Donald-Shelbourne, C., Halfon, N., et al. (1995). Factors related to immunization status among inner-city Latino and African–American preschoolers. *Pediatrics* **96**: 295–301.

Self Neglect (00193)
(2008, LOE 2.1)

Domain 1: Health Promotion
Class 2: Health Management

Definition A constellation of culturally framed behaviors involving one or more self-care activities in which there is a failure to maintain a socially accepted standard of health and well-being (Gibbons, Lauder, & Ludwick, 2006)

Defining Characteristics

- Inadequate personal hygiene
- Inadequate environmental hygiene
- Non-adherence to health activities

Related Factors

- Capgras syndrome
- Cognitive impairment (e.g., dementia)
- Depression
- Learning disability
- Fear of institutionalization
- Frontal lobe dysfunction and executive processing ability
- Functional impairment
- Lifestyle/Choice
- Maintaining control
- Malingering
- Obsessive–compulsive disorder
- Schizotypal personality disorders
- Paranoid personality disorders
- Substance abuse
- Major life stressor

References

Abrams, R.C., Lachs, M., McAvay, G., Keohane, D.J., & Bruce, M.L. (2002). Predictors of self- neglect in community-dwelling elders. *American Journal of Psychiatry* **159**: 1724–30.

Adams, J. & Johnson, J. (1998). Nurses' perceptions of gross self-neglect amongst older people living in the community. *Journal of Clinical Nursing* **7**: 547–52.

Al-Adwani, A. & Nabi, W. (2001). Coexisting Diogenes and Capgras syndromes. *International Journal of Psychiatry in Clinical Practice* **15**: 75–76.

Barocka A., Seehuber D., & Schone, D. (2004.) Messy House Syndrome. *MMW Fortschritte der Medizin* **146**(45): 36–9.

Blondell, R.D. (1999). Alcohol abuse and self-neglect in the elderly. *Journal of Elder Abuse and Neglect* **11**(2): 55–75.

Bozinovski, S.D. (2000). Older self-neglecters: Interpersonal problems and the maintenance of self-continuity. *Journal of Elder Abuse & Neglect* **12**(1): 37–56.

Branch, L. (2002). The epidemiology of elder abuse and neglect. *The Public Policy and Aging Report* **12**(2): 19–22.

Chang, B., Uman, G. & Hirsch, M. (1998). Predictive power of clinical indicators for self-care deficit. *Nursing Diagnosis*, 9(2): 71–82.

Clark, A.N.G., Mankikar, G.D., & Gray, I. (1975). Diogenes syndrome: A clinical study of gross neglect in old age. *Lancet* i: 366–368.

Daly, J.M. & Jogerst, G. (2001). Statute definitions of elder abuse. *Journal of Elder Abuse and Neglect* 13: 39–57.

Drummond, L.M., Turner, J., & Reid, S. (1997). Diogenes' syndrome: A load of old rubbish? *Irish Journal of Psychological Medicine* 14: 99–102.

Dyer, C.B., Pavlik, V.N., Murphy, K.P., & Hyman, D.J. (2000). The high prevalence of depression and dementia in elder abuse or neglect. *Journal of the American Geriatrics Society* 48: 205–8.

Esposito, D., Rouillon, F., & Limosin, F. (2003). Diogenes syndrome in a pair of siblings. *Canadian Journal of Psychiatry* 48: 571–2.

Finkel, S.I. (2003). Cognitive screening in the primary care setting: The role of physicians at the first point of entry. *Geriatrics* 58: 43–44.

Gee, A., Jones, J.S., & Brown, M.D. (1998). Self-neglect in the elderly: Emergency department assessment and crisis intervention. *Annals of Emergency Medicine,* 32(30, suppl, Part 2): S42.

Gibbons, S., Lauder, W., & Ludwick, R. (2006). Self-neglect: A proposed new NANDA diagnosis. *International Journal of Nursing Terminologies and Classification* 17(1): 10–18.

Gibbons S. (2007). Characteristics and behaviors of self-neglect in community-dwelling older adults. *Dissertation Abstracts International,* (UMI No. 3246949).

Greve, K.W., Curtis, K.L., Bianchini, K.J., & Collins, B.T. (2004). Personality disorder masquerading as dementia: a case of apparent Diogenes syndrome. *International Journal of Geriatric Psychiatry* 19: 703–5.

Gruman, C.A., Stern, A.S., & Caro, F.G. (1997). Self-neglect among the elderly: A distinct phenomenon. *Journal of Mental Health and Aging* 3: 309–23.

Gunstone, S. (2003). Risk assessment and management of patients whom self-neglect: a grey area for mental health workers. *Journal of Psychiatric and Mental Health Nursing* 10: 287–96.

Halliday, G., Banerjee, S., Philpot, M., & Macdonald, A. (2000). Community study of people who live in squalor. *The Lancet* 355: 882–6.

Jackson, G.A. (1997). Diogenes syndrome: How should we manage it? *Journal of Mental Health* 6: 113–16.

Jurgens, A. (2000). Refuse hoarding syndrome. *Psychiatrische Praxis* 27(1): 42–6.

Lachs, M.S., Williams, C.S., O'Brien, S., Pillemer, K.A., & Charlson, M.E. (1998). The mortality of elder mistreatment. *Journal of the American Medical Association* 280: 428–32.

Lachs, M.S., Williams, C.S., O'Brien, S., & Pillemer, K.A. (2002). Adult protective services use and nursing home placement. *The Gerontologist* 42: 734–9.

Lauder, W. (1999a). A survey of self-neglect in patients living in the community. *Journal of Clinical Nursing* 8: 95–102.

Lauder, W. (1999b). Constructions of self-neglect: a multiple case study design. *Nursing Inquiry* 6(1): 48–57.

Lauder, W. (2001). The utility of self-care theory as a theoretical basis for self-neglect. *Journal of Advanced Nursing* 34(4), 345–351.

Lauder, W., Anderson, I., & Barclay, A. (2002). Housing and self-neglect: Clients' and carers' perspectives. Report to the Economic and Social Research Council. Award No. R000223387.

Lauder, W., Scott, P.A., & Whyte, A. (2001). Nurses' judgments of self-neglect: A factorial survey. *International Journal of Nursing Studies* 38: 601–8.

Lauder, W., Anderson, I., & Barclay, A. (2005). Guidelines for good practice in self-neglect. *Journal of Psychiatric and Mental Health Nursing,* 12: 192–198.

Longres, J.F. (1995). Self-neglect among the elderly. *Journal of Elder Abuse & Neglect* 7(1): 69–86.

Macmillan, D. & Shaw, P. (1966). Senile breakdown in standards of personal and environmental cleanliness. *British Medical Journal* **ii**: 1032–7.

NEAIS (1998). National Elder Abuse Incidence Study. National Centre on Elder Abuse. The Administration for Children and Families and the Administration on Aging. The US Department of Health and Human Services.

O'Brien, J.G., Thibault, J.M., Turner, L.C., & Laird-Fick, H.S. (1999). Self-neglect: an overview. *Journal of Elder Abuse & Neglect* **11**(2): 1–19.

Orem, D.E. (1995). *Nursing: Concepts of practice*, 5th edn. St. Louis, MO: Mosby-Yearbook, Inc.

Orrell, M.W., Sahakin, B.J., & Bergmann, K. (1989). Self-neglect and frontal lobe dysfunction. *British Journal of Psychiatry* **155**: 101–5.

Pavlik, V.N., Hyman, D.J., Festa, N.A., & Dyer, C.B. (2001). Quantifying the problem of abuse and neglect in adults – analysis of a statewide database. *Journal of the American Geriatrics Society* **49**(1): 45–8.

Radebaugh, T.S., Hooper, F.J., & Gruenberg, E.M. (1987). The social breakdown syndrome in the elderly population living in the community: The helping study. *British Journal of Psychiatry* **151**: 341–6.

Rathbone-McCuan, E. & Bricker-Jenkins, M. (1992). A general framework for elder self-neglect. In: Rathbone-McCuan, E. & Fabian, D.R. (eds), *Self-neglecting elders: A clinical dilemma*. Westport, CT: Auburn House.

Reifler, B. (1996). Diogenes syndrome: Of omelettes and souffles. *Journal of the American Geriatrics Society* **44**: 1484–5.

Reyes-Ortiz, C.A. (2001). Diogenes syndrome: The self-neglect elderly. *Comprehensive Therapy* **27**: 117–21.

Roby, J.L. & Sullivan, R. (2000). Adult protection service laws: a comparison of state statutes from definition to case closure. *Journal of Elder Abuse and Neglect* **12**: 17–51.

Roe, P.F. (1987). Self-neglect or chosen lifestyle? [Letter]. *British Journal of Hospital Medicine* **37**(1): 83–4.

Sengstock, M.C., Thibault, J.M., & Zaranek, R. (1999). Community dimensions of elderly self-neglect. *Journal of Elder Abuse & Neglect* **11**: 77–93.

Snowdon, J. (1987). Uncleanliness among persons seen by community health workers. *Hospital & Community Psychiatry* **38**: 491–4.

Tierney, M.C., Charles, J., Naglie, G., Jaglal, S., Kiss, A., & Fisher, R.H. (2004). Risk for harm in cognitively impaired seniors who live alone: A prospective study. *Journal of the American Geriatrics Society* **52**: 1576–7.

Ungvari, G.S. & Hantz, P.M. (1991). Social breakdown in the elderly, I. Case studies and management. *Comprehensive Psychiatry* **32**: 440–4.

Vostanis, P. & Dean, C. (1992). Self-neglect in adult life. *British Journal of Psychiatry* **161**: 265–7.

Readiness for Enhanced Nutrition

(00163)

(2002, LOE 2.1)

Domain 1: Health Promotion
Class 2: Health Management

Definition A pattern of nutrient intake that is sufficient for meeting metabolic needs and can be strengthened

Defining Characteristics

- Attitude toward drinking is congruent with health goals
- Attitude toward eating is congruent with health goals
- Consumes adequate fluid
- Consumes adequate food
- Eats regularly
- Expresses knowledge of healthy fluid choices
- Expresses knowledge of healthy food choices
- Expresses willingness to enhance nutrition
- Follows an appropriate standard for intake (e.g., the food pyramid or American Diabetic Association guidelines)
- Safe preparation for fluids
- Safe preparation for food
- Safe storage for fluids
- Safe storage for food

Ineffective Family Therapeutic Regimen Management (00080)
(1992)

Domain 1: Health Promotion
Class 2: Health Management

Definition Pattern of regulating and integrating into family processes a program for treatment of illness and its sequelae that is unsatisfactory for meeting specific health goals

Defining Characteristics

- Acceleration of illness symptoms of a family member
- Inappropriate family activities for meeting health goals
- Failure to take action to reduce risk factors
- Lack of attention to illness
- Verbalizes desire to manage the illness
- Verbalizes difficulty with prescribed regimen

Related Factors

- Complexity of healthcare system
- Complexity of therapeutic regimen
- Decisional conflicts
- Economic difficulties
- Excessive demands
- Family conflict

Readiness for Enhanced Self Health Management (00162)

(2002, LOE 2.1)

Domain 1: Health Promotion
Class 2: Health Management

Definition A pattern of regulating and integrating into daily living a therapeutic regime for treatment of illness and its sequelae that is sufficient for meeting health-related goals and can be strengthened

Defining Characteristics

- Choices of daily living are appropriate for meeting goals (e.g., treatment, prevention)
- Describes reduction of risk factors
- Expresses desire to manage the illness (e.g., treatment, prevention of sequelae)

- Expresses little difficulty with prescribed regimens
- No unexpected acceleration of illness symptoms

References

Banister, N., Jastrow, S., Hodges, V., Loop, R., & Gillham, M. (2004). Diabetes self-management training program in a community clinic improves patient outcomes at modest cost. *J Am Dietetic Assoc,* **104**: 807–810.

Benavides-Vaello, S., Garcia, A., Brown, S., et al. (2004). Using focus group to plan and evaluate diabetes self-management interventions for Mexican Americans, *Diabetes Educ,* **30**(2): 238–256.

Curtin, R., Sitter, D., Schatell, D., et al. (2004). Self-management, knowledge, and functioning and well being of patients on hemodialysis, *Neph Nurs J,* **31**(4): 378–386.

Deakin, T., McShane, C., Cade, J., & Willams, R. (2005). Group-based training for self management strategies in people with type 2 diabetes mellitus. *Cochrane Database Sys Rev,* **18**(2): CD003417.

DeWalt, D., Pignone, M., Malone, R., Rawis, C., Kosnar, M., George, G., et al. (2004). Development and pilot testing of a disease management program for low literacy patients with heart failure. *Patient Educ Couns,* **55**: 78–86.

Funnel,l M. & Anderson, R. (2004). Empowerment and self-management of diabetes. *Clin Diabetes,* **22**: 123–7.

Gallant, M., Beaulieu, M. & Carnevale, F. (2002). Partnership: an analysis of the concept within the nurse-client relationship, *J Adv Nurs,* **40**(2): 149.

Georges, C., Bolton, L. & Bennett, C. (2004). Functional health literacy: an issue in African-American and other ethnic and racial communities, *J Natl Black Nurses Assoc,* **15**(1): 1–4.

Goldberg, H., Lessier, D., Mertens, K., Eytan, T. & Cheadle, A. (2004). Self management support in a web-based medical record: A pilot randomized controlled trial. *Jt Comm J Qual Saf*, **30**: 629–35, 589.

Goodwin, J., Black, S., & Satish, S. (1999). Aging versus disease: the opinions of older black, Hispanic, and non-Hispanic white Americans about the causes and treatment of common medical conditions, *J Am Geriatr Soc*, **47**(8): 973.

Gray, J. (2004). Self-management in chronic illness. *Lancet*, **364**: 1467–8.

Grey, M., Knafl, K., & McCorkle, R. (2006). A framework for the study of self- and family management of chronic conditions. *Nurs Outlook*, **54**: 278–86.

Harvey, I. (2006). Self management of a chronic illness: an exploratory study on the role of spirituality among older African American women. *J Women Aging*, **18**(3): 75–88.

Hibbard, J. (2004). Moving toward a more patient-centered health care delivery system. *Health Affairs*, Web Exclusive, VAR 133–135. Last accessed June **24**: 2008.

Kennedy, M. (2005). Education benefits women with IBS: nurses teach self management techniques. *Am J Nurs*, **105**(1): 22.

Kennedy, A., Nelson, E., Reeves, D., Richardson, G., Roberts, C., Robinson, A., et al. (2004). A randomized controlled trial to assess the effectiveness and cost of a patient oriented self–management approach to chronic inflammatory bowel disease. *Gut*, **53**: 1639–45.

Koch, T., Jenkin, P., & Kralik, D. (2004). Chronic illness self management: locating the self. *J Adv Nurs*, **48**: 484–92.

Marabini, A., Brugnami, G., Curradi, F., et al. (2002). Short term effectiveness of an asthma educational program: results of a randomized controlled trial, *Respir Med*, **96**(12): 933.

Millard, L., Hallett, C., & Luker, K. (2006). Nurse-patient interaction and decision making in care: patient involvement in community nursing. *J Adv Nurs*, **55**: 142–50.

Mohammadi, E., Abedi, H., Gofranipour, F., et al. (2002). Partnership caring: a theory of high blood pressure control in Iranian hypertensives, *Int J Nurs Pract*, **8**(6): 324.

Munir, F., Leka, S., & Griffiths, A. (2005). Dealing with self-management of chronic illness at work: predictors for self-disclosure. *Soc Sci Med*, **60**: 1397–407.

Newman, S., Steed, L., & Mulligan, K. (2004). Self management interventions for chronic illness. *Lancet*, **364**: 1523–37.

Patterson, B., Russell, C., & Thorne, S. (2003). Critical analysis of everyday self care decision making in chronic illness. *J Adv Nurs*, **35**: 335–341.

Rogers, A., Kennedy, A., Nelson, E., et al. (2005). Uncovering the limits of patient centeredness: implementing a self management trail for chronic illness, *Qual Health Res*, **15**(2): 224–239.

Stevens, S., & Sin, J. (2005). Implementing a self-management model of relapse prevention for psychosis into routine clinical practice. *J Psych Ment Health Nurs*, **12**: 495.

Domain 2
Nutrition

Ineffective Infant Feeding Pattern
(00107)
(1992, 2006, LOE 2.1)

Domain 2: Nutrition
Class 1: Ingestion

Definition Impaired ability of an infant to suck or coordinate the suck/swallow response resulting in inadequate oral nutrition for metabolic needs

Defining Characteristics

- Inability to coordinate sucking, swallowing, and breathing
- Inability to initiate an effective suck
- Inability to sustain an effective suck

Related Factors

- Anatomic abnormality
- Neurological delay
- Neurological impairment
- Oral hypersensitivity
- Prematurity
- Prolonged NPO status

References

Hazinski, M.F. (1992). *Nursing care of the critically ill child.* St Louis, MO: Mosby.

Shaker, C.S. (1991). Nipple feeding premature infants: A different perspective. *Neonatal Network: Journal of Neonatal Nursing* **8**(5): 9–17.

VandenBerg, K. (1990). Nippling management of the sick neonate in the NICU: The disorganized feeder. *Neonatal Network: Journal of Neonatal Nursing* **9**(1): 9–16.

Imbalanced Nutrition: Less Than Body Requirements (00002)
(1975, 2000)

Domain 2: Nutrition
Class 1: Ingestion

Definition
Intake of nutrients insufficient to meet metabolic needs

Defining Characteristics

- Abdominal cramping
- Abdominal pain
- Aversion to eating
- Body weight 20% or more under ideal
- Capillary fragility
- Diarrhea
- Excessive loss of hair
- Hyperactive bowel sounds
- Lack of food
- Lack of information
- Lack of interest in food
- Loss of weight with adequate food intake
- Misconceptions
- Misinformation
- Pale mucous membranes
- Perceived inability to ingest food
- Poor muscle tone
- Reported altered taste sensation
- Reported food intake less than RDA (recommended daily allowance)
- Satiety immediately after ingesting food
- Sore buccal cavity
- Steatorrhea
- Weakness of muscles required for swallowing or mastication

Related Factors

- Biological factors
- Economic factors
- Inability to absorb nutrients
- Inability to digest food
- Inability to ingest food
- Psychological factors

Imbalanced Nutrition: More Than Body Requirements (00001)
(1975, 2000)

Domain 2: Nutrition
Class 1: Ingestion

Definition   Intake of nutrients that exceeds metabolic needs

Defining Characteristics

- Concentrating food intake at the end of the day
- Dysfunctional eating pattern (e.g., pairing food with other activities)
- Eating in response to external cues (e.g., time of day, social situation)
- Eating in response to internal cues other than hunger (e.g., anxiety)
- Sedentary activity level
- Triceps skin fold >25 mm in women, >15 mm in men
- Weight 20% over ideal for height and frame

Related Factors

- Excessive intake in relation to metabolic need

Risk for Imbalanced Nutrition: More Than Body Requirements (00003)

(1980, 2000)

Domain 2: Nutrition
Class 1: Ingestion

Definition At risk for an intake of nutrients that exceeds metabolic needs

Risk Factors

- Concentrating food intake at end of day
- Dysfunctional eating patterns
- Eating in response to external cues (e.g., time of day, social situation)
- Eating in response to internal cues other than hunger (e.g., anxiety)
- Higher baseline weight at beginning of each pregnancy
- Observed use of food as comfort measure
- Observed use of food as reward
- Pairing food with other activities
- Parental obesity
- Rapid transition across growth percentiles in children
- Reported use of solid food as major food source before 5 months of age

Impaired Swallowing (00103)
(1986, 1998)

Domain 2: Nutrition
Class 1: Ingestion

Definition Abnormal functioning of the swallowing mechanism associated with deficits in oral, pharyngeal, or esophageal structure or function

Defining Characteristics

Esophageal Phase Impairment

- Abnormality in esophageal phase by swallow study
- Acidic smelling breath
- Bruxism
- Complaints of "something stuck"
- Epigastric pain
- Food refusal
- Heartburn
- Hematemesis
- Hyperextension of head (e.g., arching during or after meals)
- Nighttime awakening
- Nighttime coughing
- Observed evidence of difficulty in swallowing (e.g., stasis of food in oral cavity, coughing/choking)
- Odynophagia
- Regurgitation of gastric contents (wet burps)
- Repetitive swallowing
- Unexplained irritability surrounding mealtime
- Volume limiting
- Vomiting
- Vomitus on pillow

Oral Phase Impairment

- Abnormality in oral phase of swallow study
- Choking before a swallow
- Coughing before a swallow
- Drooling
- Food falls from mouth
- Food pushed out of mouth
- Gagging before a swallow
- Inability to clear oral cavity
- Incomplete lip closure
- Lack of chewing
- Lack of tongue action to form bolus
- Long meals with little consumption
- Nasal reflux
- Piecemeal deglutition
- Pooling in lateral sulci
- Premature entry of bolus
- Sialorrhea
- Slow bolus formation
- Weak suck resulting in inefficient nippling

Pharyngeal Phase Impairment

- Abnormality in pharyngeal phase by swallow study

- Altered head positions
- Choking
- Coughing
- Delayed swallow
- Food refusal
- Gagging
- Gurgly voice quality
- Inadequate laryngeal elevation
- Multiple swallows
- Nasal reflux
- Recurrent pulmonary infections
- Unexplained fevers

Related Factors

Congenital Deficits

- Behavioral feeding problems
- Conditions with significant hypotonia
- Congenital heart disease
- Failure to thrive
- History of tube feeding
- Mechanical obstruction (e.g., edema, tracheostomy tube, tumor)
- Neuromuscular impairment (e.g., decreased or absent gag reflex, decreased strength or excursion of muscles involved in mastication, perceptual impairment, facial paralysis)
- Protein–energy malnutrition
- Respiratory disorders
- Self-injurious behavior
- Upper airway anomalies

Neurological Problems

- Achalasia
- Acquired anatomic defects
- Cerebral palsy
- Cranial nerve involvement
- Developmental delay
- Esophageal defects
- Gastroesophageal reflux disease
- Laryngeal abnormalities
- Laryngeal defects
- Nasal defects
- Nasopharyngeal cavity defects
- Oropharynx abnormalities
- Prematurity
- Tracheal defects
- Traumas
- Traumatic head injury
- Upper airway anomalies

Risk for Unstable Blood Glucose Level
(00179)
(2006, LOE 2.1)

Domain 2: Nutrition
Class 4: Metabolism

Definition Risk for variation of blood glucose/sugar levels from the normal range

Risk Factors

- Deficient knowledge of diabetes management (e.g., action plan)
- Developmental level
- Dietary intake
- Inadequate blood glucose monitoring
- Lack of acceptance of diagnosis
- Lack of adherence to diabetes management (e.g., action plan)
- Lack of diabetes management (e.g., action plan)
- Medication management
- Mental health status
- Physical activity level
- Physical health status
- Pregnancy
- Rapid growth periods
- Stress
- Weight gain
- Weight loss

References

American Diabetes Association (2005). Standard of medical care in diabetes. *Diabetes Care* **29**: S1–36. Available at: http://care.diabetesjournals. org/cgi/content/full/28/suppl_1/s4 (accessed May 29, 2008).

Bierschbach, J., Cooper, L., & Liedl, J. (2004). Insulin pumps: What every school nurse needs to know. *Journal of School Nursing* **20**: 117–23.

US Department of Health & Human Services (2003). *Helping the student with diabetes succeed: A guide for school personnel.* http://ndep.nih.gov/resources/school.htm (accessed May 29, 2008).

Neonatal Jaundice (00194)
(2008, LOE 2.1)

Domain 2: Nutrition
Class 4: Metabolism

Definition The yellow orange tint of the neonate's skin and mucous membranes that occurs after 24 hours of life as a result of unconjugated bilirubin in the circulation

Defining Characteristics

- Abnormal blood profile (hemolysis; total serum bilirubin >2 mg/dL; inherited disorder; total serum bilirubin in high risk range on age in hour-specific nomogram)
- Abnormal skin bruising
- Yellow–orange skin
- Yellow sclera

Related Factors

- Abnormal weight loss (>7–8% in breastfeeding newborn; 15% in term infant)
- Feeding pattern not well established
- Infant experiences difficulty making transition to extrauterine life
- Neonate age 1–7 days
- Stool (meconium) passage delayed

References

American Academy of Pediatrics (2004). Management of hyperbilirubinemia in the newborn infant 35 or more weeks of gestation. *Pediatrics* **114**: 297–316.

Beachy, J.M. (2007). Investigating jaundice in the newborn. *Neonatal Network* **26**: 327–33.

Bhutani, V.K., Johnson, L.H., Schwoebel, A., & Gennaro, S. (2006). A systems approach for neonatal hyperbilirubinemia in term and near-term newborns. *J Obstet Gynecol Neonatal Nurs* **35**: 444–55.

Blackburn, S. (1995). Hyperbilirubinemia and neonatal jaundice. *Neon Netw* **14**(7): 15–25.

Boyd, S. (2004). Treatment of physiological neonatal jaundice. *Nurs Times* **100**(13): 40–3.

Cohen, S.M. (2006). Jaundice in the full-term newborn. *Pediatr Nurs* **32**: 202–7.

Gartner, L. & Herschel, M. (2001). Jaundice and breastfeeding. *Pediatric Clinics of North America*, **48**(2): 389–99.

Hillman, N. (2007). Hyperbilirubinemia in the late preterm infant. *Newborn & Infant Nursing Reviews* **7**(2): 91–4.

Porter M.L. & Dennis, B.L. (2003). Hyperbilirubinemia in the term newborn. *Am Fam Phys* **65**: 599–606, 613–14.

Risk for Impaired Liver Function (00178)
(2006, 2008 LOE 2.1)

Domain 2: Nutrition
Class 4: Metabolism

Definition At risk for a decrease in liver function that may compromise health

Domain 2

Risk Factors

- Hepatotoxic medications (e.g., acetaminophen, statins)
- HIV coinfection
- Substance abuse (e.g., alcohol, cocaine)
- Viral infection (e.g., hepatitis A, hepatitis B, hepatitis C, Epstein–Barr)

References

AASLD Practice Guideline (2004). *Diagnosis, management, and treatment of hepatitis C.* Alexandria, VA: American Association for the Study of Liver Diseases.

Fontana, R.J. & Lok, S.F. (2002). Noninvasive monitoring of patients with chronic hepatitis C. *Hepatology* **36**(5 suppl): S57–64.

Hoofnagle, J. (2002). Course and outcome of hepatitis C. *Hepatology,* **36**(5 Suppl. 1): S21–9. Review.

Laboratory Medicine Practice Guidelines (2000). *Laboratory guidelines for screening, diagnosis and monitoring of hepatic injury.* Washington DC: National Academy of Clinical Biochemistry.

National Institute of Diabetes and Digestive and Kidney Diseases (2003). *Chronic hepatitis C: Current disease management.* Washington DC: US Department of Health and Human Services.

Palmer, M. (2000). *Hepatitis Liver Disease: What you need to know.* Garden City Park, NY: Avery Publishing Group, pp. 23, 26–31, 62–7, 72–3.

Risk for Electrolyte Imbalance (00195)
(2008, LOE 2.1)

Domain 2: Nutrition
Class 5: Hydration

Definition At risk for change in serum electrolyte levels that may compromise health

Risk Factors

- Diarrhea
- Endocrine dysfunction
- Fluid imbalance (e.g., dehydration, water intoxication)
- Impaired regulatory mechanisms (e.g., diabetes insipidus, syndrome of inappropriate secretion of antidiuretic hormone
- Renal dysfunction
- Treatment-related side effects (e.g., medications, drains)
- Vomiting

References

Elgart, H.N. (2004). Assessment of fluids and electrolytes. *ACCN Clinical Issues* **15**: 607–21.

Weglicki, W., Quamme, G., Tucker, K., Haigney, M., & Resnick, L. (2005). Potassium, magnesium, and electrolyte imbalance and complications in disease management. *Clinical and Experimental Hypertension* **27**: 95–112.

Readiness for Enhanced Fluid Balance

(00160)

(2002, LOE 2.1)

Domain 2: Nutrition
Class 5: Hydration

Definition A pattern of equilibrium between fluid volume and chemical composition of body fluids that is sufficient for meeting physical needs and can be strengthened

Defining Characteristics

- Dehydration
- Expresses willingness to enhance fluid balance
- Good tissue turgor
- Intake adequate for daily needs
- Moist mucous membranes
- No evidence of edema
- No excessive thirst
- Specific gravity within normal limits
- Stable weight
- Straw-colored urine
- Urine output appropriate for intake

Deficient Fluid Volume (00027)
(1978, 1996)

Domain 2: Nutrition
Class 5: Hydration

Definition   Decreased intravascular, interstitial, and/or intracellular fluid. This refers to dehydration, water loss alone without change in sodium.

Defining Characteristics

- Change in mental state
- Decreased blood pressure
- Decreased pulse pressure
- Decreased pulse volume
- Decreased skin turgor
- Decreased tongue turgor
- Decreased urine output
- Decreased venous filling
- Dry mucous membranes

- Dry skin
- Elevated hematocrit
- Increased body temperature
- Increased pulse rate
- Increased urine concentration
- Sudden weight loss (except in third spacing)
- Thirst
- Weakness

Related Factors

- Active fluid volume loss

- Failure of regulatory mechanisms

Excess Fluid Volume (00026)

(1982, 1996)

Domain 2: Nutrition
Class 5: Hydration

Definition Increased isotonic fluid retention

Defining Characteristics

- Adventitious breath sounds
- Altered electrolytes
- Anascara
- Anxiety
- Azotemia
- Blood pressure changes
- Change in mental status
- Changes in respiratory pattern
- Decreased hematocrit
- Decreased hemoglobin
- Dyspnea
- Edema
- Increased central venous pressure
- Intake exceeds output
- Jugular vein distension
- Oliguria
- Orthopnea
- Pleural effusion
- Positive hepatojugular reflex
- Pulmonary artery pressure changes
- Pulmonary congestion
- Restlessness
- Specific gravity changes
- S3 heart sound
- Weight gain over short period of time

Related Factors

- Compromised regulatory mechanism
- Excess fluid intake
- Excess sodium intake

Risk for Deficient Fluid Volume (00028)
(1978)

Domain 2: Nutrition
Class 5: Hydration

Definition At risk for experiencing vascular, cellular, or intracellular dehydration

Risk Factors

- Deviations affecting access of fluids
- Deviations affecting intake of fluids
- Deviations affecting absorption of fluids
- Excessive losses through normal routes (e.g., diarrhea)
- Extremes of age
- Extremes of weight
- Factors influencing fluid needs (e.g., hypermetabolic state)
- Loss of fluid through abnormal routes (e.g., indwelling tubes)
- Knowledge deficiency
- Medication (e.g., diuretics)

Risk for Imbalanced Fluid Volume

(00025)

(1998, 2008, LOE 2.1)

Domain 2: Nutrition
Class 5: Hydration

Domain 2

Definition At risk for a decrease, increase, or rapid shift from one to the other of intravascular, interstitial, and/or intracellular fluid. This refers to body fluid loss, gain, or both.

Risk Factors

- Abdominal surgery
- Ascites
- Burns
- Intestinal obstruction
- Pancreatitis
- Receiving apheresis
- Sepsis
- Traumatic injury (e.g., fractured hip)

References

Batts, E. & Lazarus, H. (2007). Diagnosis and treatment of transplantation-associated trhombotic microangiopathy: Real progress or are we still waiting? *Bone Marrow Transplant*, **40**(8): 709–19. Epub 2007 Jul 2. Review. Last accessed June 24, 2008.

Boctor, F. (2005). Red blood cell exchange transfusion as an adjunct treatment for severe pediatric falciparum malaria, using automated or manual procedures. *Pediatrics* **116**: 592–5.

Burgstaler, E. (2003). Current instrumentation for apheresis. In: McLeod, B., Price, T., Weinstein, R. (eds), *Apheresis: Principles and practice,* 2nd edn. Bethesda, MD: AABB Press, pp. 961–7.

Corbin, F., Cullis, H., Freireich, E., et al. (2003). Development of apheresis instrumentation. In: McLeod, B., Price, T., Weinstein, R. (eds), *Apheresis: Principles and practice,* 2nd edn. Bethesda, MD: AABB Press, pp. 1–3.

Crookston, K. & Simon, T. (2003). Physiology of apheresis. In: McLeod, B., Price, T., Weinstein, R. (eds), *Apheresis: Principles and practice,* 2nd edn. Bethesda, MD: AABB Press, pp. 934–60.

Danielson, C. (2002). The role of red blood cell exchange transfusion in the treatment and prevention of complications of sickle cell disease. *Ther Apher* **6**(1): 24–31.

Fortenberry, J. & Paden, M. (2006). Extracorporeal therapies in the treatment of sepsis: experience and promise. *Semin Pediatr Infect Dis,* **17**(2): 72–79.

Gambro BCT (2005). *Spectra™ System Therapeutics Reference Book.* Denver: Gambro.

Hester J. (1997). Therapeutic cell depletion. In: McLeod B. & Priceth D. (eds), *Apheresis: Principles and practice.* Bethesda, MD: American Association of Blood Banks, pp. 254–259.

Kim, H. (2000). Therapeutic pediatric apheresis. *Journal of Clinical Apheresis* **15**: 129–57.

Metheny, N.M. (ed) (2000). *Fluid & Electrolyte Balance: Nursing considerations,* 4th edn. Philadelphia: Lippincott Williams & Wilkins.

Teruya, J., Styler, M., Verde, S., Topolsky, D., & Crilley, P. (2001). Questionable efficacy of plasma exchange for thrombotic thrombocytopenic purpura after bone marrow transplantation. *J Clin Apher* **16**: 169–74.

Vucic, S. & Davies, L. (1998). Safety of plasmapheresis in the treatment of neurological disease. *Aust N Z J Med.* **28**: 289–90.

Woloskie, S., Armelagos, H., Meade, J., & Haas, D. (2001). Leukodepletion for acute lymphocytic leukemia in a three-week-old infant. *J Clin Apher* **16**(1): 31–2.

Domain 3
Elimination and Exchange

Functional Urinary Incontinence (00020)

(1986, 1998)

Domain 3: Elimination and Exchange
Class 1: Urinary Function

Definition Inability of usually continent person to reach toilet in time to avoid unintentional loss of urine

Defining Characteristics

- Able to completely empty bladder
- Amount of time required to reach toilet exceeds length of time between sensing the urge to void and uncontrolled voiding
- Loss of urine before reaching toilet
- May be incontinent only in early morning
- Senses need to void

Related Factors

- Altered environmental factors
- Impaired cognition
- Impaired vision
- Neuromuscular limitations
- Psychological factors
- Weakened supporting pelvic structures

Overflow Urinary Incontinence (00176)
(2006, LOE 2.1)

Domain 3: Elimination and Exchange
Class 1: Urinary Function

Definition Involuntary loss of urine associated with overdistension of the bladder

Defining Characteristics

- Bladder distension
- High post-void residual volume
- Nocturia
- Observed involuntary leakage of small volumes of urine
- Reports involuntary leakage of small volumes of urine

Related Factors

- Bladder outlet obstruction
- Detrusor external sphincter dyssynergia
- Detrusor hypocontractility
- Fecal impaction
- Severe pelvic prolapse
- Side effects of anticholinergic medications
- Side effects of calcium channel blockers
- Side effects of decongestant medications
- Urethral obstruction

References

Agency for Health Care Policy and Research (AHCPR) (1992). *Clinical practice guideline: Urinary incontinence in adults.* AHCPR Pub. No. 92–0038. Rockville, MD: AHCPR.

National Kidney and Urologic Diseases Information Clearinghouse (NKUDIC) (2004). *Urinary incontinence in women.* Available at: http://kidney.niddk.nih.gov/kudiseases/pubs/uiwomen/index.htm (accessed May 29, 2008).

NIH consensus statements (1988). *Urinary incontinence in adults.* Available at: http://consensus.nih.gov/cons/071/071_statement.htm (accessed January 27, 2005).

Noble, J., ed. (2001). *Textbook of primary care medicine*, 3rd edn. St Louis, MO: Mosby.

Stenchever, M.A., ed. (2001). *Comprehensive gynecology.* St Louis, MO: Mosby.

Walsh, P.C., ed. (2002). *Campbell's urology*, 8th edn. Philadelphia: Saunders.

Reflex Urinary Incontinence (00018)

(1986, 1998)

Domain 3: Elimination and Exchange
Class 1: Urinary Function

Definition Involuntary loss of urine at somewhat predictable intervals when a specific bladder volume is reached

Defining Characteristics

- Inability to voluntarily inhibit voiding
- Inability to voluntarily initiate voiding
- Incomplete emptying with lesion above pontine micturition center
- Incomplete emptying with lesion above sacral micturition center
- No sensation of bladder fullness
- No sensation of urge to void
- No sensation of voiding
- Predictable pattern of voiding
- Sensation of urgency without voluntary inhibition of bladder contraction
- Sensations associated with full bladder (e.g., sweating, restlessness, abdominal discomfort)

Related Factors

- Tissue damage (e.g., due to radiation cystitis, inflammatory bladder conditions, radical pelvic surgery)
- Neurological impairment above level of pontine micturition center
- Neurological impairment above level of sacral micturition center

Stress Urinary Incontinence (00017)
(1986, 2006, LOE 2.1)

Domain 3: Elimination and Exchange
Class 1: Urinary Function

Definition Sudden leakage of urine with activities that increase intra-abdominal pressure

Defining Characteristics

- Observed involuntary leakage of small amounts of urine in the absence of detrusor contraction
- Observed involuntary leakage of small amounts of urine in the absence of an over-distended bladder
- Observed involuntary leakage of small amounts of urine on exertion
- Observed involuntary leakage of small amounts of urine with coughing
- Observed involuntary leakage of small amounts of urine with laughing
- Observed involuntary leakage of small amounts of urine with sneezing
- Reports involuntary leakage of small amounts of urine in the absence of detrusor contraction
- Reports involuntary leakage of small amounts of urine in the absence of an over-distended bladder
- Reports involuntary leakage of small amounts of urine on exertion
- Reports involuntary leakage of small amounts of urine with coughing
- Reports involuntary leakage of small amounts of urine with laughing
- Reports involuntary leakage of small amounts of urine with sneezing

Related Factors

- Degenerative changes in pelvic muscles
- High intra-abdominal pressure
- Intrinsic urethral sphincter deficiency
- Weak pelvic muscles

References

Abrams, P., Cardozo, L., Fall, M., et al. (2002). The standardisation of terminology in lower urinary tract function: Report from the Standardisation Sub-committee of the International Continence Society. *Urology* **61**: 37–49.

Agency for Health Care Policy and Research (AHCPR) (1992). *Clinical practice guideline: Urinary incontinence in adults.* AHCPR Pub. No. 92–0038. Rockville, MD: AHCPR.

National Kidney and Urologic Diseases Information Clearinghouse (NIDDK) (2004). *Urinary incontinence in women.* Available at: http://kidney.niddk.nih.gov/kudiseases/pubs/uiwomen/index.htm (accessed May 23, 2008).

NIH consensus statements (1988). *Urinary incontinence in adults.* Available at: http://consensus.nih.gov/cons/071/071_statement.htm (accessed January 27, 2005).

Noble, J., ed. (2001). *Textbook of primary care medicine*, 3rd edn. St Louis, MO: Mosby.

Sampselle, C.M. (2003). State of the science on urinary incontinence: Behavioral interventions in young and middle-age women [March supplement]. *American Journal of Nursing* **103**(3): 9–19.

Stenchever, M.A., ed. (2001). *Comprehensive gynecology.* St Louis, MO: Mosby.

Walsh, P.C., ed. (2002). *Campbell's urology*, 8th edn. Philadelphia: Saunders.

Domain 3

Urge Urinary Incontinence (00019)

(1986, 2006, LOE 2.1)

Domain 3: Elimination and Exchange
Class 1: Urinary Function

Definition Involuntary passage of urine occurring soon after a strong sense of urgency to void

Defining Characteristics

- Observed inability to reach toilet in time to avoid urine loss
- Reports urinary urgency
- Reports involuntary loss of urine with bladder contractions
- Reports involuntary loss of urine with bladder spasms
- Reports inability to reach toilet in time to avoid urine loss

Related Factors

- Alcohol intake
- Atrophic urethritis
- Atrophic vaginitis
- Bladder infection
- Caffeine intake
- Decreased bladder capacity
- Detrusor hyperactivity with impaired bladder contractility
- Fecal impaction
- Use of diuretics

References

Abrams, P., Cardozo, L., Fall, M., et al. (2002). The standardisation of terminology in lower urinary tract function: Report from the Standardisation Sub-committee of the International Continence Society. *Urology* **61**: 37–49.

Agency for Health Care Policy and Research (AHCPR) (1992). *Clinical practice guideline: Urinary incontinence in adults.* AHCPR Pub. No. 92–0038. Rockville, MD: AHCPR.

National Kidney and Urologic Diseases Information Clearinghouse (NIDDK) (2004). *Urinary incontinence in women.* Available at: http://kidney.niddk.nih.gov/kudiseases/pubs/uiwomen/index.htm (accessed May 23, 2008).

NIH consensus statements (1988). *Urinary incontinence in adults.* Available at: http://consensus.nih.gov/cons/071/071_statement.htm (accessed January 27, 2005).

Noble, J., ed. (2001). *Textbook of primary care medicine*, 3rd edn. St Louis, MO: Mosby.

Sampselle, C.M. (2003). State of the science on urinary incontinence: Behavioral interventions in young and middle-age women [March supplement]. *American Journal of Nursing* **103**(3): 9–19.

Stenchever, M.A., ed. (2001). *Comprehensive gynecology.* St Louis, MO: Mosby.

Walsh, P.C., ed. (2002). *Campbell's urology*, 8th edn. Philadelphia: Saunders.

Domain 3

Risk for Urge Urinary Incontinence

(00022)

Domain 3: Elimination and Exchange
Class 1: Urinary Function

Definition At risk for involuntary loss of urine associated with a sudden, strong sensation of urinary urgency

Risk Factors

- Effects of alcohol
- Effects of caffeine
- Effects of medications
- Detrusor hyperreflexia (e.g., from cystitis, urethritis, tumors, renal calculi, central nervous system disorders above pontine micturition center)
- Impaired bladder contractility
- Involuntary sphincter relaxation
- Ineffective toileting habits
- Small bladder capacity

Class 1: Urinary Function **97**

Impaired Urinary Elimination (00016)

(1973, 2006, LOE 2.1)

Domain 3: Elimination and Exchange
Class 1: Urinary Function

Definition Dysfunction in urine elimination

Defining Characteristics

- Dysuria
- Frequency
- Hesitancy
- Incontinence
- Nocturia
- Retention
- Urgency

Related Factors

- Anatomic obstruction
- Multiple causality
- Sensory motor impairment
- Urinary tract infection

References

Engberg, S., McDowell, B., Donovan, N., Brodak, I., & Weber, E. (1997). Treatment of urinary incontinence in homebound older adults: Interface between research and practice. *Ostomy/Wound Management* **48**(10): 18–26.

Fantl, J., Newman, D., & Colling, J. (1996). *Urinary incontinence in adults: Acute and chronic management* (clinical practice guideline No. 2). Rockville, MD: US Department of Health & Human Services.

Messick, G. & Powe, C. (1997). Applying behavioral research to incontinence. *Ostomy/ Wound management* **48**: 40–8.

Readiness for Enhanced Urinary Elimination (00166)

(2002, LOE 2.1)

Domain 3: Elimination and Exchange
Class 1: Urinary Function

Definition A pattern of urinary functions that is sufficient for meeting eliminatory needs and can be strengthened

Defining Characteristics

- Amount of output is within normal limits
- Expresses willingness to enhance urinary elimination
- Fluid intake is adequate for daily needs
- Positions self for emptying of bladder
- Specific gravity is within normal limits
- Urine is odorless
- Urine is straw colored

Domain 3

Urinary Retention (00023)

(1986)

Domain 3: Elimination and Exchange
Class 1: Urinary Function

Definition Incomplete emptying of the bladder

Defining Characteristics

- Absence of urine output
- Bladder distension
- Dribbling
- Dysuria
- Frequent voiding
- Overflow incontinence
- Residual urine
- Sensation of bladder fullness
- Small voiding

Related Factors

- Blockage
- High urethral pressure
- Inhibition of reflex arc
- Strong sphincter

Bowel Incontinence (00014)
(1975, 1998)

Domain 3: Elimination and exchange
Class 2: Gastrointestinal function

Definition Change in normal bowel habits characterized by involuntary passage of stool

Defining Characteristics

- Constant dribbling of soft stool
- Fecal odor
- Fecal staining of bedding
- Fecal staining of clothing
- Inability to delay defecation
- Inability to recognize urge to defecate
- Inattention to urge to defecate
- Recognizes rectal fullness but reports inability to expel formed stool
- Red perianal skin
- Self-report of inability to recognize rectal fullness
- Urgency

Related Factors

- Abnormally high abdominal pressure
- Abnormally high intestinal pressure
- Chronic diarrhea
- Colorectal lesions
- Dietary habits
- Environmental factors (e.g., inaccessible bathroom)
- General decline in muscle tone
- Immobility
- Impaired cognition
- Impaired reservoir capacity
- Incomplete emptying of bowel
- Laxative abuse
- Loss of rectal sphincter control
- Lower motor nerve damage
- Medications
- Rectal sphincter abnormality
- Impaction
- Stress
- Toileting self-care deficit
- Upper motor nerve damage

Domain 3

Constipation (00011)
(1975, 1998)

Domain 3: Elimination and Exchange
Class 2: Gastrointestinal Function

Definition Decrease in normal frequency of defecation accompanied by difficult or incomplete passage of stool and/or passage of excessively hard, dry stool

Defining Characteristics

- Abdominal pain
- Abdominal tenderness with palpable muscle resistance
- Abdominal tenderness without palpable muscle resistance
- Anorexia
- Atypical presentations in older adults (e.g., change in mental status, urinary incontinence, unexplained falls, elevated body temperature)
- Borborygmi
- Bright-red blood with stool
- Change in bowel pattern
- Decreased frequency
- Decreased volume of stool
- Distended abdomen
- Feeling of rectal fullness
- Feeling of rectal pressure
- Generalized fatigue
- Hard, formed stool
- Headache
- Hyperactive bowel sounds
- Hypoactive bowel sounds
- Increased abdominal pressure
- Indigestion
- Nausea
- Oozing liquid stool
- Palpable abdominal mass
- Palpable rectal mass
- Presence of soft, paste-like stool in rectum
- Percussed abdominal dullness
- Pain with defecation
- Severe flatus
- Straining with defecation
- Unable to pass stool
- Vomiting

Related Factors

Functional

- Abdominal muscle weakness
- Habitual denial
- Habitual ignoring of urge to defecate
- Inadequate toileting (e.g., timeliness, positioning for defecation, privacy)
- Irregular defecation habits
- Insufficient physical activity
- Recent environmental changes

Psychological

- Depression
- Emotional stress
- Mental confusion

Pharmacological

- Aluminum-containing antacids
- Anticholinergics
- Anticonvulsants
- Antidepressants
- Antilipemic agents
- Bismuth salts
- Calcium carbonate
- Calcium channel blockers
- Diuretics
- Iron salts
- Laxative overdose
- Nonsteroidal anti-inflammatory agents
- Opiates
- Phenothiazines
- Sedatives
- Sympathomimetics

Mechanical

- Electrolyte imbalance
- Hemorrhoids
- Hirschsprung's disease
- Neurological impairment
- Obesity
- Postsurgical obstruction
- Pregnancy
- Prostate enlargement
- Rectal abscess
- Rectal anal fissures
- Rectal anal stricture
- Rectal prolapse
- Rectal ulcer
- Rectocele
- Tumors

Physiological

- Change in eating patterns
- Change in usual foods
- Decreased motility of gastrointestinal tract
- Dehydration
- Inadequate dentition
- Inadequate oral hygiene
- Insufficient fiber intake
- Insufficient fluid intake
- Poor eating habits

Domain 3

Perceived Constipation (00012)
(1988)

Domain 3: Elimination and Exchange
Class 2: Gastrointestinal Function

Definition Self-diagnosis of constipation and abuse of laxatives, enemas, and/or suppositories to ensure a daily bowel movement

Defining Characteristics

- Expectation of a daily bowel movement
- Expectation of passage of stool at same time every day
- Overuse of laxatives
- Overuse of enemas
- Overuse of suppositories

Related Factors

- Cultural health beliefs
- Family health beliefs
- Faulty appraisal
- Impaired thought processes

Risk for Constipation (00015)
(1998)

Domain 3: Elimination and Exchange
Class 2: Gastrointestinal Function

Definition At risk for a decrease in normal frequency of defecation accompanied by difficult or incomplete passage of stool and/or passage of excessively hard, dry stool

Risk Factors

Functional

- Habitual denial of urge to defecate
- Habitual ignoring of urge to defecate
- Recent environmental changes
- Inadequate toileting (e.g., timeliness, positioning for defecation, privacy)
- Irregular defecation habits
- Insufficient physical activity
- Abdominal muscle weakness

Psychological

- Depression
- Emotional stress
- Mental confusion

Physiological

- Change in usual eating patterns
- Change in usual foods
- Decreased motility of gastrointestinal tract
- Dehydration
- Inadequate dentition
- Inadequate oral hygiene
- Insufficient fiber intake
- Insufficient fluid intake
- Poor eating habits

Pharmacological

- Aluminum-containing antacids
- Anticholinergics
- Anticonvulsants
- Antidepressants
- Antilipemic agents
- Bismuth salts
- Calcium carbonate
- Calcium channel blockers
- Diuretics
- Iron salts
- Laxative overuse
- Nonsteroidal anti-inflammatory agents
- Opiates
- Phenothiazines
- Sedatives
- Sympathomimetics

Mechanical

- Electrolyte imbalance
- Hemorrhoids
- Hirschsprung's disease
- Neurological impairment
- Obesity
- Postsurgical obstruction

- Pregnancy
- Prostate enlargement
- Rectal abscess
- Rectal anal fissures
- Rectal anal stricture
- Rectal prolapse
- Rectal ulcer
- Rectocele
- Tumors

Diarrhea (00013)

(1975, 1998)

Domain 3: Elimination and Exchange
Class 2: Gastrointestinal Function

Definition Passage of loose, unformed stools

Defining Characteristics

- Abdominal pain
- At least three loose liquid stools per day
- Cramping
- Hyperactive bowel sounds
- Urgency

Related Factors

Psychological

- Anxiety
- High stress levels

- Radiation
- Toxins
- Travel
- Tube feedings

Situational

- Adverse effects of medications
- Alcohol abuse
- Contaminants
- Laxative abuse

Physiological

- Infectious processes
- Inflammation
- Irritation
- Malabsorption
- Parasites

Dysfunctional Gastrointestinal Motility* (00196)
(2008, LOE 2.1)

Domain 3: Elimination and Exchange
Class 2: Gastrointestinal Function

Definition Increased, decreased, ineffective, or lack of peristaltic activity within the gastrointestinal system

Defining Characteristics

- Absence of flatus
- Abdominal cramping
- Abdominal distension
- Abdominal pain
- Accelerated gastric emptying
- Bile-colored gastric residual
- Change in bowel sounds (e.g., absent, hypoactive, hyperactive)
- Diarrhea
- Dry stool
- Difficulty passing stool
- Hard stool
- Increased gastric residual
- Nausea
- Regurgitation
- Vomiting

Related Factors

- Aging
- Anxiety
- Enteral feedings
- Food intolerance (e.g., gluten, lactose)
- Immobility
- Ingestion of contaminates (e.g., food, water)
- Malnutrition
- Pharmaceutical agents (e.g., narcotics/opiates, laxatives, antibiotics, anesthesia)
- Prematurity
- Sedentary lifestyle
- Surgery

References

Chial, H.J. & Camilleri, M. (2003). Motility disorders of the stomach and small intestine. In: Friedman, S.L., McQuaid, K.R., & Grendell, J.H. (eds), *Current diagnosis & treatment in gastroenterology*. New York: Lange Medical Books/McGraw Hill, pp. 355–67.

Chiantri, T. & Prabhakar, K. (2007). Diarrheal diseases in the elderly. In: *Clinics in geriatric medicine*. St Louis: Saunders Elsevier, pp. 833–56.

* This diagnosis formerly held the label, *Ineffective Tissue Perfusion (Specify Type: Gastrointestinal)*.

Holmes, H.N., Henry, K., Bilotta, K., Comerford, K., & Weinstock, D., eds (2007). *Professional guide to signs & symptoms*, 5th edn. Philadelphia: Lippincott Williams & Wilkins, pp. 112–18.

Kahrilas, P.J. (2005). Esophageal motility disorders. In: Weinstein, W.M., Hawkey, C.J., & Bosch, J. (eds), *Clinical gastroenterology and hepatology*. St Louis: Elsevier Mosby, pp. 253–9.

Madsen, D., Sebolt T., Cullen, L., et al. (2005). Listening to bowel sounds: An evidence-based practice project. *American Journal of Nursing* **105**(12): 40–9.

Ouyang, A. & Locke, R. (2007). Overview of Neurogastroenterology – gastrointestinal motility and functional GI disorders: classification, prevalence, and epidemiology. In: *Gastroenterology clinics of North America*. St Louis: Saunders Elsevier, pp. 485–98.

Quigley, E.M.M. (2006). Gastric motor and sensory function and motor disorders of the stomach. In: Feldman, M., Friedman, L.S., Brandt, L.J., Sleisenger, M.H. (eds), *Sleisinger and Fordtran's gastrointestinal and liver disease pathophysiology/diagnosis/management*. St Louis: Saunders Elsevier, pp. 999–1028.

Tack, J. (2005). Gastric motility disorders. In: Weinstein, W.M., C.J. Hawkey, C.J., & Bosch, J. (eds), *Clinical gastroenterology and hepatology*. St Louis: Elsevier Mosby, pp. 261–6.

Taylor, C., Lillis, C. LeMone, P., & Lynn, P. (2008). *Fundamentals of nursing the art and science of nursing care*, 6th edn. Philadelphia: Lippincott Williams & Wilkins, pp. 636–9.

Tursi, A. (2004). Gastrointestinal motility disturbances in celiac disease. *Journal of Clinical Gastroenterology*. Philadelphia: Lippincott Williams & Wilkins, pp. 642–5.

Watson, R.L. (2004). Gastrointestinal disorders. In: Verklan, M.T. & Walden, M. (eds), *Core curriculum for neonatal intensive care nursing*, 3rd edn. St Louis: Elsevier Saunders, pp. 654–83.

Wong, D., Hockenberry, M.J., Perry, S., Lowdermilk D., & Wilson, D. (2006). *Maternal child nursing care*, 3rd edn. St Louis: Mosby Elsevier, pp. 814–18, 859–60, 1531–7.

Risk For Dysfunctional Gastrointestinal Motility (00197)
(2008, LOE 2.1)

Domain 3: Elimination and Exchange
Class 2: Gastrointestinal Function

Definition Risk for increased, decreased, ineffective, or lack of peristaltic activity within the gastrointestinal system

Risk Factors

- Abdominal surgery
- Aging
- Anxiety
- Change in food
- Change in water
- Decreased gastrointestinal circulation
- Diabetes mellitus
- Food intolerance (e.g., gluten, lactose)
- Gastroesophageal reflux disease (GERD)
- Immobility
- Infection (e.g., bacterial, parasitic, viral)
- Pharmaceutical agents (e.g., antibiotics, laxatives, narcotics/opiates, proton pump inhibitors)
- Prematurity
- Sedentary lifestyle
- Stress
- Unsanitary food preparation

References

Chial, H.J. & Camilleri, M. (2003). Motility disorders of the stomach and small intestine. In: Friedman, S.L., McQuaid, K.R., & Grendell, J.H. (eds), *Current diagnosis & treatment in gastroenterology*. New York: Lange Medical Books/McGraw Hill, pp. 355–67.

Chiantri, T. & Prabhakar, K. (2007) Diarrheal diseases in the elderly. In: *Clinics in geriatric medicine*. St Louis: Saunders Elsevier, pp. 833–56.

Holmes, H.N., Henry, K., Bilotta, K., Comerford, K., & D. Weinstock, eds (2007). *Professional guide to signs & symptoms*, 5th edn. Philadelphia: Lippincott Williams & Wilkins, pp. 112–18.

Kahrilas, P.J. (2005). Esophageal motility disorders. In: Weinstein, W.M., Hawkey, C.J., & Bosch, J. (eds), *Clinical gastroenterology and hepatology*. St Louis: Elsevier Mosby, pp. 253–9.

Madsen, D., Sebolt T., Cullen, L., et al. (2005). Listening to bowel sounds: An evidence-based practice project. *American Journal of Nursing* **105**(12): 40–9.

Ouyang, A. & Locke, R. (2007). Overview of Neurogastroenterology – gastrointestinal motility and functional GI disorders: classification, prevalence, and epidemiology. In: *Gastroenterology clinics of North America*. St Louis: Saunders Elsevier, pp. 485–98.

Quigley, E.M.M. (2006). Gastric motor and sensory function and motor disorders of the stomach. In: Feldman, M., Friedman, L.S., Brandt, L.J., Sleisenger, M.H. (eds), *Sleisinger and Fordtran's gastrointestinal and liver disease pathophysiology/diagnosis/management*. St Louis: Saunders Elsevier, pp. 999–1028.

Tack, J. (2005). Gastric motility disorders. In: Weinstein, W.M., C.J. Hawkey, C.J., & Bosch, J. (eds), *Clinical gastroenterology and hepatology*.. St Louis: Elsevier Mosby, pp. 261–6.

Taylor, C., Lillis, C. LeMone, P., & Lynn, P. (2008). *Fundamentals of nursing the art and science of nursing care*, 6th edn. Philadelphia: Lippincott Williams &Wilkins, pp. 636–9.

Tursi, A, (2004). Gastrointestinal motility disturbances in celiac disease. *Journal of Clinical Gastroenterology*. Philadelphia: Lippincott Williams & Wilkins, pp. 642–5.

Watson, R.L. (2004). Gastrointestinal disorders. In: Verklan, M.T. & Walden, M. (eds), *Core curriculum for neonatal intensive care nursing*, 3rd edn. St Louis: Elsevier Saunders, pp. 654–83.

Wong, D., Hockenberry, M.J., Perry, S., Lowdermilk D., & Wilson, D. (2006). *Maternal child nursing care*, 3rd edn. St Louis: Mosby Elsevier, pp. 814–18, 859–60,1531–7.

Impaired Gas Exchange (00030)
(1980, 1996, 1998)

Domain 3: Elimination and Exchange
Class 4: Respiratory Function

Definition Excess or deficit in oxygenation and/or carbon dioxide elimination at the alveolar–capillary membrane

Defining Characteristics

- Abnormal arterial blood gases
- Abnormal arterial pH
- Abnormal breathing (e.g., rate, rhythm, depth)
- Abnormal skin color (e.g., pale, dusky)
- Confusion
- Cyanosis (in neonates only)
- Decreased carbon dioxide
- Diaphoresis
- Dyspnea
- Headache upon awakening
- Hypercapnia
- Hypoxemia
- Hypoxia
- Irritability
- Nasal flaring
- Restlessness
- Somnolence
- Tachycardia
- Visual disturbances

Related Factors

- Alveolar–capillary membrane changes
- Ventilation–perfusion

Domain 4
Activity/Rest

Insomnia (00095)
(2006, LOE 2.1)

Domain 4: Activity/Rest
Class 1: Sleep/Rest

Definition A disruption in amount and quality of sleep that impairs functioning

Defining Characteristics

- Observed changes in affect
- Observed lack of energy
- Increased absenteeism (e.g., work/school)
- Patient reports changes in mood
- Patient reports decreased health status
- Patient reports decreased quality of life
- Patient reports difficulty concentrating
- Patient reports difficulty falling asleep
- Patient reports difficulty staying asleep
- Patient reports dissatisfaction with sleep (current)
- Patient reports increased accidents
- Patient reports lack of energy
- Patient reports nonrestorative sleep
- Patient reports sleep disturbances that produce next-day consequences
- Patient reports waking up too early

Related Factors

- Activity pattern (e.g., timing, amount)
- Anxiety
- Depression
- Environmental factors (e.g., ambient noise, daylight/darkness exposure, ambient temperature/humidity, unfamiliar setting)
- Fear
- Frequent daytime naps
- Gender-related hormonal shifts
- Grief
- Inadequate sleep hygiene (current)
- Intake of stimulants
- Intake of alcohol
- Impairment of normal sleep pattern (e.g., travel, shift work)
- Interrupted Sleep
- Medications
- Parental responsibilities
- Physical discomfort (e.g., pain, shortness of breath, cough, gastroesophageal reflux, nausea, incontinence/urgency)
- Stress (e.g., ruminative pre-sleep pattern)

References

Attarian, H. (2000). Helping patients who say they cannot sleep. *Postgraduate Medicine* **107**: 127–42.

Becker, P., Dement, W., Erman, M., & Glazer, W. (2004). Poor Sleep: The impact on the health of our patients. Available at: Medscape.com: www.medscape.com/viewarticle/475291_1 (accessed May 29, 2008).

Buysse, D.J., Reynolds III, C.F., Monk, T.H., Berman, S.R., & Kupfer, D.J. (1989). The Pittsburgh Sleep Quality Index: A new instrument for psychiatric practice and research. *Psychiatry Research* **28**: 193–213.

Cochran, H. (2003). Diagnose and treat primary insomnia. *The Nurse Practitioner* **28**(9): 13–27.

Doran, C.M. (2003). *Prescribing mental health medication*. New York: Routledge.

First, M.B., ed. (2000). *Diagnostic and statistical manual – text revision (DSM-IV-TR, 2000)* [Electronic version]. Washington DC: American Psychiatric Association.

Fogel, J. (2003). Behavioral treatments for insomnia in primary care settings. *Advanced Practice Nursing E journal* **3**(4): 1–8.

Hoffman, S. (2003). Sleep in the older adult: implications for nurses. *Geriatric Nursing* **24**: 210–16.

Krahn, L. (2003). Sleep disorders. *Seminars in Neurology* **23**: 307–14.

Linton, S. & Bryngelsson, I. (2000). Insomnia and its relationship to work and health in a working age population. *Journal of Occupational Rehabilitation* **10**: 169–83.

Lippmann, S.L., Mazour, I., & Shahab, H. (2001). Insomnia: therapeutic approach. *Southern Medical Journal* **94**: 866–73.

McCall, V. & Rakel, R. (1999). *A practical guide to insomnia*. Minneapolis, MN: McGraw-Hill Co., Inc.

Mahowald, M. (2000). What is causing excessive daytime sleepiness? *Postgraduate Medicine* **107**: 108–23.

Medscape (2004). *Understanding sleep problems – the basics*. Available at: www.medscape.com/viewarticle/474122 (accessed May 29, 2008).

Merriam-Webster Online (2004). Insomnia. Available at: www.m-w.com/cgi-bin/dictionary?book=Dictionary&va=insomnia (accessed May 29, 2008).

Sateia, M. & Nowell, P. (2004). Insomnia. *Lancet* **364**: 1959–73.

Simon, R. (1999). Diagnosis of insomnia: A primary care perspective. *Family Practice Recertification* **21**(10): 12–19.

Sleep Health. Ineffective activity planning. Are you resting easy? [Electronic version]. *Nursing* 2004;**34**(4): 74.

Smith, M., Perlis, M., Park, A., et al. (2002). Comparative meta-analysis of pharmacotherapy and behavior therapy for persistent insomnia. *American Journal of Psychiatry* **159**: 5–11.

Walsh, J. (1999). Insomnia: Prevalence and clinical and public health considerations. *Family Practice Recertification* **21**(10): 4–11.

Disturbed Sleep Pattern (00198)
(2006, LOE 2.1)

Domain 4: Activity/Rest
Class 1: Sleep/Rest

Definition
Time-limited interruptions of sleep amount and quality due to external factors

Defining Characteristics

- Change in normal sleep pattern
- Verbal complaints of not feeling well rested
- Dissatisfaction with sleep
- Decreased ability to function
- Reports being awakened
- Reports no difficulty falling asleep

Related Factors

- Ambient temperature, humidity
- Caregiving responsibilities
- Change in daylight–darkness exposure
- Interruptions (e.g., for therapeutics, monitoring, lab tests)
- Lack of sleep privacy/ control
- Lighting
- Noise
- Noxious odors
- Physical restraint
- Sleep partner
- Unfamiliar sleep furnishings

Sleep Deprivation (00096)
(1998)

Domain 4: Activity/Rest
Class 1: Sleep/Rest

Definition Prolonged periods of time without sleep (sustained natural, periodic suspension of relative consciousness)

Defining Characteristics

- Acute confusion
- Agitation
- Anxiety
- Apathy
- Combativeness
- Daytime drowsiness
- Decreased ability to function
- Fatigue
- Fleeting nystagmus
- Hallucinations
- Hand tremors
- Heightened sensitivity to pain
- Inability to concentrate
- Irritability
- Lethargy
- Listlessness
- Malaise
- Perceptual disorders (e.g., disturbed body sensation, delusions, feeling afloat)
- Restlessness
- Slowed reaction
- Transient paranoia

Related Factors

- Aging-related sleep stage shifts
- Dementia
- Familial sleep paralysis
- Inadequate daytime activity
- Idiopathic central nervous system hypersomnolence
- Narcolepsy
- Nightmares
- Nonsleep-inducing parenting practices
- Periodic limb movement (e.g., restless leg syndrome, nocturnal myoclonus)
- Prolonged discomfort (e.g., physical, psychological)
- Sustained inadequate sleep hygiene
- Prolonged use of pharmacologic or dietary antisoporifics
- Sleep apnea
- Sleep terror
- Sleep walking
- Sleep-related enuresis
- Sleep-related painful erections
- Sundowner's syndrome
- Sustained circadian asynchrony
- Sustained environmental stimulation
- Sustained uncomfortable sleep environment

Domain 4: Activity/Rest
Class 1: Sleep/Rest

Definition A pattern of natural, periodic suspension of consciousness that provides adequate rest, sustains a desired lifestyle, and can be strengthened

Defining Characteristics

- Amount of sleep is congruent with developmental needs
- Expresses a feeling of being rested after sleep
- Expresses willingness to enhance sleep
- Follows sleep routines that promote sleep habits
- Occasional use of medications to induce sleep

Domain 4

Risk for Disuse Syndrome (00040)

(1988)

Domain 4: Activity/Rest
Class 2: Activity/Exercise

Definition At risk for deterioration of body systems as the result of prescribed or unavoidable musculoskeletal inactivity

Risk Factors

- Altered level of consciousness
- Mechanical immobilization
- Paralysis
- Prescribed immobilization
- Severe pain

Note: complications from immobility can include pressure ulcer, constipation, stasis of pulmonary secretions, thrombosis, urinary tract infection and/or retention, decreased strength or endurance, orthostatic hypotension, decreased range of joint motion, disorientation, body-image disturbance, and powerlessness.

Deficient Diversional Activity (00097)

(1980)

Domain 4: Activity/Rest
Class 2: Activity/Exercise

Definition Decreased stimulation from (or interest or engagement in) recreational or leisure activities

Defining Characteristics

- Patient's statements regarding boredom (e.g., wish there was something to do, to read)
- Usual hobbies cannot be undertaken in hospital

Related Factors

- Environmental lack of diversional activity

Sedentary Lifestyle (00168)

(2004, LOE 2.1)

Domain 4: Activity/Rest
Class 2: Activity/Exercise

Definition Reports a habit of life that is characterized by a low physical activity level

Defining Characteristics

- Chooses a daily routine lacking physical exercise
- Demonstrates physical deconditioning
- Verbalizes preference for activities low in physical activity

Related Factors

- Deficient knowledge of health benefits of physical exercise
- Lack of interest
- Lack of motivation
- Lack of resources (e.g., time, money, companionship, facilities)
- Lack of training for accomplishment of physical exercise

Impaired Bed Mobility (00091)
(1998, 2006, LOE 2.1)

Domain 4: Activity/Rest
Class 2: Activity/Exercise

Definition Limitation of independent movement from one bed position to another

Defining Characteristics

- Impaired ability to move from supine to sitting
- Impaired ability to move from sitting to supine
- Impaired ability to move from supine to prone
- Impaired ability to move from prone to supine
- Impaired ability to move from supine to long sitting
- Impaired ability to move from long sitting to supine
- Impaired ability to reposition self in bed
- Impaired ability to turn from side to side

Related Factors

- Cognitive impairment
- Deconditioning
- Deficient knowledge
- Environmental constraints (e.g., bed size, bed type, treatment equipment, restraints)
- Insufficient muscle strength
- Musculoskeletal impairment
- Neuromuscular impairment
- Obesity
- Pain
- Sedating medications

References

Brouwer, K., Nysseknabm, J., & Culham, E. (2004). Physical function and health status among seniors with and without fear of falling. *Gerontology* **50**: 15–141.

Goldstein, S. (1993). The biology of aging: Looking to defuse the time bomb. *Geriatrics* **48**(9): 76–81.

Lewis, C.L., Moutoux, M., Slaughter, M., & Bailey, S.P. (2004). Characteristics of individuals who fell while receiving home health services. *Physical Therapy* **84**(1): 23–32.

Matsouka, O., Harahousou, Y., Kabiatis, C., & Trigonis, I. (2003). Effects of a physical activity program: The study of selected physical abilities among elderly women. *Journal of Gerontological Nursing* **29**(7): 50–5.

Tinetti., M.E. & Ginter, S.F. (1988). Identifying mobility dysfunction in elderly persons. *Journal of American Medical Association* **259**: 1190–3.

Note: specify level of independence using a standardized functional scale.

Domain 4

Impaired Physical Mobility (00085)
(1973, 1998)

Domain 4: Activity/Rest
Class 2: Activity/Exercise

Definition Limitation in independent, purposeful physical movement of the body or of one or more extremities

Defining Characteristics

- Decreased reaction time
- Difficulty turning
- Engages in substitutions for movement (e.g., increased attention to other's activity, controlling behavior, focus on pre-illness disability/activity)
- Exertional dyspnea
- Gait changes
- Jerky movements
- Limited ability to perform gross motor skills
- Limited ability to perform fine motor skills
- Limited range of motion
- Movement-induced tremor
- Postural instability
- Slowed movement
- Uncoordinated movements

Related Factors

- Activity intolerance
- Altered cellular metabolism
- Anxiety
- Body mass index above 75th age-appropriate percentile
- Cognitive impairment
- Contractures
- Cultural beliefs regarding age-appropriate activity
- Deconditioning
- Decreased endurance
- Depressive mood state
- Decreased muscle control
- Decreased muscle mass
- Decreased muscle strength
- Deficient knowledge regarding value of physical activity
- Developmental delay
- Discomfort
- Disuse
- Joint stiffness
- Lack of environmental supports (e.g., physical or social)
- Limited cardiovascular endurance
- Loss of integrity of bone structures
- Malnutrition
- Medications
- Musculoskeletal impairment
- Neuromuscular impairment
- Pain
- Prescribed movement restrictions
- Reluctance to initiate movement
- Sedentary lifestyle
- Sensoriperceptual impairments

Note: specify level of independence using a standardized functional scale.

Impaired Wheelchair Mobility (00089)
(1998, 2006, LOE 2.1)

Domain 4: Activity/Rest
Class 2: Activity/Exercise

Definition Limitation of independent operation of wheelchair within environment

Defining Characteristics

- Impaired ability to operate manual wheelchair on curbs
- Impaired ability to operate power wheelchair on curbs
- Impaired ability to operate manual wheelchair on even surface
- Impaired ability to operate power wheelchair on even surface
- Impaired ability to operate manual wheelchair on uneven surface
- Impaired ability to operate power wheelchair on uneven surface
- Impaired ability to operate manual wheelchair on an incline
- Impaired ability to operate power wheelchair on an incline
- Impaired ability to operate manual wheelchair on a decline
- Impaired ability to operate power wheelchair on a decline

Related Factors

- Cognitive impairment
- Deconditioning
- Deficient knowledge
- Depressed mood
- Environmental constraints (e.g., stairs, inclines, uneven surfaces, unsafe obstacles, distances, lack of assistive devices or person, wheelchair type)
- Impaired vision
- Insufficient muscle strength
- Limited endurance
- Musculoskeletal impairment (e.g., contractures)
- Neuromuscular impairment
- Obesity
- Pain

References

Brouwer, K., Nysseknabm, J., & Culham, E. (2004). Physical function and health status among seniors with and without fear of falling. *Gerontology* **50**: 15–141.

Goldstein, S. (1993). The biology of aging: Looking to defuse the time bomb. *Geriatrics* **48**(9): 76–81.

Lewis, C.L., Moutoux, M., Slaughter, M., & Bailey, S.P. (2004). Characteristics of individuals who fell while receiving home health services. *Physical Therapy* **84**(1): 23–32.

Matsouka, O., Harahousou, Y., Kabiatis, C., & Trigonis, I. (2003). Effects of a physical activity program: The study of selected physical abilities among elderly women. *Journal of Gerontological Nursing* **29**(7): 50–5.

Tinetti., M.E. & Ginter, S.F. (1988). Identifying mobility dysfunction in elderly persons. *Journal of American Medical Association* **259**: 1190–3.

Note: specify level of independence using a standardized functional scale.

Delayed Surgical Recovery (00100)
(1998, 2006, LOE 2.1)

Domain 4: Activity/Rest
Class 2: Activity/Exercise

Definition Extension of the number of postoperative days required to initiate and perform activities that maintain life, health, and well-being

Defining Characteristics

- Difficulty in moving about
- Evidence of interrupted healing of surgical area (e.g., red, indurated, draining, immobilized)
- Fatigue
- Loss of appetite with nausea
- Loss of appetite without nausea
- Perception that more time is needed to recover
- Postpones resumption of work/employment activities
- Requires help to complete self-care
- Report of discomfort
- Report of pain

Related Factors

- Extensive surgical procedure
- Obesity
- Pain
- Postoperative surgical site infection
- Preoperative expectations
- Prolonged surgical procedure

References

Bruggeman N., Turner N., Dahm D., Voll A., Hoskin T., Jacofsky D., & Haidukewych, G. (2004). Wound complications after open Achilles tendon repair: an analysis of risk factors. *Clinical Orthopedics* **427**: 63–6.

Burger J., Luijendijk R., Hop W., Halm J., Verdaasdonk E., & Jeekel, J. (2004). Long-term follow-up of a randomized controlled trial of suture versus mesh repair of incisional hernia. *Annals of Surgery* **240**: 578–83.

Callesen T. (2003). Inguinal hernia repair: Anaesthesia, pain and convalescence. *Danish Medical Bulletin* **50**: 203–18.

Chung, F. (1995). Recovery pattern and home-readiness after ambulatory surgery. *Anesthesia & Analgesia* **80**: 896–902.

Fallis, W. & Scurrah, D. (2001). Outpatient laparoscopic cholecystectomy: home visit versus telephone follow-up. *Canadian Journal of Surgery* **44**(1): 39–44.

Harrington, G., Russo, P., Spelman, D., et al. (2004). Surgical-site infection rates and risk factor analysis in coronary artery bypass graft surgery. *Infection Control and Hospital Epidemiology* **25**: 472–6.

Hollington, P., Toogood, G., & Padbury, R. (1999). A prospective randomized trial of day-stay only versus overnight-stay laparoscopic cholecystectomy. *Australia & New Zealand Journal of Surgery* **69**: 841–3.

Horvath K.J. (2003). Postoperative recovery at home after ambulatory gynecologic laparoscopic surgery. *Journal of Perianesthesia Nursing* **18**: 324–34.

Jibodh, S., Gurkan, I., & Wenz, J. (2004). In-hospital outcome and resource use in hip arthroplasty: influence of body mass. *Orthopedics* **27**: 594–601.

Kabon, B., Nagele, A., Reddy, D., et al. (2004). Obesity decreases perioperative tissue oxygenation. *Anesthesiology* **100**: 274–80.

Kleinbeck, S.V. (2000). Self-reported at-home postoperative recovery. *Research in Nursing & Health* **23**: 461–72.

Kotiniemi, L., Ryhanen, P., Valanne, J., Jokela, R., Mustonen, A., & Poukkula, E. (1997). Postoperative symptoms at home following day-case surgery in children: a multicentre survey of 551 children. *Anaesthesia* **52**: 963–9.

Kuo, C., Wang, S., Yu, W., Chang, M., Liu, C., & Chen, T. (2004). Postoperative spinal deep wound infection: a six-year review of 3230 selective procedures. *Journal of the Chinese Medical Association* **67**: 398–402.

Lehmann, H., Fleisher, L., Lam, J., Frink, B., & Bass, E. (1999). Patient preferences for early discharge after laparoscopic cholecystectomy. *Anesthesia & Analgesia* **88**: 1280–85.

Levy, B., Rosson, J., & A. Blake (2004). MRSA in patients presenting with femoral fractures. *Surgeon* **2**: 171–2.

Lofgren, M., Poromaa, I., Stjerndahl, J., & Renstrom, B. (2004). Postoperative infections and antibiotic prophylaxis for hysterectomy in Sweden: A study by the Swedish National Register for Gynecologic Surgery. *Acta Obstetrica et Gynaecologica Scandinavica* **83**: 1202–7.

Morales, CH, Villegas, MI, Villavicencio, R., et al. (2004). Intra-abdominal infection in patients with abdominal trauma. *Archives of Surgery* **9**: 1278–85 (peroperative contamination leads to infection).

Mortenson, M., Schneider, P., Khatri, V., et al. (2004). Immediate breast reconstruction after mastectomy increases wound complications: however, initiation of adjuvant chemotherapy is not delayed. *Archives of Surgery* **139**: 988–91.

Muschik, M., Luck, W., & Schlenzka, D. (2004). Implant removal for late-developing infection alter instrumented posterior spinal fusion for scoliosis: reinstrumentation reduces loss of correction. A retrospective analysis of 45 cases. *European Spine Journal* **13**: 645–51.

Nguyen, N., Nguyen, C., Stevens, C., Steward, E., & Paya, M. (2004). The efficacy of fibrin sealant in prevention of anastomotic leak after laparoscopic gastric bypass. *Journal of the Surgical Resident* **122**: 218–24.

Phillips, C., Kiyak, H., Bloomquist, D., & Turvey, T. (2004). Perceptions of recovery and satisfaction in the short term after orthognathic surgery. *Journal of Oral Maxillofacial Surgery* **62**: 535–44.

Smith, R., Bohl, J., McElearney, S., Friel, C., Barclay, M., Sawyer, R., & Foley, E. (2004). Wound infection after elective colorectal resection. *Annals of Surgery* **239**: 599–605.

Watt-Watson, J., Chung, F., Chan, V., & McGillion, M. (2004). Pain management following discharge after ambulatory same-day surgery. *Journal of Nurse Management* **12**: 153–61.

Young, J. & O'Connell, B. (2001). Recovery following laparoscopic cholecystectomy in either a 23 hour or an 8 hour facility. *Journal of Quality Clinical Practice* **21**(1–2): 2–7.

Zalon, M. (2004). Correlates of recovery among older adults after major abdominal surgery. *Nursing Research* **53**: 99–106.

Impaired Transfer Ability (00090)

(1998, 2006, LOE 2.1)

Domain 4: Activity/Rest
Class 2: Activity/Exercise

Definition Limitation of independent movement between two nearby surfaces

Defining Characteristics

- Inability to transfer between uneven levels
- Inability to transfer from bed to chair
- Inability to transfer from chair to bed
- Inability to transfer on or off a toilet
- Inability to transfer on or off a commode
- Inability to transfer in or out of bath tub
- Inability to transfer in or out of shower
- Inability to transfer from chair to car
- Inability to transfer from car to chair
- Inability to transfer from chair to floor
- Inability to transfer from floor to chair
- Inability to transfer from standing to floor
- Inability to transfer from floor to standing
- Inability to transfer from bed to standing
- Inability to transfer from standing to bed
- Inability to transfer from chair to standing
- Inability to transfer from standing to chair

Related Factors

- Cognitive impairment
- Deconditioning
- Environmental constraints (e.g., bed height, inadequate space, wheel chair type, treatment equipment, restraints)
- Impaired balance
- Impaired vision
- Insufficient muscle strength
- Lack of knowledge
- Musculoskeletal impairment (e.g., contractures)
- Neuromuscular impairment
- Obesity
- Pain

Domain 4

References

Brouwer, K., Nysseknabm, J., & Culham, E. (2004). Physical function and health status among seniors with and without fear of falling. *Gerontology* **50**: 15–141.

Lewis, C.L., Moutoux, M., Slaughter, M., & Bailey, S.P. (2004). Characteristics of individuals who fell while receiving home health services. *Physical Therapy* **84**(1): 23–32.

Tinetti., M.E. & Ginter, S.F. (1988). Identifying mobility dysfunction in elderly persons. *Journal of American Medical Association* **259**: 1190–3.

Note: specify level of independence using a standardized functional scale.

Impaired Walking (00088)

(1998, 2006, LOE 2.1)

Domain 4: Activity/Rest
Class 2: Activity/Exercise

Definition
Limitation of independent movement within the environment on foot

Defining Characteristics

- Impaired ability to climb stairs
- Impaired ability to navigate curbs
- Impaired ability to walk required distances
- Impaired ability to walk on incline
- Impaired ability to walk on decline
- Impaired ability to walk on uneven surfaces

Related Factors

- Cognitive impairment
- Deconditioning
- Depressed mood
- Environmental constraints (e.g., stairs, inclines, uneven surfaces, unsafe obstacles, distances, lack of assistive devices or person, restraints)
- Fear of falling
- Impaired balance
- Impaired vision
- Insufficient muscle strength
- Lack of knowledge
- Limited endurance
- Musculoskeletal impairment (e.g., contractures)
- Neuromuscular impairment
- Obesity
- Pain

References

Brouwer, K., Nysseknabm, J., & Culham, E. (2004). Physical function and health status among seniors with and without fear of falling. *Gerontology* **50**: 15–141.

Lewis, C.L., Moutoux, M., Slaughter, M., & Bailey, S.P. (2004). Characteristics of individuals who fell while receiving home health services. *Physical Therapy* **84**(1): 23–32.

Tinetti., M.E. & Ginter, S.F. (1988). Identifying mobility dysfunction in elderly persons. *Journal of American Medical Association* **259**: 1190–3.

Note: specify level of independence using a standardized functional scale.

Disturbed Energy Field (00050)
(1994, 2004, LOE 2.1)

Domain 4: Activity/Rest
Class 3: Energy Balance

Definition Disruption of the flow of energy surrounding a person's being results in disharmony of the body, mind, and/or spirit

Defining Characteristics

- Perceptions of changes in patterns of energy flow, such as:
  - Movement (wave, spike, tingling, dense, flowing)
  - Sounds (tone, words)
  - Temperature change (warmth, coolness)
  - Visual changes (image, color)
  - Disruption of the field (deficit, hole, spike, bulge, obstruction, congestion, diminished flow in energy field)

Related Factors

Slowing or blocking of energy flows seconday to:

Maturational factors

- Age-related developmental crisis
- Age-related developmental difficulties

Pathophysiologic factors

- Illness
- Injury
- Pregnancy

Situational factors

- Anxiety
- Fear
- Grieving
- Pain

Treatment-related factors

- Chemotherapy
- Immobility
- Labor and delivery
- Perioperative experience

Fatigue (00093)

(1988, 1998)

Domain 4: Activity/Rest
Class 3: Energy Balance

Definition An overwhelming sustained sense of exhaustion and decreased capacity for physical and mental work at usual level

Defining Characteristics

- Compromised concentration
- Compromised libido
- Decreased performance
- Disinterest in surroundings
- Drowsy
- Feelings of guilt for not keeping up with responsibilities
- Inability to maintain usual level of physical activity
- Inability to maintain usual routines
- Inability to restore energy even after sleep
- Increase in physical complaints
- Increase in rest requirements
- Introspection
- Lack of energy
- Lethargic
- Listless
- Perceived need for additional energy to accomplish routine tasks
- Tired
- Verbalization of an unremitting lack of energy
- Verbalization of an overwhelming lack of energy

Related Factors

Psychological

- Anxiety
- Boring lifestyle
- Depression
- Stress

Physiological

- Anemia
- Disease states
- Increased physical exertion
- Malnutrition
- Poor physical condition

- Pregnancy
- Sleep deprivation

Environmental

- Humidity
- Lights
- Noise
- Temperature

Situational

- Negative life events
- Occupation

Domain 4: Activity/Rest
Class 4: Cardiovascular/Pulmonary Responses

Definition Insufficient physiological or psychological energy to endure or complete required or desired daily activities

Defining Characteristics

- Abnormal blood pressure response to activity
- Abnormal heart rate response to activity
- EKG changes reflecting arrhythmias
- EKG changes reflecting ischemia
- Exertional discomfort
- Exertional dyspnea
- Verbal report of fatigue
- Verbal report of weakness

Related Factors

- Bed rest
- Generalized weakness
- Imbalance between oxygen supply/demand
- Immobility
- Sedentary lifestyle

Risk for Activity Intolerance (00094)
(1982)

Domain 4: Activity/Rest
Class 4: Cardiovascular/Pulmonary Responses

Definition At risk for experiencing insufficient physiological or psychological energy to endure or complete required or desired daily activities

Risk Factors

- Deconditioned status
- History of previous intolerance
- Inexperience with the activity
- Presence of circulatory problems
- Presence of respiratory problems

Risk for Bleeding (00206)
(2008, LOE 2.1)

Domain 4: Activity/Rest
Class 4: Cardiovascular/Pulmonary Responses

Definition At risk for a decrease in blood volume that may compromise health

Risk Factors

- Aneurysm
- Circumcision
- Deficient knowledge
- Disseminated intravascular coagulopathy
- History of falls
- Gastrointestinal disorders (e.g., gastric ulcer disease, polyps, varices)
- Impaired liver function (e.g., cirrhosis, hepatitis)
- Inherent coagulopathies (e.g., thrombocytopenia)
- Postpartum complications (e.g., uterine atony, retained placenta)
- Pregnancy-related complications (e.g., placenta previa, molar pregnancy, abruption placenta)
- Trauma
- Treatment-related side effects (e.g., surgery, medications, administration of platelet deficient blood products, chemotherapy)

References

Brozenec, S.A. (2007). Hepatic Problems. In F.D. Monahan, J.K. Sands, M. Neighbors, J.F. Marek, & C.J. Green, (Eds.), *Phipp's Medical-Surgical Nursing: Health and Illness Perspectives* (8th ed., pp. 1209–1212). St Louis: Mosby Elsevier.

Callahan, L. (2004). Surgery in Pregnancy. In S. Mattson & J.E. Smith (Eds.), *Core Curriculum for Maternal-Newborn Nursing* (3rd ed., pp.727–749). St. Louis: Elsevier Saunders.

Deitch, E.A. & Dayal, S.D. (2006). Intensive care unit management of the trauma patient. *Critical Care Medicine* **34**: 2294–301.

Erickson, J. & Field, R. (2007). Cancer. In F.D. Monahan, J.K. Sands, M. Neighbors, J.F. Marek, & C.J. Green, (Eds.), *Phipp's Medical-Surgical Nursing: Health and Illness Perspectives* (8th ed., pp. 1209–1212). St Louis: Mosby Elsevier.

Garrigues, A.L. (2007). Hematologic problems. In: Monahan, F.D., Sands, J.K., Neighbors, M., Marek, J.F., & Green, C.J. (eds), *Phipp's medical-surgical nursing: Health and illness perspectives*, 8th edn. St Louis: Mosby Elsevier, pp. 923–8.

Haney, S. (2004). Trauma in Pregnancy. In S. Mattson & J.E. Smith (Eds.), *Core Curriculum for Maternal-Newborn Nursing* (3rd ed., pp.703–726). St Louis: Elsevier Saunders.

Higgins, P.G. (2004). Postpartum complications. In: Mattson, S. & Smith, J.E. (eds), *Core curriculum for maternal-newborn nursing*, 3rd edn.. St Louis: Elsevier Saunders, pp. 850–4.

Lowdermilk, D. & Perry, S. (2006). *Maternity Nursing* (7th ed.). St. Louis: Mosby Elsevier, pp. 599–601.

Maxwell-Thompson, C. & Reid, K. (2007). Vascular Problems. In F. Monahan, J. Sands, M. Neighbors, J. Marek, & C. Green, (Eds.), *Phipp's Medical-Surgical Nursing: Health and Illness Perspectives* (8th ed., pp. 1209–1212). St Louis: Mosby Elsevier.

Marek, J. & Boehnlein, M. (2007). Postoperative Nursing. In F. Monahan, J. Sands, M. Neighbors, J. Marek, & C. Green, (Eds.), *Phipp's Medical-Surgical Nursing: Health and Illness Perspectives* (8th ed., pp. 1209–1212). St Louis: Mosby Elsevier.

Poole, J. (2004). Hemorrhagic Disorders. In S. Mattson & J. Smith (Eds.), *Core Curriculum for Maternal-Newborn Nursing* (3rd ed., pp.630–659). St Louis: Elsevier Saunders.

Sands, J.K. (2007). Stomach and duodenal problems. In: Monahan, F.D., Sands, J.K., Neighbors, M., Marek, J.F., & Green, C.J. (eds), *Phipp's medical-surgical nursing: Health and illness perspectives*, 8th edn. St Louis: Mosby Elsevier, pp. 1209–12.

Warshaw, M. (2007). Male Reproductive Problems. In F. Monahan, J. Sands, M. Neighbors, J. Marek, & C. Green, (Eds.), *Phipp's Medical-Surgical Nursing: Health and Illness Perspectives* (8th ed., pp. 1209–1212). St Louis: Mosby Elsevier.

Domain 4

Ineffective Breathing Pattern (00032)
(1980, 1996, 1998)

Domain 4: Activity/Rest
Class 4: Cardiovascular/Pulmonary Responses

Definition Inspiration and/or expiration that does not provide adequate ventilation

Defining Characteristics

- Alterations in depth of breathing
- Altered chest excursion
- Assumption of three-point position
- Bradypnea
- Decreased expiratory pressure
- Decreased inspiratory pressure
- Decreased minute ventilation
- Decreased vital capacity

- Dyspnea
- Increased anterior-posterior diameter
- Nasal flaring
- Orthopnea
- Prolonged expiration phase
- Pursed-lip breathing
- Tachypnea
- Use of accessory muscles to breathe

Related Factors

- Anxiety
- Body position
- Bony deformity
- Chest wall deformity
- Cognitive impairment
- Fatigue
- Hyperventilation
- Hypoventilation syndrome

- Musculoskeletal impairment
- Neurological immaturity
- Neuromuscular dysfunction
- Obesity
- Pain
- Perception impairment
- Respiratory muscle fatigue
- Spinal cord injury

Decreased Cardiac Output (00029)

(1975, 1996, 2000)

Domain 4: Activity/Rest
Class 4: Cardiovascular/Pulmonary Responses

Definition Inadequate blood pumped by the heart to meet metabolic demands of the body

Defining Characteristics

Altered Heart Rate/ Rhythm

- Arrhythmias
- Bradycardia
- EKG changes
- Palpitations
- Tachycardia

Altered Preload

- Edema
- Decreased central venous pressure (CVP)
- Decreased pulmonary artery wedge pressure (PAWP)
- Fatigue
- Increased CVP
- Increased PAWP
- Jugular vein distension
- Murmurs
- Weight gain

Altered Afterload

- Clammy skin
- Dyspnea
- Decreased peripheral pulses
- Decreased pulmonary vascular resistance (PVR)

- Decreased systemic vascular resistance (SVR)
- Increased PVR
- Increased SVR
- Oliguria
- Prolonged capillary refill
- Skin color changes
- Variations in blood pressure readings

Altered Contractility

- Crackles
- Cough
- Decreased ejection fraction
- Decreased left ventricular stroke work index (LVSWI)
- Decreased stroke volume index (SVI)
- Decreased cardiac index
- Orthopnea
- Paroxysmal nocturnal dyspnea
- S3 sounds
- S4 sounds

Behavioral/Emotional

- Anxiety
- Restlessness

Domain 4

Related Factors

- Altered heart rate
- Altered rhythm
- Altered stroke volume

- Altered afterload
- Altered contractility
- Altered preload

Ineffective Peripheral Tissue Perfusion (00204)

(2008, LOE 2.1)

Domain 4: Activity/Rest
Class 4: Cardiovascular/Pulmonary Responses

Definition Decrease in blood circulation to the periphery that may compromise health

Defining Characteristics

- Absent pulses
- Altered motor function
- Altered skin characteristics (color, elasticity, hair, moisture, nails, sensation, temperature)
- Blood pressure changes in extremities
- Claudication
- Color does not return to leg on lowering it
- Delayed peripheral wound healing
- Diminished pulses
- Edema
- Extremity pain
- Paraesthesia
- Skin color pale on elevation

Related Factors

- Deficient knowledge of aggravating factors (e.g., smoking, sedentary lifestyle, trauma, obesity, salt intake, immobility)
- Deficient knowledge of disease process (e.g., diabetes, hyperlipidemia)
- Diabetes mellitus
- Hypertension
- Sedentary lifestyle
- Smoking

References

Lopez Rowe, V. (2005). Peripheral arterial occlusive disease. *eMedicine,* Available at: www.emedicine.com/med/topic391.htm (accessed May 23, 2008).

O'Donnell, J.M. & N'acul, F., eds (2001). *Surgical intensive care medicine.* Boston: Kluwer Academic Publishers.

Silva, R.C.G., Cruz, D.A.L.M., Bortolotto, L.A., et al. (2006). Ineffective peripheral tissue perfusion: Clinical validation in patients with hypertensive cardiomyopathy. *International Journal of Nursing Terminologies and Classifications,* **17**(2): 97–107.

Stephens, E. (2005). Peripheral vascular disease. *eMedicine.* Available at: www.emedicine.com/emerg/topic862.htm (accessed May 23, 2008).

Swearingen, P.L. & Hicks Keen, J. eds (2001). *Manual of critical care nursing: Nursing interventions and collaborative management,* 4th edn. St Louis: Mosby.

Domain 4

Risk for Decreased Cardiac Tissue Perfusion* (00200)
(2008, LOE 2.1)

Domain 4: Activity/Rest
Class 4: Cardiovascular/Pulmonary Responses

Definition   Risk for a decrease in cardiac (coronary) circulation

Risk Factors

- Birth control pills
- Cardiac surgery
- Cardiac tamponade
- Coronary artery spasm
- Diabetes mellitus
- Drug abuse
- Elevated C-reactive protein
- Family history of coronary artery disease
- Hyperlipidemia
- Hypertension
- Hypovolemia
- Hypoxemia
- Hypoxia
- Lack of knowledge of modifiable risk factors (e.g., smoking, sedentary lifestyle, obesity)

References

Alzamora, M.T., Bena-Diez, J.M., Sorribes, M., et al. (2007). Peripheral arterial disease study (PERART): Prevalence and predictive values of asymptomatic peripheral arterial occlusive disease related to cardiovascular morbidity and mortality. *BMC Public Health* 7: 348.

Dogan, A., Ozgul, M., Oxaydin, M., Suleyman, M.A., Gedikli, O., & Altinbas, A. (2005). Effect of clopidogrel plus aspirin on tissue perfusion and coronary flow in patients with ST-segment elevation myocardial infarction: A new reperfusion strategy. *American Heart Journal* 149: 1037–42.

Hung, J., Knuiman, M., Divitini, M., Davis, T., & Beiby, J. (2008, January). Prevalence and risk factor correlates of elevated c-reactive protein in an adult Australian population. *The American Journal of Cardiology,* 101(2): 193–8.

O'Donnell, J.M. & N'acul, F., eds (2001). *Surgical intensive care medicine.* Boston: Kluwer Academic Publishers.

Sharma, S. (2006). Pulmonary embolism. *eMedicine.* Available at: www.emedicine.com/med/TOPIC1958.HTM (accessed May 23, 2007).

Steen, H., Lehrke, S., Wiegand, U.K.H., et al. (2005). Very early cardiac magnetic resonance imaging for quantification of myocardial tissue perfusion in patients receiving tirofiban before percutaneous coronary intervention for ST-elevation myocardial infarction. *American Heart Journal,*149: 564.

Swearingen, P.L. & Hicks Keen, J., eds (2001). *Manual of critical care nursing: Nursing interventions and collaborative management,* 4th edn. St Louis: Mosby.

* This diagnosis formerly held the label, *Ineffective Tissue Perfusion (Specify Type: Cerebral).*

Risk for Ineffective Cerebral Tissue Perfusion* (00201)

(2008, LOE 2.1)

Domain 4: Activity/Rest
Class 4: Cardiovascular/Pulmonary Responses

Definition
Risk for a decrease in cerebral tissue circulation

Risk Factors

- Abnormal partial thromboplastin time
- Abnormal prothrombin time
- Akinetic left ventricular segment
- Aortic atherosclerosis
- Arterial dissection
- Atrial fibrillation
- Atrial myxoma
- Brain tumor
- Carotid stenosis
- Cerebral aneurysm
- Coagulopathy (e.g., sickle cell anemia)
- Dilated cardiomyopathy
- Disseminated intravascular coagulation
- Embolism
- Head trauma
- Hypercholesterolemia
- Hypertension
- Infective endocarditis
- Left atrial appendage thrombosis
- Mechanical prosthetic valve
- Mitral stenosis
- Neoplasm of the brain
- Recent myocardial infarction
- Sick sinus syndrome
- Substance abuse
- Thrombolytic therapy
- Treated-related side effects (cardiopulmonary bypass, medications)

References

Asante-Siaw, J., Tyrrell, J., & Hoschtitzky, A. (2006). Does the use of a centrifugal pump offer any additional benefit for patients having open heart surgery? *Best BETS*, Record 01148. Available at: www.bestbets.org/cgi-bin/bets.pl?record=01148 (accessed May 23, 2008).

Barnard, J., Musleh, G., & Bitta, M. (2004). In aortic arch surgery is there any benefit in using antegrade cerebral perfusion or retrograde cerebral perfusion as an adjunct to hypothermic circulatory arrest? *BestBETS*, Record 00690. Available at: www.bestbets.org/cgi-bin/bets.pl?record = 00690 (accessed October 23, 2006).

O'Donnell, J.M. & N'acul, F., eds (2001). *Surgical intensive care medicine*. Boston: Kluwer Academic Publishers.

* This diagnosis formerly held the label, *Ineffective Tissue Perfusion (Specify Type: Cerebral)*.

Domain 4

Sharma, M., Clark, H., Armour, T., Stotts, G., Cote, R., & Hill, M.D. (2005). *Acute stroke: Evaluation and treatment*. Agency for Healthcare Research and Quality, 127. Publication number 05-E023–1.

Swearingen, P.L. & Hicks Keen, J., eds (2001). *Manual of critical care nursing: Nursing interventions and collaborative management*, 4th edn. St Louis: Mosby.

Risk for Ineffective Gastrointestinal Perfusion* (00202)

(2008, LOE 2.1)

Domain 4: Activity/Rest
Class 4: Cardiovascular/Pulmonary Responses

Definition At risk for decrease in gastrointestinal circulation

Risk Factors

- Abdominal aortic aneurysm
- Abdominal compartment syndrome
- Abnormal partial thromboplastin time
- Abnormal prothrombin time
- Acute gastrointestinal bleed
- Acute gastrointestinal hemorrhage
- Age >60 years
- Anemia
- Coagulopathy (e.g., sickle cell anemia)
- Diabetes melitus
- Disseminated intravascular coagulation
- Female gender
- Gastric paresis (e.g., diabetes mellitus)
- Gastroesophageal varicies
- Gastrointestinal disease (e.g., duodenal or gastric ulcer, ischemic colitis, ischemic pancreatitis)
- Hemodynamic instability
- Liver dysfunction
- Myocardial infarction
- Poor left ventricular performance
- Renal failure
- Stroke
- Trauma
- Smoking
- Treatment-related side effects (e.g., cardiopulmonary bypass, medication, anesthesia, gastric surgery)
- Vascular disease (e.g., peripheral vascular disease, aortoiliac occlusive disease)

References

McSweeney, M.E., Garwood, S., et al. (2004). Adverse gastrointestinal complications after cardiopulmonary bypass: Can outcome be predicted from preoperative risk factors? [Electronic version] *Anesthesia & Analgesia* **98**: 1610–17.

O'Donnell, J.M. & N'acul, F., eds (2001). *Surgical intensive care medicine*. Boston: Kluwer Academic Publishers.

Scott-Conner, C.E.H. & Ballinger, B. (2005). Abdominal angina. eMedicine, Available at: www.emedicine.com/med/topic2.htm (accessed May 23, 2008).

Swearingen, P.L. & Hicks Keen, J., eds (2001). *Manual of critical care nursing: Nursing interventions and collaborative management*, 4th edn. St Louis: Mosby.

*This diagnosis formerly held the label, *Ineffective Tissue Perfusion (Specify Type: Peripheral)*.

Risk for Ineffective Renal Perfusion*
(00203)
(2008, LOE 2.1)

Domain 4: Activity/Rest
Class 4: Cardiovascular/Pulmonary Responses

Definition At risk for a decrease in blood circulation to the kidney that may compromise health

Risk Factors

- Abdominal compartment syndrome
- Advanced age
- Bilateral cortical necrosis
- Burns
- Cardiac surgery
- Cardiopulmonary bypass
- Diabetes mellitus
- Exposure to toxins
- Female glomerulonephritis
- Hyperlipidemia
- Hypertension
- Hypovolemia
- Hypoxemia
- Hypoxia
- Infection (e.g., sepsis, localized infection)
- Malignancy
- Malignant hypertension
- Metabolic acidosis
- Multitrauma
- Polynephritis
- Renal artery stenosis
- Renal disease (polycystic kidney)
- Smoking
- Systemic inflammatory response syndrome
- Treatment-related side effects (e.g., medications)
- Vascular embolism vasculitis

References

O'Donnell, J.M. & N'acul, F., eds (2001). *Surgical intensive care medicine*. Boston: Kluwer Academic Publishers.

Spinowitz, B. & Rodriguez, (J. 2006). Renal artery stenosis. Available at: www.emedicine.com/med/topic2001.htm (accessed May 23, 2008).

Swearingen, P.L. & Hicks Keen, J., eds (2001). *Manual of critical care nursing: Nursing interventions and collaborative management*, 4th edn. St Louis: Mosby.

* This diagnosis formerly held the label, *Ineffective Tissue Perfusion (Specify Type: Renal)*.

Risk for Shock (00205)

(2008, LOE 2.1)

Domain 4: Activity/Rest
Class 4: Cardiovascular/Pulmonary Responses

Definition
At risk for an inadequate blood flow to the body's tissues which may lead to life-threatening cellular dysfunction

Risk Factors

- Hypotension
- Hypovolemia
- Hypoxemia
- Hypoxia

- Infection
- Sepsis
- Systemic inflammatory response syndrome

References

Bridges, E.J. & Dukes, M.S. (2005). Cardiovascular aspects of septic shock: Pathophysiology, monitoring, and treatment. *Critical Care Nurse* **25**: 14–36.

Goodrich, C. (2006). Endpoints of resuscitation. *AACN Advanced Critical Care* **17**: 306–16.

Goodrich, D. (2006). Continuous central venous oximetry monitoring. *Critical Care Nursing Clinics* **18**: 203–9.

O'Donnell, J.M. & N'acul, F., eds (2001). *Surgical intensive care medicine*. Boston: Kluwer Academic Publishers.

Swearingen, P.L. & Hicks Keen, J., eds (2001). *Manual of critical care nursing: Nursing interventions and collaborative management*, 4th edn. St Louis: Mosby.

Domain 4

Impaired Spontaneous Ventilation

(00033)

(1992)

Domain 4: Activity/Rest
Class 4: Cardiovascular/Pulmonary Responses

Definition Decreased energy reserves result in an individual's inability to maintain breathing adequate to support life

Defining Characteristics

- Apprehension
- Decreased cooperation
- Decreased Po_2
- Decreased SaO_2
- Decreased tidal volume
- Dyspnea
- Increased heart rate
- Increased metabolic rate
- Increased Pco_2
- Increased restlessness
- Increased use of accessory muscles

Related Factors

- Metabolic factors
- Respiratory muscle fatigue

Dysfunctional Ventilatory Weaning Response (00034)

(1992)

Domain 4: Activity/Rest
Class 4: Cardiovascular/Pulmonary Responses

Definition
Inability to adjust to lowered levels of mechanical ventilator support that interrupts and prolongs the weaning process

Defining Characteristics

Mild

- Breathing discomfort
- Expressed feelings of increased need for oxygen
- Fatigue
- Increased concentration on breathing
- Queries about possible machine malfunction
- Restlessness
- Slight increase of respiratory rate from baseline
- Warmth

Moderate

- Apprehension
- Baseline increase in respiratory rate (<5 breaths/min)
- Color changes
- Decreased air entry on auscultation
- Diaphoresis
- Hypervigilance to activities
- Inability to cooperate
- Inability to respond to coaching
- Pale
- Slight cyanosis
- Slight increase from baseline blood pressure (<20 mmHg)

- Slight increase from baseline heart rate (<20 beats/min)
- Light respiratory accessory muscle use
- Wide-eyed look

Severe

- Adventitious breath sounds
- Agitation
- Asynchronized breathing with the ventilator
- Audible airway secretions
- Cyanosis
- Decreased level of consciousness
- Deterioration in arterial blood gases from current baseline
- Full respiratory accessory muscle use
- Gasping breaths
- Increase from baseline blood pressure (≥20 mmHg)
- Increase from baseline heart rate (≥20 breaths/min)
- Paradoxical abdominal breathing
- Profuse diaphoresis
- Respiratory rate increases significantly from baseline
- Shallow breaths

Related Factors

Physiological

- Inadequate nutrition
- Ineffective airway clearance
- Sleep pattern disturbance
- Uncontrolled pain

Psychological

- Anxiety
- Decreased motivation
- Decreased self-esteem
- Fear
- Hopelessness
- Insufficient trust in the nurse
- Knowledge deficit of the weaning process
- Patient perceived inefficacy about ability to wean
- Powerlessness

Situational

- Adverse environment (e.g., noisy, active environment; negative events in the room, low nurse:patient ratio, unfamiliar nursing staff)
- History of multiple unsuccessful weaning attempts
- History of ventilator dependence >4 days
- Inadequate social support
- Inappropriate pacing of diminished ventilator support
- Uncontrolled episodic energy demands

Readiness for Enhanced Self-Care

(00182)

(2006, LOE 2.1)

Domain 4: Activity/Rest
Class 5: Self-Care

Definition   A pattern of performing activities for oneself that helps to meet health-related goals and can be strengthened

Defining Characteristics

- Expresses desire to enhance independence in maintaining life
- Expresses desire to enhance independence in maintaining health
- Expresses desire to enhance independence in maintaining personal development
- Expresses desire to enhance independence in maintaining well-being
- Expresses desire to enhance knowledge of strategies for self-care
- Expresses desire to enhance responsibility for self-care
- Expresses desire to enhance self-care

References

Artinian, N.T., Magnan, M., Sloan, M., & Lange, M.P. (2002). Self care behaviors among patients with heart failure. *Heart & Lung* **31**:161–72.

Backscheider, J.E. (1974). Self care requirements, self care capabilities and nursing systems in the diabetic nurse management clinic. *American Journal of Public Health* **64**: 1138–46.

Becker, G., Gates, R. J., & E. Newsom (2004). Self-care among chronically ill African Americans: Culture, health disparities, and health insurance status. *American Journal of Public Health* **94**: 2066–73.

Biggs, A.J. (1990). Family caregiver versus nursing assessments of elderly self-care abilities. *Journal of Gerontological Nursing* **16**(8): 11–16.

Conn, V. (1991). Self care actions taken by older adults for influenza and colds. *Nursing Research* **40**: 176–81.

Dashiff, C., Bartolucci, A., Wallander, J., & Abdullatif, H. (2005). The relationship of family structure, maternal employment, and family conflict with self-care adherence of adolescents with Type 1 diabetes. *Families, Systems, & Health* **23**(1): 66–79.

Harris, J.L. & Williams, L.K. (1991). Universal self-care requisites as identified by homeless elderly men. *Journal of Gerontological Nursing* **17**(6): 39–43.

Hartweg, D.L. (1993). Self-care actions of healthy middle-aged women to promote well-being. *Nursing Research* **42**: 221–7.

Moore, J.B. & Beckwitt, A.E. (2004). Children with cancer and their parents: Self care and dependent care practices. *Issues in Comprehensive Pediatric Nursing* **27**: 1–17.

Oliver, M. (2005). Reaching positive outcomes by assessing and teaching patient self efficacy. *Home Healthcare Nurse* **23**: 559–62.

Domain 4

Orem, D.E. (2001). *Nursing: Concepts and practice*, 6th edn. St Louis: Mosby.

Richardson, A. & Ream, E.K. (1997). Self-care behaviours initiated by chemotherapy patients in response to fatigue. *International Journal of Nursing Studies* **34**(1): 35–43.

Smits, M.W. & Kee, C.C. (1992). Correlates of self-care among the independent elderly: Self care affects well-being. *Journal of Gerontological Nursing* **18**(9): 13–18.

Weston-Eborn, R. (2004). Home care and the adult learner. *Home Healthcare Nurse* **22**: 522–3.

Domain 4

Bathing Self-Care Deficit* (00108)

(1980, 1998)

Domain 4: Activity/Rest
Class 5: Self-Care

Definition Impaired ability to perform or complete bathing/hygiene activities for self

Defining Characteristics

- Inability to access bathroom
- Inability to dry body
- Inability to get bath supplies
- Inability to obtain water source
- Inability to regulate bath water
- Inability to wash body

Related Factors

- Cognitive impairment
- Decreased motivation
- Environmental barriers
- Inability to perceive body part
- Inability to perceive spatial relationship
- Musculoskeletal impairment
- Neuromuscular impairment
- Pain
- Perceptual impairment
- Severe anxiety
- Weakness

Note: specify level of independence using a standardized functional scale.

* This diagnosis formerly held the label *Bathing/Hygiene Self-care Deficit*.

Domain 4

Dressing Self-Care Deficit* (00109)
(1980, 1998)

Domain 4: Activity/Rest
Class 5: Self-Care

Definition Impaired ability to perform or complete dressing and grooming activities for self

Defining Characteristics

- Inability to choose clothing
- Inability to put clothing on lower body
- Inability to maintain appearance at a satisfactory level
- Inability to pick up clothing
- Inability to put clothing on upper body
- Inability to put on shoes
- Inability to put on socks
- Inability to remove clothes
- Inability to remove shoes
- Inability to remove socks
- Inability to use assistive devices
- Inability to use zippers
- Impaired ability to fasten clothing
- Impaired ability to obtain clothing
- Impaired ability to put on necessary items of clothing
- Impaired ability to put on shoes
- Impaired ability to put on socks
- Impaired ability to take off necessary items of clothing
- Impaired ability to take off shoes
- Impaired ability to take off socks

Related Factors

- Cognitive impairment
- Decreased motivation
- Discomfort
- Environmental barriers
- Fatigue
- Musculoskeletal impairment
- Neuromuscular impairment
- Pain
- Perceptual impairment
- Severe anxiety
- Weakness

Note: specify level of independence using a standardized functional scale.

* This diagnosis formerly held the label *Dressing/Grooming Self-care Deficit*.

Feeding Self-Care Deficit (00102)

(1980, 1998)

Domain 4: Activity/Rest
Class 5: Self-Care

Definition Impaired ability to perform or complete self-feeding activities

Defining Characteristics

- Inability to bring food from a receptacle to the mouth
- Inability to chew food
- Inability to complete a meal
- Inability to get food onto utensil
- Inability to handle utensils
- Inability to ingest food in a socially acceptable manner
- Inability to ingest food safely
- Inability to ingest sufficient food
- Inability to manipulate food in mouth
- Inability to open containers
- Inability to pick up cup or glass
- Inability to prepare food for ingestion
- Inability to swallow food
- Inability to use assistive device

Related Factors

- Cognitive impairment
- Decreased motivation
- Discomfort
- Environmental barriers
- Fatigue
- Musculoskeletal impairment
- Neuromuscular impairment
- Pain
- Perceptual impairment
- Severe anxiety
- Weakness

Note: specify level of independence using a standardized functional scale.

Domain 4

Toileting Self-Care Deficit (00110)

(1980, 1998)

Domain 4: Activity/Rest
Class 5: Self-Care

Definition Impaired ability to perform or complete toileting activities for self

Defining Characteristics

- Inability to carry out proper toilet hygiene
- Inability to flush toilet or commode
- Inability to get to toilet or commode
- Inability to manipulate clothing for toileting
- Inability to rise from toilet or commode
- Inability to sit on toilet or commode

Related Factors

- Cognitive impairment
- Decreased motivation
- Environmental barriers
- Fatigue
- Impaired mobility status
- Impaired transfer ability
- Musculoskeletal impairment
- Neuromuscular impairment
- Pain
- Perceptual impairment
- Severe anxiety
- Weakness

Note: specify level of independence using a standardized functional scale.

Domain 5
Perception/Cognition

Unilateral Neglect (00123)
(1986, 2006, LOE 2.1)

Domain 5: Perception/Cognition
Class 1: Attention

Definition Impairment in sensory and motor response, mental representation, and spatial attention of the body, and the corresponding environment characterized by inattention to one side and over-attention to the opposite side. Left side neglect is more severe and persistent than right side neglect.

Defining Characteristics

- Appears unaware of positioning of neglected limb
- Difficulty remembering details of internally represented familiar scenes that are on the neglected side
- Displacement of sounds to the non-neglected side
- Distortion of drawing on the half of the page on the neglected side
- Failure to cancel lines on the half of the page on the neglected side
- Failure to eat food from portion of the plate on the neglected side
- Failure to dress neglected side
- Failure to groom neglected side
- Failure to move eyes in the neglected hemispace despite being aware of a stimulus in that space
- Failure to move head in the neglected hemispace despite being aware of a stimulus in that space
- Failure to move limbs in the neglected hemispace despite being aware of a stimulus in that space
- Failure to move trunk in the neglected hemispace despite being aware of a stimulus in that space
- Failure to notice people approaching from the neglected side
- Lack of safety precautions with regard to the neglected side
- Marked deviation* of the eyes to the non-neglected side to stimuli and activities on that side
- Marked deviation* of the head to the non-neglected side to stimuli and activities on that side
- Marked deviation* of the trunk to the non-neglected side to stimuli and activities on that side
- Omission of drawing on the half of the page on the neglected side
- Perseveration of visual motor tasks on the non-neglected side

* As if drawn magnetically to stimuli and activities on that side.

- Substitution of letters to form alternative words that are similar to the original in length when reading
- Transfer of pain sensation to the non-neglected side
- Use of only vertical half of page when writing

Related Factors

- Brain injury from cerebrovascular problems
- Brain injury from neurological illness
- Brain injury from trauma
- Brain injury from tumor
- Left hemiplegia from cerebrovascular accident (CVA) of the right hemisphere
- Hemianopsia

References

Bartolomeo, P. & Chokron, S. (1999). Left unilateral neglect or right hyperattention? *Neurology* **53**(9): 2023–27.

Bartolomeo, P. & Chokron, S. (2002). Orienting of neglect in left unilateral neglect. *Neuroscience and Behavioral Reviews* **26**: 217–34.

Halligan, P.W. & Marshall J.C. (1993). The history and clinical presentation of neglect. In: Robertson, I.H. & Marshall, J.C. (eds), *Unilateral Neglect: Clinical and experimental studies*. Hove: Lawrence Erlbaum associates Ltd, pp. 3–19.

Rizzolati, G. & Berti, A. (1993). Neural mechanisms of spatial neglect. In: Robertson, I. H. & Marshall, J.C. (eds), *Unilateral neglect: Clinical and experimental studies*. Hove: Lawrence Erlbaum associates Ltd, pp. 87–102.

Rusconi, M.L., Maravita, A., Bottini, G., & Vallar, G (2002). Is the intact side really intact? Perseverative responses in patients with unilateral neglect: a productive manifestation. *Neuropsychologia* **40**: 594–604.

Stone, SP. Halligan, P.W, Marshall, J.C., & Greenwood, R.J. (1998). Unilateral neglect a common but heterogeneous syndrome. *Neurology* **50**: 1902–5.

Swan, L. (2001). Unilateral spatial neglect. *Physical Therapy* **81**: 1572–80.

Weitzel, E.A. (2001). Unilateral neglect. In: Maas, M., Buckwalter, K., Hardy, M., Tripp-Reimer, T., Titler, M., & Specht, J. (eds), *Nursing care of older adults: Diagnosis, outcomes, and interventions*. St Louis: Mosby, pp. 492–502.

Impaired Environmental Interpretation Syndrome (00127)

(1994)

Domain 5: Perception/Cognition
Class 2: Orientation

Definition Consistent lack of orientation to person, place, time, or circumstances over more than 3–6 months necessitating a protective environment

Defining Characteristics

- Chronic confusional states
- Consistent disorientation
- Inability to concentrate
- Inability to follow simple directions
- Inability to reason
- Loss of occupation
- Loss of social functioning
- Slow in responding to questions

Related Factors

- Dementia
- Depression
- Huntington's disease

Wandering (00154)
(2000)

Domain 5: Perception/Cognition
Class 2: Orientation

Definition   Meandering, aimless, or repetitive locomotion that exposes the individual to harm; frequently incongruent with boundaries, limits, or obstacles

Defining Characteristics

- Continuous movement from place to place
- Getting lost
- Fretful locomotion
- Frequent movement from place to place
- Haphazard locomotion
- Hyperactivity
- Inability to locate significant landmarks in a familiar setting
- Locomotion into unauthorized or private spaces
- Locomotion resulting in unintended leaving of a premise
- Locomotion that cannot be easily dissuaded
- Long periods of locomotion without an apparent destination
- Pacing
- Periods of locomotion interspersed with periods of nonlocomotion (e.g., sitting, standing, sleeping)
- Persistent locomotion in search of something
- Shadowing a caregiver's locomotion
- Trespassing
- Scanning behaviors
- Searching behaviors

Related Factors

- Cognitive impairment (e.g., memory and recall deficits, disorientation, poor visuoconstructive or visuospatial ability, language defects)
- Cortical atrophy
- Emotional state (e.g., frustration, anxiety, boredom, depression, agitation)
- Overstimulating environment
- Physiological state or need (e.g., hunger, thirst, pain, urination, constipation)
- Premorbid behavior (e.g., outgoing, sociable personality, premorbid dementia)
- Sedation
- Separation from familiar environment
- Time of day

Disturbed Sensory Perception (Specify: Visual, Auditory, Kinesthetic, Gustatory, Tactile, Olfactory) (00122)
(1978, 1980, 1998)

Domain 5: Perception/Cognition
Class 3: Sensation/Perception

Definition Change in the amount or patterning of incoming stimuli accompanied by a diminished, exaggerated, distorted, or impaired response to such stimuli

Defining Characteristics

- Change in behavior pattern
- Change in problem-solving abilities
- Change in sensory acuity
- Change in usual response to stimuli
- Disorientation
- Hallucinations
- Impaired communication
- Irritability
- Poor concentration
- Restlessness
- Sensory distortions

Related Factors

- Altered sensory integration
- Altered sensory reception
- Altered sensory transmission
- Biochemical imbalance
- Electrolyte imbalance
- Excessive environmental stimuli
- Insufficient environmental stimuli
- Psychological stress

Note: this diagnosis will retire from the NANDA-I Taxonomy in the **2012–2014** *edition unless additional work is done to bring it to a LOE of* **2.1** *or higher.*

Acute Confusion (00128)

(1994, 2006, LOE 2.1)

Domain 5: Perception/Cognition
Class 4: Cognition

Definition Abrupt onset of reversible disturbances of consciousness, attention, cognition, and perception that develop over a short period of time

Defining Characteristics

- Fluctuation in cognition
- Fluctuation in level of consciousness
- Fluctuation in psychomotor activity
- Hallucinations
- Increased agitation
- Increased restlessness
- Lack of motivation to follow through with goal-directed behavior
- Lack of motivation to follow through with purposeful behavior
- Lack of motivation to initiate goal-directed behavior
- Lack of motivation to initiate purposeful behavior
- Misperceptions

Related Factors

- Alcohol abuse
- Delirium
- Dementia
- Drug abuse
- Fluctuation in sleep–wake cycle
- Over 60 years of age

References

Agostini, J.V., Leo-Summers, L.S., & Inouye, S.K. (2001). Cognitive and other adverse effects of diphenhydramine use in hospitalized older patients. *Archives of Internal Medicine* **161**: 2091–7.

Alciati, A., Scaramelli, B., Fusi, A., Butteri, E., Cattameo, M.L., & Mellado, C. (1999). Three cases of delirium after "ecstasy" ingestion. *Journal of Psychoactive Drugs* **31**: 167–70.

Aldemir, M., Ozen, S., Kara, I.H., Sir, A., & Bac, B. (2001). Predisposing factors for delirium in the surgical intensive care unit. *Critical Care (London)* **5**: 265–70.

Bowman, A.M. (1997). Sleep satisfaction, perceived pain and acute confusion in elderly clients undergoing orthopaedic procedures. *Journal of Advanced Nursing* **26**: 550–64.

Brauer, C., Morrison, R.S., Silberzweig, S.B., & Sui, A.L. (2000). The cause of delirium in patients with hip fracture. *Archives of Internal Medicine* **160**: 1856–60.

Coyle, N., Breitbart, W., Weaver, S., & Portenoy, R. (1994). Delirium as a contributing factor to "crescendo" pain: three case reports. *Journal of Pain and Symptom Management* **9**(1): 44–7.

Edlund, A., Lundstrom, M., Brannstrom, B., Bucht, G., & Gustafson, Y. (2001). Delirium before and after operation for femoral neck fracture. *Journal of the American Geriatrics Society* **49**: 1335–40.

Elie, M., Cole, M.G., Primeau, F. J., & Bellavance, F. (1998). Delirium risks factors in elderly hospitalized patients. *Journal of General Internal Medicine* **13**: 204–12.

Erkinjuntti, T., Wikstrom, J. Palo, J., & Autio, L. (1986). Dementia among medical inpatients: Evaluation of 2000 Consecutive admissions. *Archives of Internal Medicine* **146**: 1923–6.

Fisher, B.W. & Flowerdew, G. (1995). A simple model for predicting postoperative delirium in older patients undergoing elective orthopedic surgery. *Journal of the American Geriatric Society* **43**: 175–8.

Foreman, M. (1989). Confusion in the hospitalized elderly: Incidence, onset, and associated factors. *Research in Nursing & Health* **12**: 21–9.

Francis, J., Martin, D., & Kapoor, W. (1990). A prospective study of delirium in hospitalized elderly. *Journal of the American Medical Association* **263**: 1097–101.

Grandberg, A.I., Malmros, C.W., Bergborn, I.L., & Lundberg, D.B. (2002) Intensive care syndrome/delirium is associated with anemia, drug therapy and duration of ventilation treatment. *Acta Anaesthesiologica Scandinavica* **46**: 726–31.

Gustafson, Y., Berggren, D., Brannstrom, B., et al. (1988). Acute confusional state in elderly patients treated for femoral neck fracture. *Journal of the American Geriatric Association* **36**: 525–30.

Han, L., McCusher, J., Cole, M. Abrahamowiz, M., Primeau, F., & Elie, M. (2001). Use of medications with anticholinergic effect predicts clinical severity of delirium symptoms in older medical inpatients. *Archives of Internal Medicine* **161**: 1099–105.

Haynes, C. (1999). Emergence delirium: a literature review. *British Journal of Theatre Nursing* **9**: 502–10.

Inouye, S.K. & Charpentier, P.A. (1996). Precipitating factors for delirium in hospitalized elderly persons: Predictive model and interrelationship with baseline vulnerability. *Journal of the American Medical Association* **275**: 852–7.

Jitapunkul, S., Pillay, I., & Ebrahim, S. (1992). Delirium in newly admitted elderly patients: A prospective study. *Quarterly Journal of Medicine NS* **83**(300): 307–14.

Kelly, M. (1997). The best is yet to be. Postoperative delirium in the elderly. *Today's Surgical Nurse* **19**(5): 10–12.

Koponen, H., Stenback, U., Mattila, E., Soininen, H., Reinikainen, K., & Riekkinen, P. (1989). Delirium among elderly persons admitted to a psychiatric hospital: clinical course during the acute state and one-year follow-up. *Acta Psychiatrica Scandinavica* **79**: 579–85.

Korevaar, J.C., van Munster, B.C., & de Rooij, S.E. (2005). Risk factors for delirium in acutely admitted elderly patients: a prospective cohort study. *BMC Geriatric* **5**(1): 6.

Lawlor, P.G., Gagnon, B., Mancini, I.L., et al. (2000). Occurrence, causes, and outcome of delirium in patients with advanced cancer. *Archives of Internal Medicine* **160**: 786–94.

Levkoff, S.E, Safran, C., Cleary, P.D., Gallop, J., & Phillips, R.S. (1988). Identification of factors associated with the diagnosis of delirium in elderly hospitalized patients. *Journal of the American Geriatrics Society* **36**: 1099–104.

Lipov, E.G. (1991). Emergence delirium in the PACU. *Critical Care Nursing Clinics of North America* **3**: 145–9.

Lynch, E.P., Lazor, M.A., Gellis, J.E., Orav, J., Goldman, L., & Marcantonioa, E.R. (1998). The impact of postoperative pain on the development of post operative delirium. *Anesthesia & Analgesia* **86**: 781–5.

McCuster, J., Cole, M., Abrahamowica, M., Han, L., Podoba, J., & Ramman-Haddad, L. (2001). Environmental risk factors for delirium in hospitalized older people. *Journal of the American Geriatrics Society* **49**: 1327–34.

Marcantonio, E.R., Simon, S.E., Bergmann, M.A., Jones, R.N., Murphy, K.M., & Morris, J.N. (2003). Delirium symptoms in post-acute care: Prevalent, persistent, and associated with poor functional recovery. *Journal of the American Geriatrics Society* **51**: 4–9.

Marcantonio, E.R., Goldman, L., Mangione, C.M., et al. (1994). A clinical prediction rule for delirium after elective noncardiac surgery. *Journal of the American Medical Association* **271**: 134–9.

Domain 5

Massie, M.J. & Holland, J.C. (1992). The cancer patient with pain: psychiatric complications and their management. *Journal of Pain and Symptom Management* **7**: 99–109.

Mentes, J., Culp, J., Maas, M., & Rantz, M. (1999). Acute confusion indicators: risk factors and prevalence using MDS data. *Research in Nursing & Health* **22**: 95–105.

Morita, T., Tei, Y. Tsunoda, J., Inouye, S., & Chihara, S. (2001). Underlying pathologies and their associations with clinical features in terminal delirium of cancer patients. *Journal of Pain and Symptom Management* **22**: 997–1006.

Morrison, R.S., Magaziner, J., Gilbert, M., et al. (2003). Relationship between pain and opioid analgesics on the development of delirium following hip fracture. *Journal of Gerontology Series A – A Biological Sciences & Medical Sciences* **58**: 76–81.

Nishikawa, K., Nakayama, M., Omote, K., & Namiki, A. (2004). Recovery characteristics and post operative delirium after long-duration laparoscope-assisted surgery in elderly patients: propofol-based vs. sevoflurane-based anesthesia. *Acta Anaesthesiologica Scandinavica* **48**: 162–8.

O'Brien, D. (2002). Acute postoperative delirium: definitions, incidence, recognition, and interventions. *Journal of Peri-Anesthesia Nursing* **17**: 384–92.

Pompei, P., Foreman, M., Rudberg, M., Inouye, S., Braund, V., & Cassel, C. (1994). Delirium in hospitalized older persons: Outcomes and predictors. *Journal of the American Geriatrics Society* **42**: 809–15.

Pratico, C., Quattrone, D., Lucanto, T., et al. (2005). Drugs of anesthesia acting on central cholinergic system may cause post operative cognitive dysfunction and delirium. *Medical Hypotheses* **65**: 972–82.

Rockwood, K. (1989). Acute confusion in elderly medical patients. *Journal of the American Geriatrics Society* **37**: 150–4.

Rolfson, D.B., McElhaney, J.E., Rockwood, K., et al. (1999). Incidence and risk factors for delirium and other adverse outcomes in older adults after coronary artery bypass graft surgery. *Canadian Journal of Cardiology* **15**: 771–6.

Ross, D.L. (1998). Factors associated with excited delirium, deaths in police custody. *Modern Pathology* **11**: 1127–37.

Ruttenber, A.J., McAnally, H.B., & Wetli, C.V. (1999). Cocaine-associated rhabdomyolysis and excited delirium: different stages of the same syndrome. *American Journal of Forensic Medicine & Pathology* **20**: 120–7.

Ruttenber, A.J., Lawler-Heavner, J., Yin, M., Wetli, C.V., Hearn, W.L. & Mash, D.C. (1997). Fatal excited delirium following cocaine use: epidemiological findings provide new evidence for mechanisms of cocaine toxicity. *Journal of Forensic Sciences* **42**: 25–31.

Seymour, D.G., Henschke, P.J, Cape, R.D., & Campbell, A.J. (1980). Acute confusional states and dementia in the elderly: The role of dehydration/volume depletion, physical illness and age. *Age and Ageing* **9**: 137–46.

Schor, J.D., Levkoff, S.E., Lipsitz, L.A., et al. (1992). Risk factors for delirium in hospitalized elderly. *Journal of the American Medical Association* **267**: 827–31.

Schururmans, M.J., Duursma, S.A., Shortridge-Baggett, L.M., Clevers, G., & Pel-Little, R. (2003). Elderly patients with hip fracture: the risk for delirium. *Applied Nursing Research* **16**(2): 75–84.

Seaman, J.S., Schillerstrom, J., Carroll, D., & Brown, T.M. (2006). Impaired oxidative metabolism precipitates delirium: a study of 101 ICU patients. *Psychosomatics* **47**(1): 56–61.

Seymour, D.G. & Vaz, F.G. (1989). A prospective study of elderly general surgical patients: II. Post operative complications. *Age and Ageing* **18**: 316–326.

Williams, M., Holloway, J., Winn, M., et al. (1979). Nursing activities and acute confusional states in elderly hip-fractured patients. *Nursing Research* **28**(1): 25–35.

Williams-Russo, P., Urquhart, B.L., Sharrock, N.E., & Charlson, M.E. (1992). Postoperative delirium: Prognosis in elderly orthopedic patients. *Journal of the American Geriatrics Society* **40**: 759–67.

Wilson, L.M. (1972). Intensive care delirium. *Archives of Internal Medicine* **130**: 225–6.

Chronic Confusion (00129)

(1994)

Domain 5: Perception/Cognition
Class 4: Cognition

Definition Irreversible, long-standing, and/or progressive deterioration of intellect and personality characterized by decreased ability to interpret environmental stimuli; decreased capacity for intellectual thought processes; and manifested by disturbances of memory, orientation, and behavior

Defining Characteristics

- Altered interpretation
- Altered personality
- Altered response to stimuli
- Clinical evidence of organic impairment
- Impaired long-term memory
- Impaired short-term memory
- Impaired socialization
- Long-standing cognitive impairment
- No change in level of consciousness
- Progressive cognitive impairment

Related Factors

- Alzheimer's disease
- Cerebral vascular attack
- Head injury
- Korsakoff's psychosis
- Multi-infarct dementia

Risk for Acute Confusion (00173)
(2006, LOE 2.2)

Domain 5: Perception/Cognition
Class 4: Cognition

Definition At risk for reversible disturbances of consciousness, attention, cognition, and perception that develop over a short period of time

Risk Factors

- Alcohol use
- Decreased mobility
- Decreased restraints
- Dementia
- Fluctuation in sleep–wake cycle
- History of stroke
- Impaired cognition
- Infection
- Male gender
- Medication/Drugs:
  - Anesthesia
  - Anticholinergics
  - Diphenhydramine
  - Multiple medications
  - Opioids
  - Psychoactive drugs
- Metabolic abnormalities:
  - Azotemia
  - Decreased hemoglobin
  - Dehydration
  - Electrolyte imbalances
  - Increased blood urea nitrogen (BUN)/creatinine
  - Malnutrition
- Over 60 years of age
- Pain
- Sensory deprivation
- Substance abuse
- Urinary retention

References

Agostini, J.V., Leo-Summers, L.S., & Inouye, S.K. (2001). Cognitive and other adverse effects of diphenhydramine use in hospitalized older patients. *Archives of Internal Medicine* **161**: 2091–7.

Alciati, A., Scaramelli, B., Fusi, A., Butteri, E., Cattameo, M.L., & Mellado, C. (1999). Three cases of delirium after "ecstasy" ingestion. *Journal of Psychoactive Drugs* **31**: 167–70.

Aldemir, M., Ozen, S., Kara, I.H., Sir, A., & Bac, B. (2001). Predisposing factors for delirium in the surgical intensive care unit. *Critical Care (London)* **5**: 265–70.

Bowman, A.M. (1997). Sleep satisfaction, perceived pain and acute confusion in elderly clients undergoing orthopaedic procedures. *Journal of Advanced Nursing* **26L** 550–64.

Brauer, C., Morrison, R.S., Silberzweig, S.B., & Sui, A.L. (2000). The cause of delirium in patients with hip fracture. *Archives of Internal Medicine* **160**: 1856–60.

Coyle, N., Breitbart, W., Weaver, S., & Portenoy, R. (1994). Delirium as a contributing factor to "crescendo" pain: three case reports. *Journal of Pain and Symptom Management* **9**(1): 44–7.

Edlund, A., Lundstrom, M., Brannstrom, B., Bucht, G., & Gustafson, Y. (2001). Delirium before and after operation for femoral neck fracture. *Journal of the American Geriatrics Society* **49**: 1335–40.

Elie, M., Cole, M.G. , Primeau, F. J., & Bellavance, F. (1998). Delirium risks factors in elderly hospitalized patients. *Journal of General Internal Medicine* **13**: 204–12.

Erkinjuntti, T., Wikstrom, J. Palo, J., & Autio, L. (1986). Dementia among medical inpatients: Evaluation of 2000 Consecutive admissions. *Archives of Internal Medicine* **146**: 1923–6.

Fisher, B.W. & Flowerdew, G. (1995). A simple model for predicting postoperative delirium in older patients undergoing elective orthopedic surgery. *Journal of the American Geriatric Society* **43**: 175–8.

Foreman, M. (1989). Confusion in the hospitalized elderly: Incidence, onset, and associated factors. *Research in Nursing & Health* **12**: 21–9.

Francis, J., Martin, D., & Kapoor, W. (1990). A prospective study of delirium in hospitalized elderly. *Journal of the American Medical Association* **263**:1097–101.

Grandberg, A.I., Malmros, C.W., Bergborn, I.L., & Lundberg, D.B. (2002) Intensive care syndrome/delirium is associated with anemia, drug therapy and duration of ventilation treatment. *Acta Anaesthesiologica Scandinavica* **46**: 726–31.

Gustafson, Y., Berggren, D., Brannstrom, B., et al. (1988). Acute confusional state in elderly patients treated for femoral neck fracture. *Journal of the American Geriatric Association* **36**: 525–30.

Han, L., McCusher, J., Cole, M. Abrahamowiz, M., Primeau, F., & Elie, M. (2001). Use of medications with anticholinergic effect predicts clinical severity of delirium symptoms in older medical inpatients. *Archives of Internal Medicine* **161**: 1099–105.

Haynes, C. (1999). Emergence delirium: a literature review. *British Journal of Theatre Nursing* **9**: 502–10.

Inouye, S.K. & Charpentier, P.A. (1996). Precipitating factors for delirium in hospitalized elderly persons: Predictive model and interrelationship with baseline vulnerability. *Journal of the American Medical Association* **275**: 852–7.

Jitapunkul, S., Pillay, I., & Ebrahim, S. (1992). Delirium in newly admitted elderly patients: A prospective study. *Quarterly Journal of Medicine NS* **83**(300): 307–14.

Kelly, M. (1997). The best is yet to be. Postoperative delirium in the elderly. *Today's Surgical Nurse* **19**(5): 10–12.

Koponen, H., Stenback, U., Mattila, E., Soininen, H., Reinikainen, K., & Riekkinen, P. (1989). Delirium among elderly persons admitted to a psychiatric hospital: clinical course during the acute state and one-year follow-up. *Acta Psychiatrica Scandinavica* **79**: 579–85.

Korevaar, J.C., van Munster, B.C., & de Rooij, S.E. (2005). Risk factors for delirium in acutely admitted elderly patients: a prospective cohort study. *BMC Geriatric* **5**(1): 6.

Lawlor, P.G., Gagnon, B., Mancini, I.L., et al. (2000). Occurrence, causes, and outcome of delirium in patients with advanced cancer. *Archives of Internal Medicine* **160**: 786–94.

Levkoff, S.E, Safran, C., Cleary, P.D., Gallop, J., & Phillips, R.S. (1988). Identification of factors associated with the diagnosis of delirium in elderly hospitalized patients. *Journal of the American Geriatrics Society* **36**: 1099–104.

Lipov, E.G. (1991). Emergence delirium in the PACU. *Critical Care Nursing Clinics of North America* **3**: 145–9.

Lynch, E.P., Lazor, M.A., Gellis, J.E., Orav, J., Goldman, L., & Marcantonioa, E.R. (1998). The impact of postoperative pain on the development of post operative delirium. *Anesthesia & Analgesia* **86**: 781–5.

McCuster, J., Cole, M., Abrahamowica, M., Han, L., Podoba, J., & Ramman-Haddad, L. (2001). Environmental risk factors for delirium in hospitalized older people. *Journal of the American Geriatrics Society* **49**: 1327–34.

Marcantonio, E.R., Simon, S.E., Bergmann, M.A., Jones, R.N., Murphy, K.M., & Morris, J.N. (2003). Delirium symptoms in post-acute care: Prevalent, persistent, and associated with poor functional recovery. *Journal of the American Geriatrics Society* **51**: 4–9.

Marcantonio, E.R., Goldman, L., Mangione, C.M., et al. (1994). A clinical prediction rule for delirium after elective noncardiac surgery. *Journal of the American Medical Association* **271**: 134–9.

Domain 5

Massie, M.J. & Holland, J.C. (1992). The cancer patient with pain: psychiatric complications and their management. *Journal of Pain and Symptom Management* 7: 99–109.

Mentes, J., Culp, J., Maas, M., & Rantz, M. (1999). Acute confusion indicators: risk factors and prevalence using MDS data. *Research in Nursing & Health* 22: 95–105.

Morita, T., Tei, Y. Tsunoda, J., Inouye, S., & Chihara, S. (2001). Underlying pathologies and their associations with clinical features in terminal delirium of cancer patients. *Journal of Pain and Symptom Management* 22: 997–1006.

Morrison, R.S., Magazine, J. Gilbert, M., et al. (2003). Relationship between pain and opioid analgesics on the development of delirium following hip fracture. *Journal of Gerontology Series A – A Biological Sciences & Medical Sciences* 58: 76–81.

Nishikawa, K., Nakayama, M., Omote, K., & Namiki, A. (2004). Recovery characteristics and post operative delirium after long-duration laparoscope-assisted surgery in elderly patients: propofol-based vs. sevoflurane-based anesthesia. *Acta Anaesthesiologica Scandinavica* 48: 162–8.

O'Brien, D. (2002). Acute postoperative delirium: definitions, incidence, recognition, and interventions. *Journal of Peri-Anesthesia Nursing* 17: 384–92.

Pompei, P., Foreman, M., Rudberg, M., Inouye, S., Braund, V., & Cassel, C. (1994). Delirium in hospitalized older persons: Outcomes and predictors. *Journal of the American Geriatrics Society* 42: 809–15.

Pratico, C., Quattrone, D. Lucan, T., et al. (2005). Drugs of anesthesia acting on central cholinergic system may cause post operative cognitive dysfunction and delirium. *Medical Hypotheses* 65: 972–82.

Rockwood, K. (1989). Acute confusion in elderly medical patients. *Journal of the American Geriatrics Society* 37: 150–4.

Rolfson, D.B., McElhaney, J.E., Rockwood, K., et al. (1999). Incidence and risk factors for delirium and other adverse outcomes in older adults after coronary artery bypass graft surgery. *Canadian Journal of Cardiology* 15: 771–6.

Ross, D.L. (1998). Factors associated with excited delirium, deaths in police custody. *Modern Pathology* 11: 1127–37.

Ruttenber, A.J., McAnally, H.B., & Wetli, C.V. (1999). Cocaine-associated rhabdomyolysis and excited delirium: different stages of the same syndrome. *American Journal of Forensic Medicine & Pathology* 20: 120–7.

Ruttenber, A.J., Lawler-Heavner, J., Yin, M., Wetli, C.V., Hearn, W.L. & Mash, D.C. (1997). Fatal excited delirium following cocaine use: epidemiological findings provide new evidence for mechanisms of cocaine toxicity. *Journal of Forensic Sciences* 42: 25–31.

Schor, J.D., Levkoff, S.E., Lipsitz, L.A., et al. (1992). Risk factors for delirium in hospitalized elderly. *Journal of the American Medical Association* 267: 827–31.

Schururmans, M.J., Duursma, S.A., Shortridge-Baggett, L.M., Clevers, G., & Pel-Little, R. (2003). Elderly patients with hip fracture: the risk for delirium. *Applied Nursing Research* 16(2): 75–84.

Seaman, J.S., Schillerstrom, J., Carroll, D., & Brown, T.M. (2006). Impaired oxidative metabolism precipitates delirium: a study of 101 ICU patients. *Psychosomatics* 47(1): 56–61.

Seymour, D.G. & Vaz, F.G. (1989). A prospective study of elderly general surgical patients: II. Post operative complications. *Age and Ageing* 18: 316–326.

Seymour, D.G., Henschke, P.J, Cape, R.D., & Campbell, A.J. (1980). Acute confusional states and dementia in the elderly: The role of dehydration/volume depletion, physical illness and age. *Age and Ageing* 9: 137–46.

Williams, M., Holloway, J., Winn, M., et al. (1979). Nursing activities and acute confusional states in elderly hip-fractured patients. *Nursing Research* 28(1): 25–35.

Williams-Russo, P., Urquhart, B.L., Sharrock, N.E., & Charlson, M.E. (1992). Post-operative delirium: Prognosis in elderly orthopedic patients. *Journal of the American Geriatrics Society* 40: 759–67.

Wilson, L.M. (1972). Intensive care delirium. *Archives of Internal Medicine* 130: 225–6.

Deficient Knowledge (00126)
(1980)

Domain 5: Perception/Cognition
Class 4: Cognition

Definition Absence or deficiency of cognitive information related to a specific topic

Defining Characteristics

- Exaggerated behaviors
- Inaccurate follow through of instruction
- Inaccurate performance of test
- Inappropriate behaviors (e.g., hysterical, hostile, agitated, apathetic)
- Verbalization of the problem

Related Factors

- Cognitive limitation
- Information misinterpretation
- Lack of exposure
- Lack of interest in learning
- Lack of recall
- Unfamiliarity with information resources

Domain 5

Domain 5: Perception/Cognition
Class 4: Cognition

Definition The presence or acquisition of cognitive information related to a specific topic is sufficient for meeting health-related goals and can be strengthened

Defining Characteristics

- Behaviors congruent with expressed knowledge
- Explains knowledge of the topic
- Expresses an interest in learning
- Describes previous experiences pertaining to the topic

Impaired Memory (00131)

(1994)

Domain 5: Perception/Cognition
Class 4: Cognition

Definition Inability to remember or recall bits of information or behavioral skills

Defining Characteristics

- Experience of forgetting
- Forgets to perform a behavior at a scheduled time
- Inability to determine if a behavior was performed
- Inability to learn new information
- Inability to learn new skills
- Inability to perform a previously learned skill
- Inability to recall events
- Inability to recall factual information
- Inability to retain new information
- Inability to retain new skills

Related Factors

- Anemia
- Decreased cardiac output
- Excessive environmental disturbances
- Fluid and electrolyte imbalance
- Hypoxia
- Neurological disturbances

Domain 5

Readiness for Enhanced Decision-Making (00184)
(2006, LOE 2.1)

Domain 5: Life Principles
Class 3: Value/Belief/Action Congruence

Definition A pattern of choosing courses of action that is sufficient for meeting short and long term health-related goals and can be strengthened

Defining Characteristics

- Expresses desire to enhance decision-making
- Expresses desire to enhance congruency of decisions with goals
- Expresses desire to enhance congruency of decisions with personal values
- Expresses desire to enhance congruency of decisions with sociocultural goals
- Expresses desire to enhance congruency of decisions with sociocultural values
- Expresses desire to enhance risk benefit analysis of decisions
- Expresses desire to enhance understanding of choices for decision-making
- Expresses desire to enhance understanding of the meaning of choices
- Expresses desire to enhance use of reliable evidence for decisions

References

Evans, R., Elwyn, G., & Edwards, A. (2004). Making interactive decision support for patients a reality. *Informatics in Primary Care* **12**: 109–13.

Harkness, J. (2005). Patient involvement: A vital principle for patient-centered health care. *World Hospitals and Health Services: The Official Journal of the International Hospital Federation* **41**(2): 12–16.

O'Connor, A.M., Tugwell, P., Wells, G.A., et al. (1998). A decision aid for women considering hormone therapy after menopause: Decision support framework and evaluation. *Patient Education and Counseling* **33**: 267–79.

O'Connor, A.M., Drake, E.R., Wells, G.A., Tugwell, P., Laupacis, A., & Elmslie, T. (2003). A survey of the decision-making need of Canadians faced with complex health decisions. *Health Expectations* **6**: 97–109.

Paterson, B.L., Russell, C., & Thorne, (S. 2001). Critical analysis of everyday self-care decision making in chronic illness. *Journal of Advanced Nursing* **35**: 335–41.

Pender, N.J., Murdaugh, C.L., & Parsons, M.A. (2006). *Health promotion in nursing Practice*, 5th edn. Upper Saddle River, NJ: Pearson Prentice-Hall.

Roelands, M., Van Oost, P., Stevens, V., Depoorter, A., & Buysse, A. (2004). Clinical practice guidelines to improve shared decision-making about assistive device use in home care: A pilot interventions study. *Patient Education and Counseling* **55**: 252–64.

Ross, M.M., Carswell, A., Hing, M., Hollingworth, G., & Dalziel, W.B. (2001). Seniors decision making about pain management. *Journal of Advanced Nursing* **35**: 442–51.

Rothert, M.L., Holmes-Rovner, M., Rovner, D., et al. (1997). An educational intervention as decision support for menopausal women. *Research in Nursing & Health* **20**: 377–87.

Tunis, S.R. (2005). Perspective: A clinical research strategy to support shared decision making. *Health Affairs* **24**(1): 180–4.

Domain 5: Perception/Cognition
Class 5: Cognition

Definition Inability to prepare for a set of actions fixed in time and under certain conditions.

Defining Characteristics

- Verbalization of fear toward a task to be undertaken
- Verbalization of worries toward a task to be undertaken
- Excessive anxieties toward a task to be undertaken
- Failure pattern of behavior
- Lack of plan
- Lack of resources
- Lack of sequential organization
- Procrastination
- Unmet goals for chosen activity

Related Factors

- Compromised ability to process information
- Defensive flight behavior when faced with proposed solution
- Hedonism
- Lack of family support
- Lack of friend support
- Unrealistic perception of events
- Unrealistic perception of personal competence

References

American Psychiatric Association (2004). *Mini DSM IV-TR*. Masson: Paris, p. 384.

Auger, L. (2006). *Vivre avec sa tête ou avec son cœur*. Centre la Pensée Réaliste, republication par Pierre Bovo, p. 156.

Auger, L. (2001). *Savoir vivre*. Québec: Les éditions Un monde différent ltée, p. 208.

Auger, L. (1992). *Prendre soin de soi, guide pratique de micro-thérapie*. Montréal: CIM, p. 237.

Auger, L. (1980). *S'aider soi-même d'avantage*. Québec: Les Éditions De l'Homme, p. 133.

Auger, L. (1972–2006). *Vivre avec sa tête où avec son cœur*. Montréal: Micheline Côté-Auger ed., p. 156.

Barth, B-M. (1985). Jérôme Bruner et l'innovation pédagogique. *Communication et Langages* **66**: 45–58.

Beck, A.T., et al. (1979). *Cognitive therapy of depression*. New York: Guilford Press.

Corbière, M., Laisné, F, & et Mercier, C. (2001). Élaboration du questionnaire: obstacles à l'insertion au travail et sentiment d'efficacité pour les surmonter. Manuscrit inédit,

Centre de recherche Femand-Seguin, Unité 218, Hôpital Louis-H. Lafontaine, Montréal.

Debray, Q., Kindynis, S., Leclère, M., & Seigneurie, A. (2005). *Protocoles de traitement des personnalités pathologiques, Approche cognitivo-comportementale*: Paris: Masson, p. 224.

Ellis, A. (1962). *Reason and emotion in psychotherapy*. New York: Secausus, Lyle Stuart.

Ellis, A. & Harper, R. (1992). *L'aprroche émotivo-rationnelle, Une nouvelle façon de vivre*. Québec: Les Éditions De l'Homme, p. 373.

Filion, F. (1989), *J'améliore mes plans d'action*. Québec: CAER Ed, 98 PP.

Greenberg, D. & Padesky, C. (2004). *Détression et anxiété: comprendre et surmonter par l'approche cognitive*. Québec: Décarie Éditeur, p. 264.

Ladouceur, R., Marchand, A., & Boivert, J-M. (1999). *Les troubles anxieux, Approche cognitive et comportementale*. Gaétan Morin & Paris: Masson, p. 213.

Lalonde, P., Aubut, J., & Grunberg, F., eds (2001). *Psychiatrie clinique, Une approche bio-psyco-sociale*. Québec: Tome II, p. 2091.

Lecomte, T. & Leclerc, C. (2004). *Manuel de réadaptation psychiatrique*. Québec: Presses de l'Université du Québec, p. 461.

Monastès, J.L. & Boyer, C. (2006). *Les thérapies comportementales et cognitives, Se libérer des troubles psy*. Milan: Les Essentiels Milan, p. 63.

Morin, C., Briand, C., & Lalonde, P. (1999). De la symptomatologie à la résolution de problèmes: approche intégrée pour les personnes atteintes de schizophrénie. In: *Santé Mentale au Québec; Dossier Schizophrénie, délires et thérapie cognitive*, Vol XXIV, No 1, p. 277.

Riberio, K.L. (1999). The labyrinth of community mental health: In search of meaningful occupation. *Psychiatric Rehabilitation Journal* (23): 2.

Seyle, H. (1959), *The stress of life*. New York: McGraw-Hill.

Townsend, M-C. (2004). *Soins infirmiers, Psychiatrie et santé mentale*. Québec: ERPI, p. 692.

Wilson, R. & Branch, R. (2004). *Les thérapies comportementales et cognitives pour les nulls*. Paris: First, p. 334.

Domain 5

Impaired Verbal Communication (00051)
(1983, 1996, 1998)

Domain 5: Perception/Cognition
Class 5: Communication

Definition Decreased, delayed, or absent ability to receive, process, transmit, and/or use a system of symbols

Defining Characteristics

- Absence of eye contact
- Cannot speak
- Difficulty in comprehending usual communication pattern
- Difficulty expressing thoughts verbally (e.g., aphasia, dysphasia, apraxia, dyslexia)
- Difficulty forming sentences
- Difficulty forming words (e.g., aphonia, dyslalia, dysarthria)
- Difficulty in maintaining usual communication pattern
- Difficulty in selective attending
- Difficulty in use of body expressions
- Difficulty in use of facial expressions
- Disorientation to person
- Disorientation to space
- Disorientation to time
- Does not speak
- Dyspnea
- Inability to speak language of caregiver
- Inability to use body expressions
- Inability to use facial expressions
- Inappropriate verbalization
- Partial visual deficit
- Slurring
- Speaks with difficulty
- Stuttering
- Total visual deficit
- Verbalizes with difficulty
- Willful refusal to speak

Related Factors

- Absence of significant others
- Altered perceptions
- Alteration in self-concept
- Alteration in self-esteem
- Alteration of central nervous system
- Anatomical defect (e.g., cleft palate, alteration of the neuromuscular visual system, auditory system, phonatory apparatus)
- Brain tumor
- Cultural differences
- Decrease in circulation to brain
- Differences related to developmental age
- Emotional conditions
- Environmental barriers
- Lack of information
- Physical barrier (e.g., tracheostomy, intubation)

- Physiological conditions
- Psychological barriers (e.g., psychosis, lack of stimuli)
- Side effects of medication
- Stress
- Weakening of the musculoskeletal system

Domain 5: Perception/Cognition
Class 5: Communication

Definition A pattern of exchanging information and ideas with others that is sufficient for meeting one's needs and life's goals, and can be strengthened

Defining Characteristics

- Able to speak a language
- Able to write a language
- Expresses feelings
- Expresses satisfaction with ability to share ideas with others
- Expresses satisfaction with ability to share information with others
- Expresses thoughts
- Expresses willingness to enhance communication
- Forms phrases
- Forms sentences
- Forms words
- Interprets nonverbal cues appropriately
- Uses nonverbal cues appropriately

Domain 6
Self-Perception

Seel also Readiness for Enhanced **Hope** (Domain 10, p. 291)

Risk for Compromised Human Dignity (00174)

(2006, LOE 2.1)

Domain 6: Self-perception
Class 1: Self-concept

Definition At risk for perceived loss of respect and honor

Risk Factors

- Cultural incongruity
- Disclosure of confidential information
- Exposure of the body
- Inadequate participation in decision-making
- Loss of control of body functions
- Perceived dehumanizing treatment
- Perceived humiliation
- Perceived intrusion by clinicians
- Perceived invasion of privacy
- Stigmatizing label
- Use of undefined medical terms

References

Shottom, L. & Seedhouse, D. (1998). Practical dignity in caring. *Nursing Ethics* **5**: 246–55.

Mairis, E. (1994). Concept clarification of professional practice dignity. *Journal of Advanced Nursing* **19**: 924–31.

Walsh, K. & Kowanko, I. (2002). Nurses and patients. Perceptions of dignity. *International Journal of Nursing Practice* **8**: 143–51.

Domain 6

Hopelessness (00124)
(1986)

Domain 6: Self-Perception
Class 1: Self-Concept

Definition Subjective state in which an individual sees limited or no alternatives or personal choices available and is unable to mobilize energy on own behalf

Defining Characteristics

- Closing eyes
- Decreased affect
- Decreased appetite
- Decreased response to stimuli
- Decreased verbalization
- Lack of initiative
- Lack of involvement in care
- Passivity
- Shrugging in response to speaker
- Sleep pattern disturbance
- Turning away from speaker
- Verbal cues (e.g., despondent content, "I can't", sighing)

Related Factors

- Abandonment
- Deteriorating physiological condition
- Lost belief in spiritual power
- Lost belief in transcendent values
- Long-term stress
- Prolonged activity restriction creating isolation

Domain 6: Self-Perception
Class 1: Self-Concept

Definition Inability to maintain an integrated and complete perception of self

Defining Characteristics

- Contradictory personal traits
- Delusional description of self
- Disturbed body image
- Disturbed relationships
- Feelings of emptiness
- Feelings of strangeness
- Fluctuating feelings about self
- Gender confusion
- Ineffective coping
- Ineffective role performance
- Unable to distinguish between inner and outer stimuli
- Uncertainty about goals
- Uncertainty about cultural values (e.g., beliefs, religion, and moral questions)
- Uncertainty about ideological values (e.g., beliefs, religion and moral questions)

Related Factors

- Cult indoctrination
- Cultural discontinuity
- Discrimination or prejudice
- Dysfunctional family processes
- Ingestion of toxic chemicals
- Inhalation of toxic chemicals
- Low self-esteem
- Manic states
- Multiple personality disorder
- Organic brain syndromes
- Psychiatric disorders (e.g., psychoses, depression, dissociative disorder)
- Situational crises
- Social role change
- Stages of growth
- Stages of development
- Use of psychoactive drugs

References

Bender, D. & Skodol, A. (2007). Borderline Personality as a self-other Representational Disturbance. *J Personal Disord*, **21**(5): 500–17.

Bergh, S. & Erling, A. (2006). Adolescent identity formation: a Swedish study of identity status using the EOM-EIS-II. *Adolescence* **6**: 22

Erikson, E.H. (1982). *Identitet: ungdom og kriser* [Identity: youth and crisis, (1968)]. Denmark: Hans Reitzel.

Domain 6

Evang, A. (2003). *Utvikling, personlighet og borderline* [Development, personality and borderline]. Norway: Cappelen Akademisk Forlag.

Fuchs, T. (2007). Fragmented selves: temporality and identity in borderline personality disorder. *Psychopathology,* **40**(6): 379–88, Epbu 2007 July 25. Last accessed June 24, 2008.

Mitchell A. (1985). The borderline diagnosis and integration of self. *American Journal of Psychoanalysis* **45**: 234–50.

Stuart, G.W & Laraia, M.T. (2001) *Principles and practice of psychiatric nursing.* St Louis: Mosby.

Risk for Loneliness (00054)

(1994, 2006, LOE 2.1)

Domain 6: Self-Perception
Class 1: Self-Concept

Definition At risk for experiencing discomfort associated with a desire or need for more contact with others

Risk Factors

- Affectional deprivation
- Cathectic deprivation
- Physical isolation
- Social isolation

References

Leiderman, P.H. (1969). Loneliness: A psychodynamic interpretation. In: Scheidman, E.S. & Ortega, M.J. (eds), *Aspects of depression: International psychiatry clinics*, Vol. 6. Boston: Little, Brown, pp. 155, 174.

Lien-Gieschen, T. (1993). Validation of social isolation related to maturational age: Elderly. *Nursing Diagnosis* **4**(1): 37–44.

Warren, B.J. (1993). Explaining social isolation through concept analysis. *Archives of Psychiatric Nursing* **7**: 270–6.

Domain 6

Readiness for Enhanced Power (00187)
(2006, LOE 2.1)

Domain 6: Self-Perception
Class 1: Self-Concept

Definition A pattern of participating knowingly in change that is sufficient for well-being and can be strengthened

Defining Characteristics

- Expresses readiness to enhance awareness of possible changes to be made
- Expresses readiness to enhance freedom to perform actions for change
- Expresses readiness to enhance identification of choices that can be made for change
- Expresses readiness to enhance involvement in creating change
- Expresses readiness to enhance knowledge for participation in change
- Expresses readiness to enhance participation in choices for daily living
- Expresses readiness to enhance participation in choices for health
- Expresses readiness to enhance power

References

Anderson, R.M. & Funnell, M.M. (2005). Patient empowerment: Reflections on the challenge of fostering the adoption of a new paradigm. *Patient Education and Counseling* **57**: 153–7.

Barrett, E.A.M. (1990). A measure of power as knowing participation in change. In Strickland, O. & Waltz, C. (eds), *Measurement of nursing outcomes:* Volume 4, *Measuring client self-care and coping skills* (pp. 159–180). New York: Springer.

Caroselli, C. & Barrett, E.A.M. (1998). A review of the power as knowing participation in change literature. *Nursing Science Quarterly* **11**(1): 9–16.

Cowling, W.R. (2004). Pattern, participation, praxis, and power in unitary appreciative inquiry. *Nursing Science Quarterly* **27**: 202–14.

Funnell, M.M. (2004). Patient empowerment. *Critical Care Nursing Quarterly* **27**: 201–4.

Guinn, M.J. (2004). A daughter's journey promoting geriatric self-care: Promoting positive health care interactions. *Geriatric Nursing* **25**: 267–71.

Harkness, J. (2005). Patient involvement: A vital principle for patient-centered health care. *World Hospitals & Health Services* **41**(2): 12–16, 40–3.

Hashimoto, H. & Fukuhara, S. (2003). The influence of locus of control on preferences for information and decision making. *Patient Education and Counseling* **55**: 236–40.

Jeng, C., Yang, S., Chang, P., & Tsao, L. (2004). Menopausal women: Perceiving continuous power through the experience of regular exercise. *Journal of Clinical Nursing* **13**: 447–54.

Mok, E. (2001). Empowerment of cancer patients: From a Chinese perspective. *Nursing Ethics* **8**(1): 69–76.

Pender, N.J., Murdaugh, C.L., & Parsons, M.A. (2006). *Health promotion in nursing practice,* 5th edn. Stamford, CT: Appleton & Lange.

Pibernik-Okanovic, M., Prasek, M., Poljicanin-Filipovic, T., Pavlic-Renar, I., & Metelko, Z. (2003). Effects of an empowerment-based psychosocial intervention on quality of life and metabolic control in type 2 diabetic patients. *Patient Education and Counseling* **52**: 193–9.

Shearer, N.B.C. & Reed, P.G. (2004). Empowerment: reformulation of a non-Rogerian concept. *Nursing Science Quarterly* **17**: 253–9.

Wright, B.W. (2004). Trust and power in adults: An investigation using Rogers' science of unitary human beings. *Nursing Science Quarterly* **17**: 139–46.

Note: even though power (a response) and empowerment (an intervention approach) are different concepts, the literature related to both concepts supports the defining characteristics of this diagnosis.

Powerlessness (00125)
(1982)

Domain 6: Self-Perception
Class 1: Self-Concept

Definition Perception that one's own action will not significantly affect an outcome; a perceived lack of control over a current situation or immediate happening

Defining Characteristics

Low

- Expressions of uncertainty about fluctuating energy levels
- Passivity

Moderate

- Anger
- Dependence on others that may result in irritability
- Does not defend self-care practices when challenged
- Does not monitor progress
- Expressions of dissatisfaction over inability to perform previous activities
- Expressions of dissatisfaction over inability to perform previous tasks
- Expressions of doubt regarding role performance
- Expressions of frustration over inability to perform previous activities
- Expressions of frustration over inability to perform previous tasks
- Fear of alienation from caregivers
- Guilt
- Inability to seek information regarding care
- Nonparticipation in care when opportunities are provided
- Nonparticipation in decision-making when opportunities are provided
- Passivity
- Reluctance to express true feelings
- Resentment

Severe

- Apathy
- Depression over physical deterioration
- Verbal expressions of having no control (e.g., over self-care, situation, outcome)

Related Factors

- Healthcare environment
- Illness-related regimen
- Interpersonal interaction
- Lifestyle of helplessness

Risk for Powerlessness (00152)

(2000)

Domain 6: Self-Perception
Class 1: Self-Concept

Definition At risk for perceived lack of control over a situation and/or one's ability to significantly affect an outcome

Risk Factors

Physiological

- Acute injury
- Aging
- Dying
- Illness
- Progressive debilitating disease process (e.g., spinal cord injury, multiple sclerosis)

Psychosocial

- Absence of integrality (e.g., essence of power)
- Chronic low self-esteem
- Deficient knowledge (e.g., of illness or healthcare system)
- Disturbed body image
- Inadequate coping patterns
- Lifestyle of dependency
- Situational low self-esteem

Domain 6: Self-Perception
Class 1: Self-Concept

Definition A pattern of perceptions or ideas about the self that is sufficient for well-being and can be strengthened

Defining Characteristics

- Accepts limitations
- Accepts strengths
- Actions are congruent with verbal expression
- Expresses confidence in abilities
- Expresses satisfaction with body image
- Expresses satisfaction with personal identity
- Expresses satisfaction with role performance
- Expresses satisfaction with sense of worthiness
- Expresses satisfaction with thoughts about self
- Expresses willingness to enhance self-concept

Situational Low Self-Esteem (00120)

(1988, 1996, 2000)

Domain 6: Self-Perception
Class 2: Self-Esteem

Definition Development of a negative perception of self-worth in response to a current situation (specify)

Defining Characteristics

- Evaluation of self as unable to deal with events
- Evaluation of self as unable to deal with situations
- Expressions of helplessness
- Expressions of uselessness
- Indecisive behavior
- Nonassertive behavior
- Self-negating verbalizations
- Verbally reports current situational challenge to self-worth

Related Factors

- Behavior inconsistent with values
- Developmental changes
- Disturbed body image
- Failures
- Functional impairment
- Lack of recognition
- Loss
- Rejections
- Social role changes

Domain 6

Domain 6: Self-Perception
Class 2: Self-Esteem

Definition Long-standing negative self-evaluating/feelings about self or self-capabilities

Defining Characteristics

- Dependent on others' opinions
- Evaluation of self as unable to deal with events
- Exaggerates negative feedback about self
- Excessively seeks reassurance
- Expressions of guilt
- Expressions of shame
- Frequent lack of success in life events
- Hesitant to try new situations
- Hesitant to try new things
- Indecisive behavior
- Lack of eye contact
- Nonassertive behavior
- Overly conforming
- Passive
- Rejects positive feedback about self

Related Factors

- Ineffective adaptation to loss
- Lack of affection
- Lack of approval
- Lack of membership in group
- Perceived discrepancy between self and cultural norms
- Perceived discrepancy between self and spiritual norms
- Perceived lack of belonging
- Perceived lack of respect from others
- Psychiatric disorder
- Repeated failures
- Repeated negative reinforcement
- Traumatic event
- Traumatic situation

References

Bredeholf, D. (1990). An evaluation study of the self-esteem: a family affair program with risk abuse parents. *Trans Anal J*, **20**(2): 111–117.

Brown, J., Dutton, K., Brown J., Dutton, K. The thrill of victory, the complexity of defeat: self-esteem and people's emotional reactions to success and failure. *J Pers Soc Psychol*, **68**(4): 712–22.

Buckner J., Beardslee W., Bassuk E., & Ray, S. (2004). Exposure to violence and low-income children's mental health: direct, moderated, and mediated relations. *Am J Orthopsychiatry* **74**: 413–23.

Buckner J., Mezzacappa, E., & Beardslee, W. (2003). Characteristics of resilient youths living in poverty: the role of self-regulatory processes. *Dev Psychopathol* **15**(1): 139–62.

Byers, P., Raven, L., Hill, J., & Robyak, J. (1990). Enhancing self-esteem of inpatient alcoholics. *Iss Ment Health Nurs* **11**: 337–46.

Caron-Trabut, P. (2000). Les abus sexuels chez les enfants en bas âge. *L'infirmière du Québec* Sept–Oct: 27–32.

Consoli, S. (2003). Depression and associated organic pathologies, a still under-estimated comorbidity. *Presse Med* **32**(1): 10–21.

Crowe, M. (2004). Never good enough – part 2: clinical implications. *J Psychiatr Ment Health Nurs* **11**: 335–40.

Dumas, D. & Pelletier, L. (1997). La perception de soi: La clé de voûte des interventions de l'infirmière auprès de l'enfant hyperactive. *L'infirmière du Québec* March–Apr: 28–36.

Fitts, W. (1972). *The self-concept and psychopathology*. Nashville, TN: Counselor Recordings and Tests.

Gary, F., Baker, M., & Grandbois, D. (2005). Perspectives on suicide prevention among American Indian and Alaska native children and adolescents: a call for help. *Online J Issues Nurs*, **10**(2): 6.

Hall, P. & Tarrier, N. (2003). The cognitive-behavioural treatment of low self-esteem in psychotic patients: a pilot study. *Behav Res Ther* **41**: 317–32.

Heap, J. (2004). Enuresis in children and young people: a public health nurse approach in New Zealand. *J Child Health Care* **8**(2): 92–101 (review).

Leblanc, L. & Ouellet, N. (2004). Dépistage de la violence conjugale: le role de l'infirmière. *Perspectives infirmière* May–June: 39–43.

McFarland, G.K. & McFarlane, E.A. (1995). *Traité de diagnostic infirmier* (adaptation of S. Truchon and D. Fleury). St-Laurent: ERPI, pp. 507–520.

Maslow, A. (1970). *Motivation and personality*, 2nd edn. New York: Harper & Row.

Meridith, P., Strong J., & Feeney, J. (2006). The relationship of adult attachment to emotion, catastrophizing, control, threshold and tolerance, in experimentally-induced pain. *Pain* **120**(1–2): 44–52.

Mozley P. (1976). Psychophysiologic infertility: an overview. *Clin Obstet Gynecol* **19**: 407–17.

Nishina, A. & Juvonen, J. (2005). Daily reports of witnessing and experiencing peer harassment in middle school. *Child Dev* **76**: 435–50.

Page, C. (1995). Intervenir auprès des femmes présentant un trouble dépressif. *L'infirmière du Québec* May–June: 26–33.

Ratheram-Borus, M. (1990). Adolescents' reference group choices, self-esteem, and judgment. *J Person Soc Psych* **59**: 1075–81.

Ray S. & Heap, J. (2001). Male survivors' perspectives of incest/sexual abuse. *Perspect Psychiatr Care* **37**(2): 49–59.

Rodin, J. (1993). Cultural and psychosocial determinants of weight concerns. *Ann Intern Med* **119**(7Pt2): 643–5.

Sharma, V. & Mavi, J. (2001). Self-esteem and performance on word tasks. *J Soc Psychol* **141**: 723–9.

Sloman L, Gilbert P., & Hasey, G. (2003). Evolved mechanisms in depression: the role and interaction of attachment and social rank in depression. *J Affect Disord* **74**(2): 107–21

Talf, L. (1985). Self-esteem in later life: A nursing perspective. *Adv Nursing Sci* **8**(1): 77–84.

Thorne A. & Michaelieu, Q. (1996). Situating adolescent gender and self-esteem personal memories. *Child Dev* **67**: 1374–90.

Westermeyer, J. (1989). Cross-cultural care for PTSD: research, training and service needs for the future. *J Traum Stress* **2**: 515–36.

Domain 6

Risk for Situational Low Self-Esteem (00153)

(2000)

Domain 6: Self-Perception
Class 2: Self-Esteem

Definition At risk for developing negative perception of self-worth in response to a current situation (specify)

Risk Factors

- Behavior inconsistent with values
- Decreased control over environment
- Developmental changes
- Disturbed body image
- Failures
- Functional impairment
- History of abandonment
- History of abuse
- History of learned helplessness
- History of neglect
- Lack of recognition
- Loss
- Physical illness
- Rejections
- Social role changes
- Unrealistic self-expectations

Disturbed Body Image (00118)
(1973, 1998)

Domain 6: Perception/Cognition
Class 3: Body Image

Definition Confusion in mental picture of one's physical self

Defining Characteristics

- Behaviors of acknowledgment of one's body
- Behaviors of avoidance of one's body
- Behaviors of monitoring one's body
- Nonverbal response to actual change in body (e.g., appearance, structure, function)
- Nonverbal response to perceived change in body (e.g., appearance, structure, function)
- Verbalization of feelings that reflect an altered view of one's body (e.g., appearance, structure, function)
- Verbalization of perceptions that reflect an altered view of one's body in appearance

Objective

- Actual change in function
- Actual change in structure
- Behaviors of acknowledging one's body
- Behaviors of monitoring one's body
- Change in ability to estimate spatial relationship of body to environment
- Change in social involvement

- Extension of body boundary to incorporate environmental objects
- Intentional hiding of body part
- Intentional overexposure of body part
- Missing body part
- Not looking at body part
- Not touching body part
- Trauma to nonfunctioning part
- Unintentional hiding of body part
- Unintentional overexposing of body part

Subjective

- Depersonalization of loss by impersonal pronouns
- Depersonalization of part by impersonal pronouns
- Emphasis on remaining strengths
- Fear of reaction by others
- Focus on past appearance
- Focus on past function
- Focus on past strength
- Heightened achievement
- Negative feelings about body (e.g., feelings of helplessness, hopelessness, powerlessness)

- Personalization of loss by name
- Personalization of part by name
- Preoccupation with change
- Preoccupation with loss
- Refusal to verify actual change
- Verbalization of change in lifestyle

Related Factors

- Biophysical
- Cognitive
- Cultural
- Developmental changes
- Illness
- Illness treatment
- Injury
- Perceptual
- Psychosocial
- Spiritual
- Surgery
- Trauma

Domain 7
Role Relationships

Caregiver Role Strain (00061)

(1992, 1998, 2000)

Domain 7: Role Relationships
Class 1: Caregiving Roles

Definition Difficulty in performing family caregiver role

Defining Characteristics

Caregiving Activities

- Apprehension about care receiver's care if caregiver unable to provide care
- Apprehension about the future regarding care receiver's health
- Apprehension about the future regarding caregiver's ability to provide care
- Apprehension about possible institutionalization of care receiver
- Difficulty completing required tasks
- Difficulty performing required tasks
- Dysfunctional change in caregiving activities
- Preoccupation with care routine

Caregiver Health Status

Physical

- Cardiovascular disease
- Diabetes
- Fatigue
- Gastrointestinal upset
- Headaches
- Hypertension
- Rash
- Weight change

Emotional

- Anger
- Disturbed sleep
- Feeling depressed
- Frustration
- Impaired individual coping
- Impatience
- Increased emotional lability
- Increased nervousness
- Lack of time to meet personal needs
- Somatization
- Stress

Socioeconomic

- Changes in leisure activities
- Low work productivity
- Refuses career advancement
- Withdraws from social life

Caregiver–Care Receiver Relationship

- Difficulty watching care receiver go through the illness
- Grief regarding changed relationship with care receiver
- Uncertainty regarding changed relationship with care receiver

Class 1: Caregiving Roles **201**

Domain 7

Family Processes

- Concerns about family members
- Family conflict

Related Factors

Care Receiver Health Status

- Addiction
- Co-dependency
- Cognitive problems
- Dependency
- Illness chronicity
- Illness severity
- Increasing care needs
- Instability of care receiver's health
- Problem behaviors
- Psychological problems
- Unpredictability of illness course

Caregiver Health Status

- Addiction
- Co-dependency
- Cognitive problems
- Inability to fulfill one's own expectations
- Inability to fulfill other's expectations
- Marginal coping patterns
- Physical problems
- Psychological problems
- Unrealistic expectations of self

Caregiver–Care Receiver Relationship

- History of poor relationship
- Mental status of elder inhibiting conversation

- Presence of abuse
- Presence of violence
- Unrealistic expectations of caregiver by care receiver

Caregiving Activities

- 24-hour care responsibilities
- Amount of activities
- Complexity of activities
- Discharge of family members to home with significant care needs
- Ongoing changes in activities
- Unpredictability of care situation
- Years of caregiving

Family Processes

- History of family dysfunction
- History of marginal family coping

Resources

- Caregiver is not developmentally ready for caregiver role
- Deficient knowledge about community resources
- Difficulty accessing community resources
- Emotional strength
- Formal assistance
- Formal support

- Inadequate community resources (e.g., respite services, recreational resources)
- Inadequate equipment for providing care
- Inadequate informal assistance
- Inadequate informal support
- Inadequate physical environment for providing care (e.g., housing, temperature, safety)
- Inadequate transportation

- Inexperience with caregiving
- Insufficient finances
- Insufficient time
- Lack of caregiver privacy
- Lack of support
- Physical energy

Socioeconomic

- Alienation from others
- Competing role commitments
- Insufficient recreation
- Isolation from others

Risk for Caregiver Role Strain (00062) (1992)

Domain 7: Role Relationships
Class 1: Caregiving Roles

Definition Caregiver is vulnerable for felt difficulty in performing the family caregiver role

Risk Factors

- Addiction
- Amount of caregiving tasks
- Care receiver exhibits bizarre behavior
- Care receiver exhibits deviant behavior
- Caregiver's competing role commitments
- Caregiver health impairment
- Caregiver is female
- Caregiver is spouse
- Caregiver isolation
- Caregiver not developmentally ready for caregiver role
- Co-dependency
- Cognitive problems in care receiver
- Complexity of caregiving tasks
- Congenital defect
- Developmental delay of the care receiver
- Developmental delay of the caregiver
- Discharge of family member with significant home care needs
- Duration of caregiving required
- Family dysfunction before the caregiving situation
- Family isolation
- Illness severity of the care receiver
- Inadequate physical environment for providing care (e.g., housing, transportation, community services, equipment)
- Inexperience with caregiving
- Instability in the care receiver's health
- Lack of recreation for caregiver
- Lack of respite for caregiver
- Marginal caregiver's coping patterns
- Marginal family adaptation
- Past history of poor relationship between caregiver and care receiver
- Premature birth
- Presence of abuse
- Presence of situational stressors that normally affect families (e.g., significant loss, disaster or crisis, economic vulnerability, major life events)
- Presence of violence
- Psychological problems in caregiver
- Psychological problems in care receiver
- Retardation of the care receiver
- Retardation of the caregiver
- Unpredictable illness course

Impaired Parenting (00056)

(1978, 1998)

Domain 7: Role Relationships
Class 1: Caregiving Roles

Definition Inability of the primary caretaker to create, maintain, or regain an environment that promotes the optimum growth and development of the child

Defining Characteristics

Infant or Child

- Behavioral disorders
- Failure to thrive
- Frequent accidents
- Frequent illness
- Incidence of abuse
- Incidence of trauma (e.g., physical and psychological)
- Lack of attachment
- Lack of separation anxiety
- Poor academic performance
- Poor cognitive development
- Poor social competence
- Runaway

Parental

- Abandonment
- Child abuse
- Child neglect
- Frequently punitive
- Hostility to child
- Inadequate attachment
- Inadequate child health maintenance
- Inappropriate caretaking skills
- Inappropriate stimulation (e.g., visual, tactile, auditory)
- Inappropriate child care arrangements
- Inconsistent behavior management
- Inconsistent care
- Inflexibility in meeting needs of child
- Little cuddling
- Maternal–child interaction deficit
- Negative statements about child
- Paternal–child interaction deficit
- Poor parent–child interaction
- Rejection of child
- Statements of inability to meet child's needs
- Unsafe home environment
- Verbalization of inability to control child
- Verbalization of frustration
- Verbalization of role inadequacy

Related Factors

Infant or Child

- Altered perceptual abilities
- Attention deficit hyperactivity disorder
- Developmental delay

- Difficult temperament
- Handicapping condition
- Illness
- Multiple births
- Not desired gender
- Premature birth
- Separation from parent
- Temperamental conflicts with parental expectations

Knowledge

- Deficient knowledge about child development
- Deficient knowledge about child health maintenance
- Deficient knowledge about parenting skills
- Inability to respond to infant cues
- Lack of cognitive readiness for parenthood
- Lack of education
- Limited cognitive functioning
- Poor communication skills
- Preference for physical punishment
- Unrealistic expectations

Physiological

- Physical illness

Psychological

- Closely spaced pregnancies
- Depression
- Difficult birthing process
- Disability
- High number of pregnancies
- History of mental illness
- History of substance abuse
- Lack of prenatal care

- Sleep deprivation
- Sleep disruption
- Young parental age

Social

- Change in family unit
- Chronic low self-esteem
- Father of child not involved
- Financial difficulties
- History of being abused
- History of being abusive
- Inability to put child's needs before own
- Inadequate child care arrangements
- Job problems
- Lack of family cohesiveness
- Lack of parental role model
- Lack of resources
- Lack of social support networks
- Lack of transportation
- Lack of valuing of parenthood
- Legal difficulties
- Low socioeconomic class
- Maladaptive coping strategies
- Marital conflict
- Mother of child not involved
- Single parent
- Social isolation
- Poor home environment
- Poor parental role model
- Poor problem-solving skills
- Poverty
- Presence of stress (e.g., financial, legal, recent crisis, cultural move)
- Relocations
- Role strain
- Situational low self-esteem
- Unemployment
- Unplanned pregnancy
- Unwanted pregnancy

Readiness for Enhanced Parenting (00164)

(2002, LOE 2.1)

Domain 7: Role Relationships
Class 1: Caregiving Roles

Definition A pattern of providing an environment for children or other dependent person(s) that is sufficient to nurture growth and development, and can be strengthened

Defining Characteristics

- Children express satisfaction with home environment
- Emotional support of children
- Emotional support of other dependent person(s)
- Evidence of attachment
- Exhibits realistic expectations of children
- Exhibits realistic expectations of other dependent person(s)
- Expresses willingness to enhance parenting
- Needs of children are met (e.g., physical and emotional)
- Needs of other dependent person(s) is/are met (e.g., physical and emotional)
- Other dependent person(s) express(es) satisfaction with home environment

Risk for Impaired Parenting (00057)

(1978, 1998)

Domain 7: Role Relationships
Class 1: Caregiving Roles

Definition Risk for inability of the primary caretaker to create, maintain, or regain an environment that promotes the optimum growth and development of the child

Risk Factors

Infant or Child

- Altered perceptual abilities
- Attention deficit hyperactivity disorder
- Developmental delay
- Difficult temperament
- Handicapping condition
- Illness
- Multiple births
- Not gender desired
- Premature birth
- Prolonged separation from parent
- Temperamental conflicts with parental expectation

Knowledge

- Deficient knowledge about child development
- Deficient knowledge about child health maintenance
- Deficient knowledge about parenting skills
- Inability to respond to infant cues
- Lack of cognitive readiness for parenthood
- Low cognitive functioning
- Low educational level
- Poor communication skills
- Preference for physical punishment
- Unrealistic expectations of child

Physiological

- Physical illness

Psychological

- Closely spaced pregnancies
- Depression
- Difficult birthing process
- Disability
- High number of pregnancies
- History of mental illness
- History of substance abuse
- Sleep deprivation
- Sleep disruption
- Young parental age

Social

- Change in family unit
- Chronic low self-esteem
- Father of child not involved
- Financial difficulties
- History of being abused
- History of being abusive
- Inadequate child care arrangements

- Job problems
- Lack of access to resources
- Lack of family cohesiveness
- Lack of parental role model
- Lack of prenatal care
- Lack of resources
- Lack of social support network
- Lack of transportation
- Lack of valuing of parenthood
- Late prenatal care
- Legal difficulties
- Low socioeconomic class
- Maladaptive coping strategies
- Marital conflict
- Mother of child not involved
- Parent–child separation
- Poor home environment
- Poor parental role model
- Poor problem-solving skills
- Poverty
- Role strain
- Single parent
- Situational low self-esteem
- Social isolation
- Stress
- Relocation
- Unemployment
- Unplanned pregnancy
- Unwanted pregnancy

Risk for Impaired Attachment* (00058)
(1994)

Domain 7: Role Relationships
Class 2: Family Relationships

Definition Disruption of the interactive process between parent/significant other and child/infant that fosters the development of a protective and nurturing reciprocal relationship

Risk Factors

- Anxiety associated with the parent role
- Ill child who is unable effectively to initiate parental contact as a result of altered behavioral organization
- Inability of parents to meet personal needs
- Lack of privacy
- Parental conflict resulting from altered behavioral organization
- Physical barriers
- Premature infant who is unable to effectively initiate parental contact due to altered behavioral organization
- Separation
- Substance abuse

* This diagnosis formerly held the label, *Risk for Impaired Parent/Child Attachment.*

Dysfunctional **Family** **Processes*** (00063)
(1994)

Domain 7: Role/Relationships
Class 2: Family Relationships

Definition Psychosocial, spiritual, and physiological functions of the family unit are chronically disorganized, which leads to conflict, denial of problems, resistance to change, ineffective problem-solving, and a series of self-perpetuating crises

Defining Characteristics

Behavioral

- Alcohol abuse
- Agitation
- Blaming
- Broken promises
- Chaos
- Contradictory communication
- Controlling communication
- Criticizing
- Deficient knowledge about alcoholism
- Denial of problems
- Dependency
- Difficulty having fun
- Difficulty with intimate relationships
- Difficulty with life cycle transitions
- Diminished physical contact
- Disturbances in academic performance in children
- Disturbances in concentration
- Enabling maintenance of alcohol drinking pattern
- Escalating conflict
- Failure to accomplish developmental tasks
- Family special occasions are alcohol centered

- Harsh self-judgment
- Immaturity
- Impaired communication
- Inability to accept help
- Inability to accept a wide range of feelings
- Inability to adapt to change
- Inability to deal constructively with traumatic experiences
- Inability to express a wide range of feelings
- Inability to meet emotional needs of its members
- Inability to meet security needs of its members
- Inability to meet spiritual needs of its members
- Inability to receive help appropriately
- Inadequate understanding of alcoholism
- Inappropriate expression of anger
- Ineffective problem-solving skills
- Isolation
- Lack of dealing with conflict
- Lack of reliability
- Lying

Domain 7

* This diagnosis formerly held the label, *Dysfunctional Family Processes: Alcoholism.*

- Manipulation
- Nicotine addiction
- Orientation toward tension relief rather than achievement of goals
- Paradoxical communication
- Power struggles
- Rationalization
- Refusal to get help
- Seeking affirmation
- Seeking approval
- Self-blaming
- Stress-related physical illnesses
- Substance abuse other than alcohol
- Unresolved grief
- Verbal abuse of children
- Verbal abuse of parent
- Verbal abuse of spouse

- Hurt
- Insecurity
- Lack of identity
- Lingering resentment
- Loneliness
- Loss
- Mistrust
- Misunderstood
- Moodiness
- Powerlessness
- Rejection
- Repressed emotions
- Responsibility for alcoholic's behavior
- Suppressed rage
- Shame
- Tension
- Unhappiness
- Vulnerability
- Worthlessness

Feelings

- Abandonment
- Anger
- Anxiety
- Being different from other people
- Being unloved
- Confuses love and pity
- Confusion
- Decreased self-esteem
- Depression
- Dissatisfaction
- Distress
- Embarrassment
- Emotional control by others
- Emotional isolation
- Failure
- Fear
- Frustration
- Guilt
- Hopelessness
- Hostility

Roles and Relationships

- Altered role function
- Chronic family problems
- Closed communication systems
- Deterioration in family relationships
- Disrupted family rituals
- Disrupted family roles
- Disturbed family dynamics
- Economic problems
- Family denial
- Family does not demonstrate respect for autonomy of its members
- Family does not demonstrate respect for individuality of its members
- Inconsistent parenting
- Ineffective spouse communication
- Intimacy dysfunction

- Lack of cohesiveness
- Lack of skills necessary for relationships
- Low perception of parental support
- Marital problems
- Neglected obligations
- Pattern of rejection
- Reduced ability of family members to relate to each other for mutual growth and maturation
- Triangulating family relationships

Related Factors

- Abuse of alcohol
- Addictive personality
- Biochemical influences
- Family history of alcoholism
- Family history of resistance to treatment
- Genetic predisposition
- Inadequate coping skills
- Lack of problem-solving skills

Interrupted Family Processes (00060)
(1982, 1998)

Domain 7: Role Relationships
Class 2: Family Relationships

Definition Change in family relationships and/or functioning

Defining Characteristics

- Changes in assigned tasks
- Changes in availability for affective responsiveness
- Changes in availability for emotional support
- Changes in communication patterns
- Changes in effectiveness in completing assigned tasks
- Changes in expressions of conflict with community resources
- Changes in expressions of isolation from community resources
- Changes in expressions of conflict within family
- Changes in intimacy
- Changes in mutual support
- Changes in patterns
- Changes in participation in problem-solving
- Changes in participation in decision-making
- Changes in power alliances
- Changes in rituals
- Changes in satisfaction with family
- Changes in somatic complaints
- Changes in stress-reduction behaviors

Related Factors

- Developmental crises
- Developmental transition
- Family roles shift
- Interaction with community
- Modification in family finances
- Modification in family social status
- Power shift of family members
- Shift in health status of a family member
- Situation transition
- Situational crises

Readiness for Enhanced Family Processes (00159)

(2002, LOE 2.1)

Domain 7: Role Relationships
Class 2: Family Relationships

Definition A pattern of family functioning that is sufficient to support the well-being of family members and can be strengthened

Defining Characteristics

- Activities support the growth of family members
- Activities support the safety of family members
- Balance exists between autonomy and cohesiveness
- Boundaries of family members are maintained
- Communication is adequate
- Energy level of family supports activities of daily living
- Expresses willingness to enhance family dynamics
- Family adapts to change
- Family functioning meets needs of family members
- Family resilience is evident
- Family roles are appropriate for developmental stages
- Family roles are flexible for developmental stages
- Family tasks are accomplished
- Interdependent with community
- Relationships are generally positive
- Respect for family members is evident

Domain 7

Effective Breastfeeding (00106)

(1990)

Domain 7: Role Relationships
Class 3: Role Performance

Definition   Mother–infant dyad/family exhibits adequate proficiency and satisfaction with breastfeeding process

Defining Characteristics

- Adequate infant elimination patterns for age
- Appropriate infant weight pattern for age
- Eagerness of infant to nurse
- Effective mother–infant communication patterns
- Infant content after feeding
- Maternal verbalization of satisfaction with the breastfeeding process
- Mother able to position infant at breast to promote a successful latching-on response
- Regular suckling at the breast
- Regular swallowing at the breast
- Signs of oxytocin release
- Sustained suckling at the breast
- Sustained swallowing at the breast
- Symptoms of oxytocin release

Related Factors

- Basic breastfeeding knowledge
- Infant gestational age >34 weeks
- Maternal confidence
- Normal breast structure
- Normal infant oral structure
- Support source

Ineffective Breastfeeding (00104)
(1988)

Domain 7: Role Relationships
Class 3: Role Performance

Definition Dissatisfaction or difficulty a mother, infant, or child experiences with the breastfeeding process

Defining Characteristics

- Inadequate milk supply
- Infant arching at the breast
- Infant crying at the breast
- Infant inability to latch on to maternal breast correctly
- Infant exhibiting crying within the first hour after breastfeeding
- Infant exhibiting fussiness within the first hour after breastfeeding
- Insufficient emptying of each breast per feeding
- Insufficient opportunity for suckling at the breast
- No observable signs of oxytocin release
- Nonsustained suckling at the breast
- Observable signs of inadequate infant intake
- Perceived inadequate milk supply
- Persistence of sore nipples beyond first week of breastfeeding
- Resisting latching on
- Unresponsive to other comfort measures
- Unsatisfactory breastfeeding process

Related Factors

- Infant anomaly
- Infant receiving supplemental feedings with artificial nipple
- Interruption in breastfeeding
- Knowledge deficit
- Maternal ambivalence
- Maternal anxiety
- Maternal breast anomaly
- Nonsupportive family
- Nonsupportive partner
- Poor infant sucking reflex
- Prematurity
- Previous breast surgery
- Previous history of breastfeeding failure

Domain 7

Interrupted Breastfeeding (00105)
(1992)

Domain 7: Role Relationships
Class 3: Role Performance

Definition Break in the continuity of the breastfeeding process as a result of inability or inadvisability to put baby to breast for feeding

Defining Characteristics

- Infant receives no nourishment at the breast for some or all feedings
- Lack of knowledge about expression of breast milk
- Lack of knowledge about storage of breast milk
- Maternal desire to eventually provide breast milk for child's nutritional needs
- Maternal desire to maintain breastfeeding for child's nutritional needs
- Maternal desire to provide breast milk for child's nutritional needs
- Separation of mother and child

Related Factors

- Contraindications to breastfeeding
- Infant illness
- Maternal employment
- Maternal illness
- Need to abruptly wean infant
- Prematurity

Parental Role Conflict (00064)
(1988)

Domain 7: Role Relationships
Class 3: Role Performance

Definition Parent experience of role confusion and conflict in response to crisis

Defining Characteristics

- Anxiety
- Demonstrated disruption in caretaking routines
- Expresses concern about perceived loss of control over decisions relating to his or her child
- Fear
- Parent(s) express(es) concern(s) about changes in parental role
- Parent(s) express(es) concern(s) about family (e.g., functioning, communication, health)
- Parent(s) express(es) feeling(s) of inadequacy to provide for child's needs (e.g., physical, emotional)
- Reluctant to participate in usual caretaking activities
- Verbalizes feelings of frustration
- Verbalizes feelings of guilt

Related Factors

- Change in marital status
- Home care of a child with special needs
- Interruptions of family life due to home care regimen (e. g., treatments, caregivers, lack of respite)
- Intimidation with invasive modalities (e.g., intubation)
- Intimidation with restrictive modalities (e.g., isolation)
- Separation from child because of chronic illness
- Specialized care center

Readiness for Enhanced Relationship (00207)

(2006, LOE 2.1)

Domain 7: Role Relationships
Class 3: Role Performance

Definition A pattern of mutual partnership that is sufficient to provide each other's needs and can be strengthened

Defining Characteristics

- Express desire to enhance communication between partners
- Express satisfaction with sharing of information and ideas between partners
- Express satisfaction with fulfilling physical and emotional needs by one's partner
- Demonstrates mutual respect between partners
- Meets developmental goals appropriate for family life-cycle stage
- Demonstrates well-balanced autonomy and collaboration between partners
- Demonstrates mutual support in daily activities between partners
- Identifies each other as a key person
- Demonstrates understanding of partner's insufficient (physical, social, psychological) function
- Express satisfaction with complementary relation between partners

References

Aoki, Y., Kato, N., & Hirasawa, M., eds (2002). *Josangaku Taikei 5 Boshi no Shinri Shakaigaku* [*Midwifery System* Vol. 5 *Psychosociology for mother and child*]. Tokyo: Japanese Nursing Association Publishing Co.

Kanbara, F. (1991). *Gendai no Kekkon to Fufu Kankei* [today's marriage and marital relationship]. Tokyo: Baifukan.

Kawano M. (1999). *Sexuality no Kango* [*Nursing for sexuality*]. Tokyo: Medical Friend.

Mochizuki, T. (1996). *Kazoku Shyakai-gaku Nyumon* [*Introduction to family sociology*]. Tokyo: Baifukan.

Muramoto, J. & Mori, A., eds (2007). *Bosei Kango-gaku Joron* [*Introduction to maternal nursing*, 2nd edn]. Tokyo: Ishiyaku Publishing Co.

Nojima, S. & Suzuki, K., eds (2005). *Kazoku Kango-gaku* [*Family nursing*]. Tokyo: Kenpansha.

Roy, C. (1984). *Introduction to Nursing: Adaptation model*, 2nd edn. Upper Saddle River: Prentice-Hall.

Domain 7

Ineffective Role Performance (00055)
(1978, 1996, 1998)

Domain 7: Role Relationships
Class 3: Role Performance

Definition Patterns of behavior and self-expression that do not match the environmental context, norms, and expectations

Defining Characteristics

- Altered role perceptions
- Anxiety
- Change in capacity to resume role
- Change in other's perception of role
- Change in self-perception of role
- Change in usual patterns of responsibility
- Deficient knowledge
- Depression
- Discrimination
- Domestic violence
- Harassment
- Inadequate adaptation to change
- Inadequate confidence
- Inadequate coping
- Inadequate external support for role enactment
- Inadequate motivation
- Inadequate opportunities for role enactment
- Inadequate role competency
- Inadequate self-management
- Inadequate skills
- Inappropriate developmental expectations
- Pessimism
- Powerlessness
- Role ambivalence
- Role confusion
- Role conflict
- Role denial
- Role dissatisfaction
- Role overload
- Role strain
- System conflict
- Uncertainty

Related Factors

Knowledge

- Inadequate role model
- Inadequate role preparation (e.g., role transition, skill rehearsal, validation)
- Lack of education
- Lack of role model
- Unrealistic role expectations

Physiological

- Body image alteration
- Cognitive deficits
- Depression
- Fatigue
- Low self-esteem
- Mental illness
- Neurological defects

Domain 7

- Pain
- Physical illness
- Substance abuse

Social

- Conflict
- Developmental level
- Domestic violence

- Inadequate role socialization
- Inadequate support system
- Inappropriate linkage with the healthcare system
- Job schedule demands
- Lack of resources
- Lack of rewards
- Low socioeconomic status
- Stress
- Young age

Impaired Social Interaction (00052)
(1986)

Domain 7: Role Relationships
Class 3: Role Performance

Definition Insufficient or excessive quantity or ineffective quality of social exchange

Defining Characteristics

- Discomfort in social situations
- Dysfunctional interaction with others
- Family report of changes in interaction (e.g., style, pattern)
- Inability to communicate a satisfying sense of social engagement (e.g., belonging, caring, interest, shared history)
- Inability to receive a satisfying sense of social engagement (e.g., belonging, caring, interest, shared history)
- Use of unsuccessful social interaction behaviors

Related Factors

- Absence of significant others
- Communication barriers
- Deficit about ways to enhance mutuality (e.g., knowledge, skills)
- Disturbed thought processes
- Environmental barriers
- Limited physical mobility
- Self-concept disturbance
- Sociocultural dissonance
- Therapeutic isolation

Domain 7

Domain 8
Sexuality

Sexual Dysfunction (00059)
(1980, 2006, LOE 2.1)

Domain 8: Sexuality
Class 2: Sexual Function

Definition The state in which an individual experiences a change in sexual function during the sexual response phases of desire, excitation, and/or orgasm, which is viewed as unsatisfying, unrewarding, or inadequate

Defining Characteristics

- Alterations in achieving sexual satisfaction
- Alterations in achieving perceived sex role
- Actual limitations imposed by disease
- Actual limitations imposed by therapy
- Change of interest in others
- Change of interest in self
- Inability to achieve desired satisfaction
- Perceived alteration in sexual excitation
- Perceived deficiency of sexual desire
- Perceived limitations imposed by disease
- Perceived limitations imposed by therapy
- Seeking confirmation of desirability
- Verbalization of problem

Related Factors

- Absent role models
- Altered body function (e.g., pregnancy, recent childbirth, drugs, surgery, anomalies, disease process, trauma, radiation)
- Altered body structure (e.g., pregnancy, recent childbirth, surgery, anomalies, disease process, trauma, radiation)
- Biopsychosocial alteration of sexuality
- Deficient knowledge
- Ineffectual role models
- Lack of privacy
- Lack of significant other
- Misinformation
- Values conflict
- Psychosocial abuse (e.g., harmful relationships)
- Physical abuse
- Vulnerability

References

Cavalcanti, R. & Cavalcanti, M. (1996). *Tratamento clínico das inadequacies sexuals*, 2nd edn. São Paulo: Roca.

Domain 8

Fehring, R.J. (1994). The Fehring model. In: Carrol-Johnson, R.M. & Paquete, M. (eds). *Classification of nursing diagnoses: Proceedings of the Tenth Conference*. Philadelphia: J.B. Lippincott, pp. 55–62

Hogan, R.M. (1985). *Human sexuality: A nursing perspective*. New York: Appleton-Century-Crofts.

Hoskins, L.M. (1989). Clinical validation, methodologies for nursing diagnoses research. In: Carrol Johnson, R.M. et al. (eds), *Classification of nursing diagnoses: Proceedings of the eighth conference of North American Nursing Diagnosis Association*. Philadelphia: Lippincott, pp. 126–31.

Kaplan, H.S. (1977). *A nova terapia do sexo: tratamento dinâmico das disfuncões sexuals*. Rio de Janeiro: Nova Fronteira.

Kaplan, H.S. (1983). *O desejo sexual – e novos conceitos etécnicas da terapia do sexo*. Rio de Janeiro: Nova Fronteira.

Domain 8

Domain 8: Sexuality
Class 2: Sexual Function

Definition   Expressions of concern regarding own sexuality

Defining Characteristics

- Alterations in achieving perceived sex role
- Alteration in relationship with significant other
- Conflicts involving values
- Reported changes in sexual activities
- Reported changes in sexual behaviors
- Reported difficulties in sexual activities
- Reported difficulties in sexual behaviors
- Reported limitations in sexual activities
- Reported limitations in sexual behaviors

Related Factors

- Absent role model
- Conflicts with sexual orientation preferences
- Conflicts with variant preferences
- Fear of acquiring a sexually transmitted infection
- Fear of pregnancy
- Impaired relationship with a significant other
- Ineffective role model
- Knowledge about alternative responses to health related transitions, altered body function or structure, illness, or medical treatment
- Lack of privacy
- Lack of significant other
- Skill deficit about alternative responses to health-related transitions, altered body function or structure, illness, or medical treatment

References

Cavalcanti, R. & Cavalcanti, M. (1996). *Tratamento clinico das inadequacies sexuals*, 2nd edn. São Paulo: Roca.

Fehring, R.J. (1994). The Fehring model. In: Carrol-Johnson, R.M. & Paquete, M. (eds), *Classification of nursing diagnoses: Proceedings of the Tenth Conference*. Philadelphia: J.B. Lippincott, pp. 55–62

Hogan, R.M. (1985). *Human sexuality: A nursing perspective*. New York: Appleton-Century-Crofts.

Domain 8

Hoskins, L.M. (1989). Clinical validation, methodologies for nursing diagnoses research. In: Carrol Johnson, R.M. et al. (eds), *Classification of nursing diagnoses: Proceedings of the eighth conference of North American Nursing Diagnosis Association*. Philadelphia: Lippincott, pp. 126–31.

Kaplan, H.S. (1977). *A nova terapia do sexo: tratamento dinâmico das disfuncões sexuals*. Rio de Janeiro: Nova Fronteira.

Kaplan, H.S. (1983). *O desejo sexual – e novos conceitos etécnicas da terapia do sexo*. Rio de Janeiro: Nova Fronteira.

Domain 8

Domain 8: Sexuality
Class 3: Reproduction

Definition   A pattern of preparing for, maintaining and strengthening a healthy pregnancy and childbirth process and care of newborn*

Defining Characteristics

During Pregnancy

■ Reports appropriate prenatal lifestyle (e.g., diet, elimination, sleep, bodily movement, exercise, personal hygiene)
■ Reports appropriate physical preparations
■ Reports managing unpleasant symptoms in pregnancy
■ Demonstrates respect for unborn baby
■ Reports a realistic birth plan
■ Prepares necessary newborn care items
■ Seeks necessary knowledge (e.g., of labor and delivery, newborn care)
■ Reports availability of support systems
■ Has regular prenatal health visits

During Labor and Delivery

■ Reports lifestyle (e.g., diet, elimination, sleep, bodily movement, personal hygiene) that is appropriate for the stage of labor
■ Responds appropriately to onset of labor
■ Is proactive in labor and delivery
■ Uses relaxation techniques appropriate for the stage of labor
■ Demonstrates attachment behavior to the newborn baby
■ Utilizes support systems appropriately

After Birth*

■ Demonstrates appropriate baby feeding techniques
■ Demonstrates appropriate breast care
■ Demonstrates attachment behavior to the baby
■ Demonstrates basic baby care techniques
■ Provides safe environment for the baby

* The original Japanese term for "Childbearing" is "Shussan Ikuji Koudou" which encompasses both childbirth and rearing of neonate. It is one of the main concepts of Japanese midwifrey.

Domain 8

- Reports appropriate postpartum lifestyle (e.g. diet, elimination, sleep, bodily movement, exercise, personal hygiene)
- Utilizes support system appropriately

References

Aoki, Y., ed. (1998). *Bosei Hoken wo meguru Shidou Kyouiku Soudan 2* [*Coaching, education, and counseling in maternal health*, Vol. 2]. Tokyo: Life Science Co.

Aoki, Y., Kato, N., & Hirasawa, M., eds (2002). *Josangaku Taikei 5 Boshi no Shinri Shakaigaku* [*Midwifery System* Vol. 5 *Psychosociology for mother and child*]. Tokyo: Japanese Nursing Association Publishing Co.

Aoki, Y., Kato, N., & Hirasawa, M., eds (2003). *Josangaku Taikei 8 Josan Shindan Gijyutsu-gaku 2* [*Midwifery System* Vol. 8 *Maternity diagnoses and techniques* 2]. Tokyo: Japanese Nursing Association Publishing Co.

Japan Society for Maternity Diagnoses, ed. (2004). *Maternity Shindan guidebook* [*Guidebook of maternity diagnoses*]. Tokyo: Igakushoin.

Kabeyama, K., ed. (2006). *Rinsho Josanfu Hikkei: Seimei to Bunka wo Fumaeta Shigen* [*Essentials of clinical midwifery: Caring based on life and culture*, 2nd edn)]. Tokyo: Igakushoin.

Okayama National Hospital, ed. (2000). *Akachan ni Yasashii Byouin no Bonyuu Ikuji Shidou* [*Breast-feeding and newborn-care teaching manuals from a baby-friendly hospital*]. Tokyo: Medica Publishing Co.

Taketani, Y. & Kabeyama, S., eds)(2007). *Josangaku Kouza 6* [*Midwifery Course* Vol. 6]. Tokyo: Igakushoin.

Domain 8

Risk for Disturbed Maternal/Fetal Dyad (00209)

Domain 8: Sexuality
Class 3: Reproduction

Definition   At risk for disruption of the symbiotic maternal/fetal dyad as a result of comorbid or pregnancy-related conditions

Risk Factors

- Complications of pregnancy (e.g., premature rupture of membranes, placenta previa or abruption, late prenatal care, multiple gestation)
- Compromised O_2 transport (e.g., anemia, cardiac disease, asthma, hypertension, seizures, premature labor, hemorrhage)
- Impaired glucose metabolism (e.g., diabetes, steroid use)
- Physical abuse
- Substance abuse (e.g., tobacco, alcohol, drugs)
- Treatment related side effects (e.g., medications, surgery, chemotherapy)

References

Berg, M. (2005). Pregnancy and diabetes: How women handle the challenges. *Journal of Perinatal Education* **14**(3): 23–32.

Curran, C.A. (2003). Intrapartum emergencies. *Journal of Obstetric, Gynecologic, & Neonatal Nursing* **32**: 802–13.

Higgins, L.P. & Hawkins, J.W. (2005). Screening for abuse during pregnancy: Implementing a multisite program. *American Journal of Maternal/Child Nursing* **30**: 109–14.

Lange, S.S. & Jenner, M. (2004). Myocardial infarction in the obstetric patient. In: Campbell, P.T. (ed.), *Critical care nursing clinics of North America: Obstetric and neonatal intensive care*, Vol. 16(2). Philadelphia: Elsevier Saunders, pp. 211–19.

McCarter-Spaulding, D.E. (2005). Medications in pregnancy and lactation. *American Journal of Maternal/Child Nursing* **30**: 10–17.

Poole, J.H. (2004). Multiorgan dysfunction in the perinatal patient. In: Campbell, P.T. (ed.), *Critical care nursing clinics of North America: Obstetric and neonatal intensive care*, Vol. 16(2). Philadelphia: Elsevier Saunders, pp. 193–204.

Rudisill, P.T. (2004). Amniotic fluid embolism. In: Campbell, P.T. (ed.), *Critical care nursing clinics of North America: Obstetric and neonatal intensive care*, Vol. 16(2). Philadelphia: Elsevier Saunders, pp. 221–5

Shannon, M., King, T.L., & Kennedy, H.P. (2007). Allostasis: A theoretical framework for understanding and evaluating perinatal health outcomes. *Journal of Obstetric, Gynecologic, & Neonatal Nursing* **36**: 125–34.

Simpson, K.R. (2004). Monitoring the preterm fetus during labor. *American Journal of Maternal/Child Nursing* **29**: 380–8.

Domain 8

Stark, C.J. & Stepans, M.B.F. (2004). A comparison of blood pressure in term, low birth weight infants of smoking and nonsmoking mothers. *Journal of Perinatal Education* **13**(4): 17–26.

Stringer, M., Miesnik, S. R., Brown, L., Martz, A.H., & Macones, G. (2004). Nursing care of the patient with preterm premature rupture of membranes. *American Journal of Maternal/Child Nursing* **29**: 144–150.

Torgersen, K.L. & Curran, C.A. (2006). A systematic approach to the physiologic adaptations of pregnancy. *Critical Care Nursing Quarterly* **29**(1): 2–19.

Wolfe, B.E. (2005). Reproductive health in women with eating disorders. *Journal of Obstetric, Gynecologic, & Neonatal Nursing* **34**: 255–63.

Domain 8

Domain 9
Coping/Stress Tolerance

Post-Trauma Syndrome (00141)
(1986, 1998)

Domain 9: Coping/Stress Tolerance
Class 1: Post-Trauma Responses

Definition Sustained maladaptive response to a traumatic, overwhelming event

Defining Characteristics

- Aggression
- Alienation
- Altered mood states
- Anger
- Anxiety
- Avoidance
- Compulsive behavior
- Denial
- Depression
- Detachment
- Difficulty concentrating
- Enuresis (in children)
- Exaggerated startle response
- Fear
- Flashbacks
- Gastric irritability
- Grieving
- Guilt
- Headaches
- Hopelessness
- Horror
- Hypervigilance
- Intrusive dreams
- Intrusive thoughts
- Irritability
- Neurosensory irritability
- Nightmares
- Palpitations
- Panic attacks
- Psychogenic amnesia
- Rage
- Rape
- Reports feeling numb
- Repression
- Shame
- Substance abuse

Related Factors

- Abuse (physical and/or psychosocial)
- Being held prisoner of war
- Criminal victimization
- Disasters
- Epidemics
- Events outside the range of usual human experience
- Serious accidents (e.g., industrial, motor vehicle)
- Serious injury to loved ones
- Serious injury to self
- Serious threat to loved ones
- Serious threat to self
- Sudden destruction of one's community
- Sudden destruction of one's home
- Torture
- Tragic occurrence involving multiple deaths
- Wars
- Witnessing mutilation
- Witnessing violent death

Domain 9

Domain 9: Coping/Stress Tolerance
Class 1: Post-Trauma Responses

Definition At risk for sustained maladaptive response to a traumatic, overwhelming event

Risk Factors

- Diminished ego strength
- Displacement from home
- Duration of the event
- Exaggerated sense of responsibility
- Inadequate social support
- Occupation (e.g., police, fire, rescue, corrections, emergency room staff, mental health worker)
- Perception of event
- Survivor's role in the event
- Unsupportive environment

Domain 9: Coping/Stress Tolerance
Class 1: Post-Trauma Responses

Definition Sustained maladaptive response to a forced, violent sexual penetration against the victim's will and consent

Defining Characteristics

- Aggression
- Agitation
- Anger
- Anxiety
- Change in relationships
- Confusion
- Denial
- Dependence
- Depression
- Disorganization
- Dissociative disorders
- Embarrassment
- Fear
- Guilt
- Helplessness
- Humiliation
- Hyperalertness
- Impaired decision-making
- Loss of self-esteem
- Mood swings
- Muscle spasms
- Muscle tension
- Nightmares
- Paranoia
- Phobias
- Physical trauma
- Powerlessness
- Revenge
- Self-blame
- Sexual dysfunction
- Shame
- Shock
- Sleep disturbances
- Substance abuse
- Suicide attempts
- Vulnerability

Related Factors

- Rape

Domain 9

Relocation Stress Syndrome (00114)
(1992, 2000)

Domain 9: Coping/Stress Tolerance
Class 1: Post-Trauma Responses

Definition Physiological and/or psychosocial disturbance following transfer from one environment to another

Defining Characteristics

- Alienation
- Aloneness
- Anger
- Anxiety (e.g., separation)
- Concern over relocation
- Dependency
- Depression
- Fear
- Frustration
- Increased illness
- Increased physical symptoms
- Increased verbalization of needs
- Insecurity
- Loneliness
- Loss of identity
- Loss of self-esteem
- Loss of self-worth
- Pessimism
- Sleep disturbance
- Verbalizes unwillingness to move
- Withdrawal
- Worry

Related Factors

- Decreased health status
- Feelings of powerlessness
- Unpredictability of experience
- Impaired psychosocial health
- Isolation
- Lack of adequate support system
- Lack of predeparture counseling
- Language barrier
- Losses
- Move from one environment to another
- Passive coping

Risk for Relocation Stress Syndrome

(00149)

(2000)

Domain 9: Coping/Stress Tolerance
Class 1: Post-Trauma Responses

Definition   At risk for physiological and/or psychosocial disturbance following transfer from one environment to another

Risk Factors

- Decreased health status
- Lack of adequate support system
- Lack of predeparture counseling
- Losses
- Moderate-to-high degree of environmental change
- Moderate mental competence
- Move from one environment to another
- Passive coping
- Unpredictability of experiences
- Verbal expression of powerlessness

Domain 9

Anxiety (00146)
(1973, 1982, 1998)

Domain 9: Coping/Stress Tolerance
Class 2: Coping Responses

Definition Vague uneasy feeling of discomfort or dread accompanied by an autonomic response (the source often nonspecific or unknown to the individual); a feeling of apprehension caused by anticipation of danger. It is an alerting signal that warns of impending danger and enables the individual to take measures to deal with threat

Defining Characteristics

Behavioral

- Diminished productivity
- Expressed concerns due to change in life events
- Extraneous movement
- Fidgeting
- Glancing about
- Insomnia
- Poor eye contact
- Restlessness
- Scanning
- Vigilance

Affective

- Apprehensive
- Anguish
- Distressed
- Fearful
- Feelings of inadequacy
- Focus on self
- Increased wariness
- Irritability
- Jittery
- Overexcited
- Painful increased helplessness
- Persistent increased helplessness
- Rattled

- Regretful
- Uncertainty
- Worried

Physiological

- Facial tension
- Hand tremors
- Increased perspiration
- Increased tension
- Shakiness
- Trembling
- Voice quivering

Sympathetic

- Anorexia
- Cardiovascular excitation
- Diarrhea
- Dry mouth
- Facial flushing
- Heart pounding
- Increased blood pressure
- Increased pulse
- Increased reflexes
- Increased respiration
- Pupil dilation
- Respiratory difficulties
- Superficial vasoconstriction

- Twitching
- Weakness

Parasympathetic

- Abdominal pain
- Decreased blood pressure
- Decreased pulse
- Diarrhea
- Faintness
- Fatigue
- Nausea
- Sleep disturbance
- Tingling in extremities
- Urinary frequency
- Urinary hesitancy
- Urinary urgency

Cognitive

- Awareness of physiologic symptoms
- Blocking of thought
- Confusion
- Decreased perceptual field
- Difficulty concentrating
- Diminished ability to learn
- Diminished ability to problem solve
- Fear of unspecified consequences
- Forgetfulness
- Impaired attention
- Preoccupation
- Rumination
- Tendency to blame others

Related Factors

- Change in:
  - Economic status
  - Environment
  - Health status
  - Interaction patterns
  - Role function
  - Role status
- Exposure to toxins
- Familial association
- Heredity
- Interpersonal contagion
- Interpersonal transmission
- Maturational crises
- Situational crises
- Stress

- Substance abuse
- Threat of death
- Threat to:
  - Economic status
  - Environment
  - Health status
  - Interaction patterns
  - Role function
  - Role status
  - Self-concept
- Unconscious conflict about essential goals of life
- Unconscious conflict about essential values
- Unmet needs

Domain 9

Death Anxiety (00147)

(1998, 2006, LOE 2.1)

Domain 9: Coping/Stress Tolerance
Class 2: Coping Responses

Definition Vague uneasy feeling of discomfort or dread generated by perceptions of a real or imagined threat to one's existence

Defining Characteristics

- Reports concerns of overworking the caregiver
- Reports deep sadness
- Reports fear of developing terminal illness
- Reports fear of loss of mental abilities when dying
- Reports fear of pain related to dying
- Reports fear of premature death
- Reports fear of the process of dying
- Reports fear of prolonged dying
- Reports fear of suffering related to dying
- Reports feeling powerless over dying
- Reports negative thoughts related to death and dying
- Reports worry about the impact of one's own death on significant others

Related Factors

- Anticipating adverse consequences of general anesthesia
- Anticipating impact of death on others
- Anticipating pain
- Anticipating suffering
- Confronting reality of terminal disease
- Discussions on topic of death
- Experiencing dying process
- Near death experience
- Nonacceptance of own mortality
- Observations related to death
- Perceived proximity of death
- Uncertainty about an encounter with a higher power
- Uncertainty about the existence of a higher power
- Uncertainty about life after death
- Uncertainty of prognosis

References

Abdel-Khalek, AM. & Tomàs-Sàbado, J. (2005). Anxiety and death anxiety in Egyptian and Spanish nursing students, *Death Studies* **29**: 157–69.

Aday, R.H. (1984–85). Belief in afterlife and death anxiety: correlates and comparisons. *Omega: Journal of Death and Dying* **15**: 67–75.

Adelbratt, S. & Strang, P. (2000). Death anxiety in brain tumour patients and their spouses. *Palliative Medicine* **14**: 499–507.

Alvarado, J.A., Templer, D.I., Bresler, C., & Thomas-Dobson, S. (1995). The relationship of religious variables to death depresión and death anxiety. *Journal of Clinical Psychology* **51**: 202–4.

Amenta, M.M. (1984). Death anxiety purpose in life and duration of service in hospice volunteers. *Psychological Reports* **54**: 979–84.

Angst, J., Angst, F., & Stassen, H.H. (1999). Suicide risk in patients with major depressive disorder. *Journal of Clinical Psychiatry* **60**: 57–72.

Bay, E. & Algase, D.L. (1999). Fear and anxiety: a simultaneous concept analysis. *Nursing Diagnosis* **10**: 103–11.

Beck, C.T. (1997). Nursing students' experiences caring for dying patients. *Journal of Nursing Education* **36**: 408–15.

Bene, B. & Foxall, M.J. (1991). Death anxiety and job stress in hospice and medical-surgical nurses. *Hospice Journal* **7**: 25–41.

Bolt, M. (1977). Religious orientation and death fears. *Review of Religious Research* **19**: 73–6.

Braunstein, J.W. (2000). An investigation of irrational beliefs and death anxiety as a function of HIV status in homosexual men (immune deficiency). *The Sciences and Engineering* **61**: 1626.

Brockopp, D.Y,. King, D.B., & Hamilton, J.E. (1991). The dying patient: a comparative study of nurse caregiver characteristics. *Death Studies* **15**: 245–8.

Chiappetta, W., Floyd, H.H., & McSeveney, D.R. (1977). Sex differences in coping with death anxiety. *Psychological Reports* **39**: 945–6.

Clements, R. (1998). Intrinsic religious motivation and attitudes toward death among the elderly. *Current Psychology* **17**: 237–48.

Cully, J.A., La Voie, D., & Gfeller, J.D. (2001). Reminiscence, personality, and psychological functioning in older adults. *Gerontologist* **41**: 89–95.

Hunt, B. & Rosenthal, D.A. (2000). Rehabilitation counselors' experiences with client death anxiety. *Journal of Rehabilitation* **66**: 44–50.

Kuuppelomaky, M. (2000). Cancer patients', family members' and professional helpers' conceptions and beliefs concerning death. *European Journal of Oncology Nursing* **4**(1): 39–47.

Kastenbaum, R, (1992). *The psychology of death*. New York: The Guilford Press

Matalon, T.H. (2000). The relationship among children's conceptualization of death, parental communication about death, and parental death anxiety. *Humanities and Social Sciences* **61**: 510.

Mok, E., Lee, W.M., & Wong, F.K. (2002). The issue of death and dying: employing problem-based learning in nursing education. *Nurse Education Today* **22**: 319–29.

Nelson, L.D. & Cantrell, C.H. (1980). Religiosity and death anxiety: A multi-dimensional Analysis. *Review of religious Research* **21**: 148–57.

Rasmussen, C.A. & Brems, C. (1996). The relationship of death anxiety with age psychosocial maturity. *Journal of Psychology* **130**: 141–4.

Rasmussen, C.H. & Johnson, M.E. (1994). Spirituality and religiosity: Relative relationships to death anxiety. *Omega: Journal of Death and Dying* **29**: 313–18.

Robbins, R.A. (1992). Death competency: a study of hospice volunteers. *Death Studies* **16**: 557–69.

Domain 9

Rosenhein, E. & Muchnick, B. (1984–85). Death concerns in differential levels of consciousness as functions of defence strategy and religious belief. *Omega: Journal of Death and Dying* **15**: 15–24.

Sanders, J.F., Poole, T.E., & Rivero, W.T. (1980). Death anxiety among the elderly. *Psychological Reports* **46**: 53–4.

Sherman, D.W. (1996). Nurses' willingness to care for AIDS patients and spirituality, social support, and death anxiety. *Image: Journal of Nursing Scholarship* **28**: 205–13.

Stoller, E.P. (1980–81). The impact of death-related fears on attitudes of nurses in hospital work setting. *Omega: Journal of Death and Dying* **11**: 85–96.

Straub, S.H., & Roberts, J.M. (2001). Fear of death in widows: Effects of age at widowhood and suddenness of death. *Omega: Journal of Death and Dying* **43**: 25–41.

Sulmasy, D.P. & McIlvane, J.M. (2002). Patients' ratings of quality and satisfaction with care at the end of life. *Archive of Internal Medicine* **162**: 2098–104.

Whitley, G.G. (1994). Expert validation and differentiation of the nursing diagnosis anxiety and fear. *Nursing Diagnosis* **5**: 143–50.

Whitley, G.G. & Tousman, S.A. (1996). A multivariate approach for validation of anxiety and fear. *Nursing Diagnosis* **7**: 116–24.

Whitley, G.G. (1997). Three phases of research in validating nursing diagnoses. *Western Journal of Nursing Research* **19**: 379–99.

Whitley, G.G. (1999). Processes and methodologies for research validation of nursing diagnoses. *Nursing Diagnosis* **10**(1): 5–14.

Domain 9: Coping/Stress Tolerance
Class 2: Coping Responses

Definition
Impaired ability to modify lifestyle/behaviors in a manner that improves health status

Defining Characteristics

- Demonstrates nonacceptance of health status change
- Failure to achieve optimal sense of control
- Failure to take action that prevents health problems
- Minimizes health status change

Related Factors

- Excessive alcohol
- Inadequate comprehension
- Inadequate social support
- Low self-efficacy
- Low socioeconomic status
- Multiple stressors
- Negative attitude toward healthcare
- Smoking

References

Alder, J. & Bitzer, J. (2003). Retrospective evaluation of the treatment for breast cancer: How does the patient's personal experience of the treatment affect later adjustment to the illness? [Electronic version]. *Archives of Women's Mental Health* **6**: 91–7.

American Medical Association (2001). Executive summary of the third report of the national cholesterol education program (NCEP) expert panel on detection, evaluation, and treatment of high blood cholesterol in adults (adult treatment panel III). *Journal of the American Medical Association* **285**: 2486–97.

Bandura A. (1982). Self Efficacy Mechanism in human agency. *American Psychologist* **37**: 122–7.

Bornstein, J. & Bahat-Sterensus, H. (2004). Predictive factors for noncompliance with follow-up among women treated for cervical intraepithelial neoplasia. *Gynecologic and Obstetric investigation* **58**: 202–6.

DiMatteo, R.M., Lepper, H.S., & Croghan, T.W. (2000). Depression is a risk factor for non-compliance with medical treatment. *Archives of Internal Medicine* **160**: 2101–7.

Jager, B., Liedtke, R., Lamprecht, F., & Freyberger, H. (2004). Social and health adjustment of bulimic women 7–9 years following therapy. [Electronic version] *Acta Psychiatrica Scandinavia* **110**: 138–45.

* This diagnosis formerly held the label, *Impaired Adjustment*.

Domain 9

Kiefe, C.L., Heudebert, G., Box, J.B., Farmer, R.M., Micahel, M., & Clancy, C.M. (1999). Compliance with post-hospitalization follow-up visits: rationing by inconvenience? [Electronic version] *Ethnicity & disease* **19**: 387–95.

Koenigsberg, M., Barlett, D. & Carmer, J.S. (2004). Facilitating treatment adherence with lifestyle changes in diabetes. [Electronic version] *American Family Physician* **69**: 309–16, 319–20, 323–4.

Lifshitz, H. & Glaubman, R. (2004). Caring for the people with disabilities in the Haredi community: Adjustment mechanism in action. [Electronic version] *Disability and Society* **19**: 469–86.

Medline. *Medline plus medical encyclopedia.* Available at: www/nlm.nih.gov/medline-plus/ency/article/000932.htm (accessed October 21, 2004).

Merriam-Webster (1993). *Webster's third new international dictionary, unabridged.* Springfield, MA: Merriam-Webster.

National Heart, Lung, and Blood Institute. *How you can lower your cholesterol level?* Available at: www.nhlbi.nih.gov/chd/lifestyles.htm (accessed May 23, 2008).

National Heart, Lung, and Blood Institute (2003). *Seventh report of the Joint National Committee of the Prevention, Detection, Evaluation, and Treatment of High Blood Pressure (JNC 7).* Available at: www.nhlbi.nih.gov/guidelines/hypertension/jnc7full.htm (accessed May 23, 2008).

National Kidney Foundation/Kidney Disease Outcomes Institute Guidelines (2002). *K/DOQI Clinical practice guidelines for chronic kidney disease: Evaluation, classification, and stratification.* Available at: www.kidney.org/professionals/kdoqi/p4_class_g2.htm (accessed May 1, 2005).

Newsom, J.T., Kaplan, M. S., Huguet, N. & Mcfarland, B.H. (2004). Health behaviors in a representative sample of older Canadians: Prevalences, reported change, motivation to change, and perceived barriers [Electronic version]. *The Gerontologist* **44**:193–205.

Nose, M. & Barbui, C. (2003). Systematic review of clinical interventions for reducing treatment non adherence in psychosis. [Electronic version]. *Epidemiologia e psichiatria sociale* **12**: 272–86.

Pinto, M.B., Maruyama, N.C., Clark, M.M., Cruess, D.G., Park, E., & Roberts, M. (2002). Motivation to modify lifestyle risk behaviors in women treated for breast cancer [Electronic version]. *Mayo Foundation for Medical Education and Research* **77**: 122–9.

Prelow, H.M., Danoff-Burg, S., Swenson, R.R., & Pulgiano, D. (2004). The impact of ecological risk and perceived discrimination on the psychological adjustment of African American and European youth [Electronic version]. *Journal of Community Psychology* **32**: 375–89.

Psyweb. *Adjustment disorders.* Available at: www.psyweb.com/Mdisord/adjd.html (accessed May 23, 2008).

Shemesh, E. (2004). Non-adherence to medications following pediatric liver transplantation. [Electronic version]. *Pediatric Transplantation* **8**: 600–5.

Uphold C.R. & Graham, M.R. (2003) *Clinical guidelines in family practice,* 4th edn. Gainesville, FL: Barmarrae Books.

Compromised Family Coping (00074)
(1980, 1996)

Domain 9: Coping/Stress Tolerance
Class 2: Coping Responses

Definition Usually supportive primary person (family member or close friend) provides insufficient, ineffective, or compromised support, comfort, assistance, or encouragement that may be needed by the client to manage or master adaptive tasks related to his or her health challenge

Defining Characteristics

Objective

- Significant person attempts assistive behaviors with unsatisfactory results
- Significant person attempts supportive behaviors with unsatisfactory results
- Significant person displays protective behavior disproportionate to client's abilities
- Significant person displays protective behavior disproportionate to client's need for autonomy
- Significant person enters into limited personal communication with client
- Significant person withdraws from client

Subjective

- Client expresses a complaint about significant person's response to health problem
- Client expresses a concern about significant person's response to health problem
- Significant person expresses an inadequate knowledge base, which interferes with effective supportive behaviors
- Significant person expresses an inadequate understanding, which interferes with supportive behaviors
- Significant person describes preoccupation with personal reaction (e.g., fear, anticipatory grief, guilt, anxiety) to client's need

Related Factors

- Coexisting situations affecting the significant person
- Developmental crises that the significant person may be facing
- Exhaustion of supportive capacity of significant people
- Inadequate information by a primary person
- Inadequate understanding of information by a primary person
- Incorrect information by a primary person

Domain 9

- Incorrect understanding of information by a primary person
- Lack of reciprocal support
- Little support provided by client, in turn, for primary person
- Prolonged disease that exhausts supportive capacity of significant people
- Situational crises that the significant person may be facing
- Temporary family disorganization
- Temporary family role changes
- Temporary preoccupation by a significant person

Defensive Coping (00071)
(1988, 2008, LOE 2.1)

Domain 9: Coping/Stress Tolerance
Class 2: Coping Responses

Definition Repeated projection of falsely positive self-evaluation based on a self-protective pattern that defends against underlying perceived threats to positive self-regard

Defining Characteristics

- Denial of obvious problems
- Denial of obvious weaknesses
- Difficulty establishing relationships
- Difficulty maintaining relationships
- Difficulty in perception of reality testing
- Grandiosity
- Hostile laughter
- Hypersensitivity to criticism
- Hypersensitivity to slight
- Lack of follow-through in therapy
- Lack of follow-through in treatment
- Lack of participation in therapy
- Lack of participation in treatment
- Projection of blame
- Projection of responsibility
- Rationalization of failures
- Reality distortion
- Ridicule of others
- Superior attitude toward others

Related Factors

- Conflict between self-perception and value system
- Deficient support system
- Fear of failure
- Fear of humiliation
- Fear of repercussions
- Lack of resilience
- Low level of confidence in others
- Low level of self confidence
- Uncertainty
- Unrealistic expectations of self

References

Balder, L. & Denour, A.K. (1984). Couples' reactions and adjustments to mastectomy. *Int J Psychiatry in Men* **14**: 265–70.

Bartek S.E., Krebs D.L., & Taylor, M.C. (1993). Coping, defending, and the relations between moral judgment and moral behavior in prostitutes and other female juvenile delinquents. *J Abnorm Psychol* **102**(1): 66–73.

Domain 9

Bean, G., Cooper, S., Alpert, R., & Kipnis, D. (1980). Coping mechanisms of cancer patients: a study of 33 patients receiving chemotherapy. *CA* **30**: 257–9.

Brown J.D. & Dutton, K.A. (1995). The thrill of victory, the complexity of defeat: self-esteem and people's emotional reactions to success and failure. *J Pers Soc Psychol* **68**: 712–22.

Cassileth, B.R., Lusk, E.J., Strouse, T.B., Miller, D.S., Brown, L.L., & Cross, P.A. (1985). Psychological analysis of cancer patients and their next of kin. *Cancer* **55**: 72–6.

Coelho, G.V., Hamburg, D.A. & Adams, J.E. (1974). *Coping and Adaptation.* New York: Basic Books.

Coopersmith, S. (1967). *Antecedents of self-esteem.* San Francisco, CA: Freeman, Cooper.

Creswell C. & Chalder, T. (2001). Defensive coping styles in chronic fatigue syndrome. *J Psychosom Res* **51**: 607–10.

Cyspouw-Guitouni, A. (2001). L'avenir et la sauvegarde des valeurs. *Psychologie Préventive* **37**:18–23.

Dalle Grave R., Calugi S., Molinari E., et al. & QUOVADIS Study Group (2005). Weight loss expectations in obese patients and treatment attrition: an observational multi-center study. *Obese Res* **13**: 1961–9.

George, J.M., Scott, D.S., Turner, S.P., & Gregg, J.M. (1980). The effects of psychological factors of physical trauma on recovery from oral surgery. *J Behav Med* **3**: 291–310.

Guitouni, M. (2002). Le choix d'une génération: démisionner ou résister. *Psychologie Préventive* **38**: 25–9.

Jaramillo-Velez D.E., Ospina-Munoz D.E., Cabarcas-Iglesias G., & Humphreys, J. (2005). Resilience, spirituality, distress and tactics for battered women's conflict resolution. *Rev Salud Publica* **7**: 281–92 (Spanish).

Kools S. (1999). Self-protection in adolescents in foster care. *J Child Adolesc Psychiatr Nurs* **12**: 139–52.

Lazarus, R.S. (1966). *Psychological stress and the coping process.* New York: McGraw-Hill.

Lindstrom, T.C. (1989). Defence mechanisms and some notes on their relevance for the caring professions. *Scand J Caring Sci* **3**(3): 99–104.

McFarland, G.K. and McFarlane, E.A. (1995). *Traité de diagnostic infirmier* (adaptation of S. Truchon & D. Fleury). St-Laurent: ERPI, pp. 741–52.

Meredith P.J., Strong J., & Feeney, J.A. (2006) The relationship of adult attachment to emotion, catastrophizing, control, threshold and tolerance, in experimentally-induced pain. *Pain* **120**(1–2): 44–52. Epub 2005 Dec 13.

Morris, C.A. (1985). Self-concept as altered by the diagnosis of cancer. *Nurs Clin North Am* **20**: 611–30.

Noy, S. (2004). Minimizing casualties in biological and chemical threats (war and terrorism): the importance of information to the public in a prevention program. *Prehospital Disaster Med* **19**(1): 29–36.

Perez-Sales, P. & Vazquez Valverde, C. (2003). Support psychotherapy in traumatic situations. *Rev Enferm* **26**(12): 44–52 (Spanish).

Taubes, I. (2002). Tout commence par une confiance primitive dans la vie: entretien avec Boris Cyulnik. *Psychologies* March: 90–4.

Taubes, I. (2005). Je fuis les responsabilités. *Psychologies* March: 88–9.

Tod, A.M. & Lacey, A. (2004). Overweight and obesity: helping clients to take action. *Br J Community Nurs* **9**(2): 59–66.

Tromp, D.M., Brouha, X.D., De Leeuw, J.R., Hordijk, G.J., & Winnubst, J.A (2004). Psychological factors and patient delay in patients with head and neck cancer. *Eur J Cancer* **40**: 1509–16.

Worder, J.W. & Sobel. J. (1978). Ego strength and psychosocial adaptation to cancer. *Psychosom Med* **40**: 585–92.

Yehuda, R., McFarlane, A.C., & Shalev, A.Y. (1998). Predicting the development of post-traumatic stress disorder from the acute response to a traumatic event. *Biol Psychiatry* **44**: 1305–13.

Domain 9

Domain 9: Coping/Stress Tolerance
Class 2: Coping Responses

Definition Behavior of significant person (family member or other primary person) that disables his or her capacities and the client's capacities to effectively address tasks essential to either person's adaptation to the health challenge

Defining Characteristics

- Abandonment
- Aggression
- Agitation
- Carrying on usual routines without regard for client's needs
- Client's development of dependence
- Depression
- Desertion
- Disregarding client's needs
- Distortion of reality regarding client's health problem
- Family behaviors that are detrimental to well-being
- Hostility
- Impaired individualization
- Impaired restructuring of a meaningful life for self
- Intolerance
- Neglectful care of client in regard to basic human needs
- Neglectful care of client in regard to illness treatment
- Neglectful relationships with other family members
- Prolonged over-concern for client
- Psychosomaticism
- Rejection
- Taking on illness signs of client

Related Factors

- Arbitrary handling of family's resistance to treatment
- Dissonant coping styles for dealing with adaptive tasks by the significant person and client
- Dissonant coping styles among significant people
- Highly ambivalent family relationships
- Significant person with chronically unexpressed feelings (e.g., guilt, anxiety, hostility, despair)

Domain 9

Ineffective Coping (00069)
(1978, 1998)

Domain 9: Coping/Stress Tolerance
Class 2: Coping Responses

Definition Inability to form a valid appraisal of the stressors, inadequate choices of practiced responses, and/or inability to use available resources

Defining Characteristics

- Abuse of chemical agents
- Change in usual communication patterns
- Decreased use of social support
- Destructive behavior toward others
- Destructive behavior toward self
- Difficulty organizing information
- Fatigue
- High illness rate
- Inability to attend to information
- Inability to meet basic needs
- Inability to meet role expectations
- Inadequate problem solving
- Lack of goal-directed behavior
- Lack of resolution of problem
- Poor concentration
- Risk taking
- Sleep disturbance
- Use of forms of coping that impede adaptive behavior
- Verbalization of inability to ask for help
- Verbalization of inability to cope

Related Factors

- Disturbance in pattern of appraisal of threat
- Disturbance in pattern of tension release
- Gender differences in coping strategies
- High degree of threat
- Inability to conserve adaptive energies
- Inadequate level of confidence in ability to cope
- Inadequate level of perception of control
- Inadequate opportunity to prepare for stressor
- Inadequate resources available
- Inadequate social support created by characteristics of relationships
- Maturational crisis
- Situational crisis
- Uncertainty

Ineffective Community Coping (00077)
(1994, 1998)

Domain 9: Coping/Stress Tolerance
Class 2: Coping Responses

Definition Pattern of community activities for adaptation and problem-solving that is unsatisfactory for meeting the demands or needs of the community

Defining Characteristics

- Community does not meet its own expectations
- Deficits in community participation
- Excessive community conflicts
- Expressed community powerlessness
- Expressed vulnerability
- High illness rates
- Increased social problems (e.g., homicides, vandalism, arson, terrorism, robbery, infanticide, abuse, divorce, unemployment, poverty, militancy, mental illness)
- Stressors perceived as excessive

Related Factors

- Deficits in community social support services
- Deficits in community social support resources
- Natural disasters
- Man-made disasters
- Inadequate resources for problem solving
- Ineffective community systems (e.g., lack of emergency medical system, transportation system, disaster planning systems)
- Nonexistent community systems

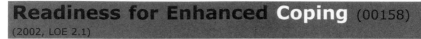

Domain 9: Coping/Stress Tolerance
Class 2: Coping Responses

Definition A pattern of cognitive and behavioral efforts to manage demands that is sufficient for well-being and can be strengthened

Defining Characteristics

- Acknowledges power
- Aware of possible environmental changes
- Defines stressors as manageable
- Seeks knowledge of new strategies
- Seeks social support
- Uses a broad range of emotion-oriented strategies
- Uses a broad range of problem-oriented strategies
- Uses spiritual resources

Domain 9

Readiness for Enhanced Community Coping (00076)

(1994)

Domain 9: Coping/Stress Tolerance
Class 2: Coping Responses

Definition Pattern of community activities for adaptation and problem-solving that is satisfactory for meeting the demands or needs of the community but can be improved for management of current and future problems/stressors

Defining Characteristics

One or more characteristics that indicate effective coping:

- Active planning by community for predicted stressors
- Active problem solving by community when faced with issues
- Agreement that community is responsible for stress management
- Positive communication among community members
- Positive communication between community/ aggregates and larger community
- Programs available for recreation
- Programs available for relaxation
- Resources sufficient for managing stressors

Domain 9

Readiness for Enhanced Family Coping (00075)
(1980)

Domain 9: Coping/Stress Tolerance
Class 2: Coping Responses

Definition Effective management of adaptive tasks by family member involved with the client's health challenge, who now exhibits desire and readiness for enhanced health and growth in regard to self and in relation to the client

Defining Characteristics

- Chooses experiences that optimize wellness
- Family member attempts to describe growth impact of crisis
- Family member moves in direction of enriching lifestyle

- Family member moves in direction of health promotion
- Individual expresses interest in making contact with others who have experienced a similar situation

Ineffective Denial (00072)

(1988, 2006, LOE 2.1)

Domain 9: Coping/Stress Tolerance
Class 2: Coping Responses

Definition Conscious or unconscious attempt to disavow the knowledge or meaning of an event to reduce anxiety/fear, but leading to the detriment of health

Defining Characteristics

- Delays seeking healthcare attention to the detriment of health
- Displaces fear of impact of the condition
- Displaces source of symptoms to other organs
- Displays inappropriate affect
- Does not admit fear of death
- Does not admit fear of invalidism
- Does not perceive personal relevance of danger
- Does not perceive personal relevance of symptoms
- Makes dismissive comments when speaking of distressing events
- Makes dismissive gestures when speaking of distressing events
- Minimizes symptoms
- Refuses healthcare attention to the detriment of health
- Unable to admit impact of disease on life pattern
- Uses self-treatment

Related Factors

- Anxiety
- Fear of death
- Fear of loss of autonomy
- Fear of separation
- Lack of competency in using effective coping mechanisms
- Lack of control of life situation
- Lack of emotional support from others
- Overwhelming stress
- Threat of inadequacy in dealing with strong emotions
- Threat of unpleasant reality

References

Bartle, S.H. (1980). Denial of cardiac warnings. *Psychosomatics* **12**(1): 74–7.
Bennet, D.H. & Holmes, D.S. (1975). Influence of denial (situation redefinition) and projection on anxiety associated with threat to self-esteem. *J Pers Soc Psychol* **32**: 915–21.

Byrne, B (2000). Relationships between anxiety, fear, self-esteem, and coping strategies in adolescence. *Adolescence* **35**: 201–15.

Davey, G.C., Burgess, I. & Rashes, R. (1995). Coping strategies and phobias: the relationship between fears, phobias and methods of coping with stressors. *Br J Clin Psychol* **34**(Pt 3): 423–34.

Fryer, S., Waller, G., & Kroese, B.S (1997). Stress, coping, and disturbed eating attitudes in teenage girls. *Int J Eat Disord* **22**: 427–36.

Gammon, J. (1998). Analysis of the stressful effects of hospitalisation and source isolation coping and psychological constructs. *Int J Nurs Pract* **4**(2): 84–96.

Gottschalk, L.A., Fronczek, J., Abel, L., Buchsbaum, M.S., & Fallon, J.H. (2001). The cerebral neurobiology of anxiety, anxiety displacement, and anxiety denial. *Psychother Psychosom* **70**(1): 17–24.

Greenberg, J., Solomon, S., Pyszczynski, T., et al. (1992). Why do people need self-esteem? Converging evidence that self-esteem serves an anxiety-buffering function. *J Pers Soc Psychol* **63**: 913–22.

Heilbrun, A.B. & Pepe, V. 91985). Awareness of cognitive defences and stress management. *Br J Med Psychol* **58**(Pt 1): 9–17.

Hobfoll, S.E. & Walfisch, S. (1984). Coping with a threat to life: a longitudinal study of self-concept, social support, and psychological distress. *Am J Community Psychol* **12**(1): 87–100.

Hovey, J.D. & Magana, C.G. (2002). Exploring the mental health of Mexican migrant farm workers in Midwest: psychosocial predictors of psychological distress and suggestions for prevention and treatment. *J Psychol* **136**: 493–513.

Kennedy, P., Duff, J., Evans, M., & Beedie, A. (2003). Coping effectiveness training reduces depression and anxiety following traumatic spinal cord injuries. *Br J Clin Psychol* **42**(pt 1): 41–52.

Kollbrunner, J., Zbaren, P., & Quack, K. (2001). Quality of life stress in patients with large tumors of the mouth. Dealing with the illness: coping, anxiety and depressive symptoms. *HNO* **49**: 998–1007.

Leserman, J., Perkins, D.O., & Evans, D.L. (1992). Coping with the threat of AIDS: the role of social support. *Am J Psychiatry* **149**: 1514–20.

Mogg, K., Mathews, A., Bird, C., & Macgregor-Morris, R. (1990). Effects of stress and anxiety on the processing of threat stimuli. *J Pers Soc Psychol* **59**: 1230–7.

Monat, A. & Lazarus, R.S. (1991). *Stress and Coping: An anthology*, 3rd edn. New York: Columbia University Press.

Muller, L. & Spitz, E. (2003). Multidimensional assessment of coping: validation of the Brief COPE among French population. *Encephale* **29**: 507–18.

Sandstrom, M.J. & Cramer, P. (2003). Defense mechanisms and psychological adjustment in childhood. *J Nerv Ment Dis* **191**: 487–95.

Schimel, J., Greenberg, J., & Martens, A. (2003). Evidence that projection of a feared trait can serve a defensive function. *Pers Soc Psychol Bull* **29**: 969–79.

Skinner, N. & Brewer, N. (2002). The dynamics of threat and challenge appraisals prior to stressful achievement events. *J Pers Soc Psychol* **83**: 678–92.

Westman, A.S. (1992). Existential anxiety as related to conceptualization of self and of death, denial of death, and religiosity. *Psychol Rep* **71**(3 Pt 2): 1064–6.

Domain 9: Coping/Stress Tolerance
Class 2: Coping Responses

Definition Response to perceived threat that is consciously recognized as a danger

Defining Characteristics

- Report of alarm
- Report of apprehension
- Report of being scared
- Report of decreased self-assurance
- Report of dread
- Report of excitement
- Report of increased tension
- Report of jitteriness
- Report of panic
- Report of terror

Cognitive

- Diminished productivity
- Diminished learning ability
- Diminished problem-solving ability
- Identifies object of fear
- Stimulus believed to be a threat

Behaviors

- Attack behaviors

- Avoidance behaviors
- Impulsiveness
- Increased alertness
- Narrowed focus on the source of the fear

Physiological

- Anorexia
- Diarrhea
- Dry mouth
- Dyspnea
- Fatigue
- Increased perspiration
- Increased pulse
- Increased respiratory rate
- Increased systolic blood pressure
- Muscle tightness
- Nausea
- Pallor
- Pupil dilation
- Vomiting

Related Factors

- Innate origin (e.g., sudden noise, height, pain, loss of physical support)

- Innate releasers (neurotransmitters)
- Language barrier

Domain 9

- Learned response (e.g., conditioning, modeling from or identification with others)
- Phobic stimulus
- Sensory impairment
- Separation from support system in potentially stressful situation (e.g., hospitalization, hospital procedures)
- Unfamiliarity with environmental experience(s)

Grieving* (00136)

(1980, 1996, 2006, LOE 2.1)

Domain 9: Coping/Stress Tolerance
Class 2: Coping Responses

Definition A normal complex process that includes emotional, physical, spiritual, social, and intellectual responses and behaviors by which individuals, families, and communities incorporate an actual, anticipated, or perceived loss into their daily lives

Defining Characteristics

- Alteration in activity level
- Alterations in dream patterns
- Alterations in immune function
- Alterations in neuroendocrine function
- Alterations in sleep patterns
- Anger
- Blame
- Detachment
- Despair
- Disorganization
- Experiencing relief
- Maintaining the connection to the deceased
- Making meaning of the loss
- Pain
- Panic behavior
- Personal growth
- Psychological distress
- Suffering

Related Factors

- Anticipatory loss of significant object (e.g., possession, job, status, home, parts and processes of body)
- Anticipatory loss of a significant other
- Death of a significant other
- Loss of significant object (e.g., possession, job, status, home, parts and processes of body)

References

Center for the Advancement of Health (2004). Report on bereavement and grief research. Themes in research on bereavement and grief. *Death Studies* **28**: 498–505.

Center for the Advancement of Health (2004). Report on bereavement and grief research Outcomes of bereavement. *Death Studies* **28**: 520–42.

Christ, G., Bonnano, G., Malkinson, R., & Rubin, S. (2003). Bereavement experiences after the death of a child. In: Field, M. & Berhman, R. (eds), *When children die: Improving*

* This diagnosis formerly held the label *Anticipatory Grieving*.

palliative and end-of-life care for children and their families. Washington DC: National Academy Press, pp. 553–79.

Davis, C. & Nolen-Hocksema, S. (2001). Loss and meaning: How do people make sense of loss? *American Behavioral Scientist,***44**: 726–41.

Gamino, L., Sewell, K., & Easterling, L. (2000). Scott and White Grief Study – Phase 2: Toward an adaptive model of grief. *Death Studies* **24**: 633–60.

Gamino, L., Hogan, N., & Sewell, K. (2002). Feeling the absence: A content analysis from the Scott and White grief study. *Death Studies* **26**: 793–813.

Hall, M. & Irwin, M. (2001). Physiological indices of functioning in bereavement. In: Stroebe, M., Hannson, R., Stroebe, W. & Schut, H. (eds), *Handbook of bereavement research: Consequences, coping and care.* Washington DC: American Psychological Association, pp. 473–93.

Hansson, R. & Stroebe, (M. 2003). Grief, older adulthood. In: Gullotta, T. & Bloom, M. (eds), *Encyclopedia of primary prevention and health promotion.* New York: Plenum, pp. 515–21.

Hogan, N., Worden, J.W., & Schmidt, L. (2004). An empirical study of the proposed complicated grief disorder criteria. *OMEGA* **48**: 263–77.

Jacobs, S. (1999). *Traumatic grief: Diagnosis, treatment, and prevention.* Caselton, NY: Brunner/Mazel.

Matthews, L. & Marwit, S. (2004). Complicated grief and the trend toward cognitive-behavioral therapy. *Death Studies* **28**: 849–63.

Ogrodniczuk, J., Piper, W., Joyce, A., et al. (2003). Differentiating symptoms of complicated grief and depression among psychiatric outpatients. *Canadian Journal of Psychiatry* **48**(2): 87–93.

Ott, C. (2003). The impact of complicated grief on mental and physical health at various points in the bereavement process. *Death Studies* **27**: 249–72.

Prigerson, H. & Jacobs, S. (2001). Traumatic grief as a distinct disorder: A rationale, consensus criteria, and a preliminary empirical test. In: Stroebe, M., Hannson, R., Stroebe, W. & Schut, H. (eds)., *Handbook of bereavement research: Consequences, coping and care.* Washington DC: American Psychological Association, pp. 613–46.

Complicated Grieving* (00135)
(1980, 1986, 2004, 2006, LOE 2.1)

Domain 9: Coping/Stress Tolerance
Class 2: Coping Responses

Definition A disorder that occurs after the death of a significant other, in which the experience of distress accompanying bereavement fails to follow normative expectations and manifests in functional impairment

Defining Characteristics

- Decreased functioning in life roles
- Decreased sense of wellbeing
- Depression
- Experiencing somatic symptoms of the deceased
- Fatigue
- Grief avoidance
- Longing for the deceased
- Low levels of intimacy
- Persistent emotional distress
- Preoccupation with thoughts of the deceased
- Rumination
- Searching for the deceased
- Self-blame
- Separation distress
- Traumatic distress
- Verbalizes anxiety
- Verbalizes distressful feelings about the deceased
- Verbalizes feeling dazed
- Verbalizes feeling empty
- Verbalizes feeling in shock
- Verbalizes feeling stunned
- Verbalizes feelings of anger
- Verbalizes feelings of detachment from others
- Verbalizes feelings of disbelief
- Verbalizes feelings of mistrust
- Verbalizes lack of acceptance of the death
- Verbalizes persistent painful memories
- Verbalizes self-blame
- Yearning

Related Factors

- Death of a significant other
- Emotional instability
- Lack of social support
- Sudden death of significant other

References

Center for the Advancement of Health (2004). Report on bereavement and grief research. Themes in research on bereavement and grief. *Death Studies* **28**: 498–505.

* This diagnosis formerly held the label *Dysfunctional Grieving*.

Domain 9

Center for the Advancement of Health (2004). Report on bereavement and grief research Outcomes of bereavement. *Death Studies* **28**: 520–42.

Christ, G., Bonnano, G., Malkinson, R., & Rubin, S. (2003). Bereavement experiences after the death of a child. In: Field, M. & Berhman, R. (eds), *When children die: Improving palliative and end-of-life care for children and their families*. Washington DC: National Academy Press, pp. 553–79.

Davis, C. & Nolen-Hocksema, S. (2001). Loss and meaning: How do people make sense of loss? *American Behavioral Scientist* **44**: 726–41.

Gamino, L., Sewell, K., & Easterling, L. (2000). Scott and White Grief Study – Phase 2: Toward an adaptive model of grief. *Death Studies* **24**: 633–60.

Gamino, L., Hogan, N., & Sewell, K. (2002). Feeling the absence: A content analysis from the Scott and White grief study. *Death Studies* **26**: 793–813.

Hall, M. & Irwin, M. (2001). Physiological indices of functioning in bereavement. In: Stroebe, M., Hannson, R., Stroebe, W. & Schut, H. (eds)., *Handbook of bereavement research: Consequences, coping and care*. Washington DC: American Psychological Association, pp. 473–93.

Hansson, R. & Stroebe, (M. 2003). Grief, older adulthood. In: Gullotta, T. & Bloom, M. (eds), *Encyclopedia of primary prevention and health promotion*. New York: Plenum, pp. 515–21.

Hogan, N., Worden, J.W., & Schmidt, L. (2004). An empirical study of the proposed complicated grief disorder criteria. *OMEGA* **48**: 263–77.

Jacobs, S. (1999). *Traumatic grief: Diagnosis, treatment, and prevention*. Caselton, NY: Brunner/Mazel.

Matthews, L. & Marwit, S. (2004). Complicated grief and the trend toward cognitive–behavioral therapy. *Death Studies* **28**: 849–63.

Ogrodniczuk, J., Piper, W., Joyce, A., et al. (2003). Differentiating symptoms of complicated grief and depression among psychiatric outpatients. *Canadian Journal of Psychiatry* **48**(2): 87–93.

Ott, C. (2003). The impact of complicated grief on mental and physical health at various points in the bereavement process. *Death Studies* **27**: 249–72.

Prigerson, H. & Jacobs, S. (2001). Traumatic grief as a distinct disorder: A rationale, consensus criteria, and a preliminary empirical test. In: Stroebe, M., Hannson, R., Stroebe, W. & Schut, H. (eds)., *Handbook of bereavement research: Consequences, coping and care*. Washington DC: American Psychological Association, pp. 613–46.

Domain 9: Coping/Stress Tolerance
Class 2: Coping Responses

Definition

At risk for a disorder that occurs after the death of a significant other, in which the experience of distress accompanying bereavement fails to follow normative expectations and manifests in functional impairment

Risk Factors

- Death of a significant other
- Emotional instability
- Lack of social support

References

Center for the Advancement of Health (2004). Report on bereavement and grief research. Themes in research on bereavement and grief. *Death Studies* **28**: 498–505.

Center for the Advancement of Health (2004). Report on bereavement and grief research Outcomes of bereavement. *Death Studies* **28**: 520–42.

Christ, G., Bonnano, G., Malkinson, R., & Rubin, S. (2003). Bereavement experiences after the death of a child. In: Field, M. & Berhman, R. (eds), *When children die: Improving palliative and end-of-life care for children and their families*. Washington DC: National Academy Press, pp. 553–79.

Davis, C. & Nolen-Hocksema, S. (2001). Loss and meaning: How do people make sense of loss? *American Behavioral Scientist* **44**: 726–41.

Gamino, L., Sewell, K., & Easterling, L. (2000). Scott and White Grief Study – Phase 2: Toward an adaptive model of grief. *Death Studies* **24**: 633–60.

Gamino, L., Hogan, N., & Sewell, K. (2002). Feeling the absence: A content analysis from the Scott and White grief study. *Death Studies* **26**: 793–813.

Hall, M. & Irwin, M. (2001). Physiological indices of functioning in bereavement. In: Stroebe, M., Hannson, R., Stroebe, W. & Schut, H. (eds)., *Handbook of bereavement research: Consequences, coping and care*. Washington DC: American Psychological Association, pp. 473–93.

Hansson, R. & Stroebe, (M. 2003). Grief, older adulthood. In: Gullotta, T. & Bloom, M. (eds), *Encyclopedia of primary prevention and health promotion*. New York: Plenum, pp. 515–21.

Hogan, N., Worden, J.W., & Schmidt, L. (2004). An empirical study of the proposed complicated grief disorder criteria. *OMEGA* **48**: 263–77.

Jacobs, S. (1999). *Traumatic grief: Diagnosis, treatment, and prevention*. Caselton, NY: Brunner/Mazel.

Matthews, L. & Marwit, S. (2004). Complicated grief and the trend toward cognitive–behavioral therapy. *Death Studies* **28**: 849–63.

Ogrodniczuk, J., Piper, W., Joyce, A., et al. (2003). Differentiating symptoms of complicated grief and depression among psychiatric outpatients. *Canadian Journal of Psychiatry* **48**(2): 87–93.

* This diagnosis formerly held the label *Risk for Dysfunctional Grieving*.

Domain 9

Ott, C. (2003). The impact of complicated grief on mental and physical health at various points in the bereavement process. *Death Studies* **27**: 249–72.

Prigerson, H. & Jacobs, S. (2001). Traumatic grief as a distinct disorder: A rationale, consensus criteria, and a preliminary empirical test. In: Stroebe, M., Hannson, R., Stroebe, W. & Schut, H. (eds)., *Handbook of bereavement research: Consequences, coping and care*. Washington DC: American Psychological Association, pp. 613–46.

Domain 9: Coping/Stress Tolerance
Class 2: Coping Responses

Definition Decreased ability to sustain a pattern of positive responses to an adverse situation or crisis

Defining Characteristics

- Decreased interest in academic activities
- Decreased interest in vocational activities
- Depression
- Guilt
- Isolation
- Low self-esteem
- Lower perceived health status
- Renewed elevation of distress
- Shame
- Social isolation
- Using maladaptive coping skills (i.e., drug use, violence, etc.)

Related Factors

- Demographics that increase chance of maladjustment
- Drug use
- Gender
- Inconsistent parenting
- Low intelligence
- Low maternal education
- Large family size
- Minority status
- Parental mental illness
- Poor impulse control
- Poverty
- Psychological disorders
- Vulnerability factors which encompass indices that exacerbate the negative effects of the risk condition
- Violence
- Violence in neighborhood

References

Armstrong, M., Birnie-Lefcovitch, S., & Ungar, M (2005) Pathways between social support family wellbeing, quality of parenting and child resilience: What we know. *Journal of Child and Family Studies* 14: 269–81.

Bonanno, G.A. (2005). Clarifying and extending the construct of adult resilience. *American Psychologist* 60: 265.

Brown, J.H. & Brown, D. (2005). Why 'at risk' is at risk. *American School Board Journal* 192(11): 44.

Crosnoe, R. & Elder, G. (2004). Family dynamics, supportive relationships, and educational resilience during adolescence. *Journal of Family Issues* 25: 571–602.

Domain 9

Kaylor, G. & Otis, M. (2003). The effect of childhood maltreatment on adult criminality: a tobit regression analysis. *Child Maltreatment* **8**: 129–137.

Luthar, S.S. & Cicchetti, D. (2000). The construct of resilience: implications for interventions and social policies. *Developmental Psychopathology* **12**: 857–85.

Richardson, G.E. (2002). The metatheory of resilience and resiliency. *Journal of Clinical Psychology* **58**: 307–21.

Rutter, M. & Sroufe, A. (2000). Developmental psychopathology: concepts and challenges. *Developmental Psychopathology* **12**: 265–96.

Taylor, J. (2000). Sisters of the yam: African American women's healing and self-recovery from intimate male partner violence. *Issues in Mental Health Nursing* **21**: 515–31.

Readiness for Enhanced Resilience (00212)
(2008, LOE 2.1)

Domain 9: Coping/Stress Tolerance
Class 2: Coping Responses

Definition A pattern of positive responses to an adverse situation or crisis that can be strengthened to optimize human potential

Defining Characteristics

- Access to resources
- Demonstrates positive outlook
- Effective use of conflict management strategies
- Enhances personal coping skills
- Expressed desire to enhance resilience
- Identifies available resources
- Identifies support systems
- Increases positive relationships with others
- Involvement in activities
- Makes progress toward goals
- Presence of a crisis
- Safe environment is maintained
- Sets goals
- Takes responsibilities for actions
- Use of effective communication skills
- Verbalizes an enhanced sense of control
- Verbalizes self esteem

Related Factors

- Demographics that increase chance of maladjustment
- Drug use
- Gender
- Inconsistent parenting
- Low intelligence
- Low maternal education
- Large family size
- Minority status
- Parental mental illness
- Poor impulse control
- Poverty
- Psychological disorders
- Vulnerability factors which encompass indices that exacerbate the negative effects of the risk condition
- Violence

References

Bolger, K. & Patterso, C. (2003). Sequelae of child maltreatment: Vulnerability and resilience. In Luthar, S. (Eds.), *Resilience and vulnerability: Adaptation in the context of childhood adversities*. (Pp. 156–181) United Kingdom: Cambridge University Press.

Bolger, K., Patterson, C., & Kupersmidt, J. (1998). Peer relationships and self-esteem among children who have been maltreated. *Child Development*, **69**(4): 1171–97.

Bonanno, G.A. (2005). Clarifying and extending the construct of adult resilience. *American Psychologist* **60**: 265.

Brown, J.H. & Brown, D. (2005). Why 'at risk' is at risk. *American School Board Journal* **192**(11): 44.

Crosnoe, R. & Elder, G. (2004). Family dynamics, supportive relationships, and educational resilience during adolescence. *Journal of Family Issues*, **25**(5): 571–602.

Evans, G.W. & Kantrowitz, E. (2002). Socioeconomic status and health: the potential role of environmental risk exposure. *Annual Review of Public Health* **23**: 303–1.

Fergus, S. & Zimmerman, M. (2005). Adolescent resilience: a framework for understanding healthy development in the face of risk. *Annual Review of Public Health* **26**: 399–419.

Haskett, M. & Willoughby, M. (2007). Paths to child social adjustment: Parenting quality and children's processing of social information. *Child: Care, Health and Development*, **33**(1): 67–77.

Kelley, T.M. (2005). Natural resilience and innate mental health. *American Psychologist* **60**: 265.

Kim, J. & Cicchetti, D. (2003). Social self-efficacy and behavior problems in maltreated children. *Journal of Clinical Child and Adolescent Psychology*, **32**(1): 106–17.

Luthar, S., Cicchetti, D., & Becker, B. (2000). The construct of resilience: a critical evaluation and guidelines for future work. *Child Dev*, **71**(3): 543–62.

Luthar, S. S. & Cicchetti, D. (2000). The construct of resilience: implications for interventions and social policies. *Developmental Psychopathology* **12**: 857–85.

Manly, J.T., Kim, J.E., Rogosch, F.A., & Cicchetti, D. (2001). Dimensions of child maltreatment and children's adjustment: contributions of developmental timing and subtype. *Developmental Psychopathology* **13**: 759–82.

Masten, A.S. (2004). Regulatory processes, risk and resilience in adolescent development. *Annuals of the New York Academy of Science*, **1021**: 310–19.

Masten, A., Burt, K., Roisman, G., Obradovic, J., Long, J., & Tellegen, A. (2004). Resources and resilience in the transition to adulthood: Continuity and Change. *Development and Psychopathology*, **16**: 1071–94.

Masten, A., & Powell, J. (2003). A resilience framework for research policy and practice. In S. Luthar (Ed.), *Resilience and vulnerability: Adaptation in the context of childhood adversities* (pp. 1–25). United Kingdom: Cambridge University Press.

Masten, A.S. (2001). Ordinary Magic: Resilience processes in development. *American Psychologist* **56**: 227–38.

Richardson, G.E. (2002). The metatheory of resilience and resiliency. *Journal of Clinical Psychology*, **58**(3): 307–21.

Rutter, M. (1987). Psychosocial resilience and protective mechanism. *American Journal of Orthopsychiatry*, **57**(3): 316–31.

Rutter, M. & O'Conner, T. (2004). Are there biological programming effects of psychological development? Findings from a study of Romanian Adoptees. *Developmental Psychology*, **40**(1): 81–94.

Rutter, M. & Sroufe, A. (2000). Developmental psychopathology: concepts and challenges. *Developmental Psychopathology*, **12**: 265–296.

Sinclair, V.G. & Wallston, K.A. (2004). The development and psychometric evaluation of the brief resilient coping scale. *Assessment* **11**(1): 94–101.

Tusaie, K., & J. Dyer (2004). Resilience: a historical review of the construct. *Holistic Nursing Practice*, **18**(1), 3–8.

Werner, E.E. (1996a). Protective factors and individual resilience. In: Meisels, S. & Shonkoff, J. (eds), *Handbook of early childhood interventions*. New York: Cambridge University Press.

Werner, E.E. (1996b). Vulnerable but invincible. *European Child and Adolescent Psychiatry* **5**: 47–51.

Domain 9

Domain 9: Coping/Stress Tolerance
Class 2: Coping Responses

Definition At risk for decreased ability to sustain a pattern of positive responses to an adverse situation or crisis

Risk factors

- Chronicity of existing crises
- Multiple coexisting adverse situations
- Presence of an additional new crisis (e.g., unplanned pregnancy, death of a spouse, loss of job, illness, loss of housing, death of family member)

References

Armstrong, M., Birnie-Lefcovitch, S., & Ungar, M (2005) Pathways between social support family wellbeing, quality of parenting and child resilience: What we know. *Journal of Child and Family Studies* **14**: 269–81.

Black, C. & Ford-Gilboe, M. (2004). Adolescent mothers: Resilience, family health, work and health promoting practices. *Journal of Advanced Nursing* **48**: 351–60.

Bonanno, G.A. (2005). Clarifying and extending the construct of adult resilience. *American Psychologist* **60**: 265.

Brown, J.H. & Brown, D. (2005). Why 'at risk' is at risk. *American School Board Journal* **192**(11): 44.

Evans, G.W. & Kantrowitz, E. (2002). Socioeconomic status and health: the potential role of environmental risk exposure. *Annual Review of Public Health* **23**: 303–1.

Fergus, S. & Zimmerman, M. (2005). Adolescent resilience: a framework for understanding healthy development in the face of risk. *Annual Review of Public Health* **26**: 399–419.

Gorman, C., Dale, S. S., Grossman, W., Klarreich, K., McDowell, J., & Whitaker, L. (2005). The Importance of RESILIENCE. *Time* **165**(3): A52.

Greef, A. & Ritman, I. (2005). Individual characteristics associated with resilience in single-parent families. *Psychological Reports* **96**(1): 36–42.

Kelley, T.M. (2005). Natural resilience and innate mental health. *American Psychologist* **60**: 265.

Luthar, S. S. & Cicchetti, (D. 2000). The construct of resilience: implications for interventions and social policies. *Developmental Psychopathology* **12**: 857–85.

Manly, J.T., Kim, J.E., Rogosch, F.A., & Cicchetti, D. (2001). Dimensions of child maltreatment and children's adjustment: contributions of developmental timing and subtype. *Developmental Psychopathology* **13**: 759–82.

Martin, A.J. & Marsh, H.W. (2006). Academic resilience and its psychological and educational correlates: A construct validity approach. *Psychology in the Schools* **43**: 267–81

Masten, A.S. (2001). Ordinary Magic: Resilience processes in development. *American Psychologist* **56**: 227–38.

Domain 9

Rogers, S., Muir, K., & Evenson, C.R. (2003). Signs of resilience: assets that support deaf adults' success in bridging the deaf and hearing worlds. *American Annals of the Deaf* **148**: 222.

Sinclair, V.G. & Wallston, K.A. (2004). The development and psychometric evaluation of the brief resilient coping scale. *Assessment* **11**(1): 94–101.

Taylor, J. (2000). Sisters of the yam: African American women's healing and self-recovery from intimate male partner violence. *Issues in Mental Health Nursing* **21**: 515–31.

Werner, E.E. (1996a). Protective factors and individual resilience. In: Meisels, S. & Shonkoff;, J. (eds), *Handbook of early childhood interventions*. New York: Cambridge University Press.

Werner, E.E. (1996b). Vulnerable but invincible. *European Child and Adolescent Psychiatry* **5**: 47–51.

Domain 9

Chronic Sorrow (00137)
(1998)

Domain 9: Coping/Stress Tolerance
Class 2: Coping Responses

Definition Cyclical, recurring, and potentially progressive pattern of pervasive sadness experienced (by a parent, caregiver, individual with chronic illness or disability) in response to continual loss, throughout the trajectory of an illness or disability

Defining Characteristics

- Expresses negative feelings (e.g., anger, being misunderstood, confusion, depression, disappointment, emptiness, fear, frustration, guilt, self-blame, helplessness, hopelessness, loneliness, low self-esteem, recurring loss, overwhelmed)
- Expresses feelings of sadness (e.g., periodic, recurrent)
- Expresses feelings that interfere with ability to reach highest level of personal wellbeing
- Expresses feelings that interfere with ability to reach highest level of social wellbeing

Related Factors

- Death of a loved one
- Experiences chronic disability (e.g., physical or mental)
- Experiences chronic illness (e.g., physical or mental)
- Crises in management of the disability
- Crises in management of the illness
- Crises related to developmental stages
- Missed opportunities
- Missed milestones
- Unending caregiving

Stress Overload (00177)

(2006, LOE 3.2)

Domain 9: Coping/Stress Tolerance
Class 2: Coping Responses

Definition Excessive amounts and types of demands that require action

Defining Characteristics

- Demonstrates increased feelings of anger
- Demonstrates increased feelings of impatience
- Expresses difficulty in functioning
- Expresses a feeling of pressure
- Expresses a feeling of tension
- Expresses increased feelings of anger
- Expresses increased feelings of impatience
- Expresses problems with decision making
- Reports negative impact from stress (e.g., physical symptoms, psychological distress, feeling of being sick or of going to get sick)
- Reports excessive situational stress (e.g., rates stress level as seven or above on a 10-point scale)

Related Factors

- Inadequate resources (e.g., financial, social, education/ knowledge level)
- Intense stressors (e.g., family violence, chronic illness, terminal illness)
- Multiple coexisting stressors (e.g., environmental threats/ demands; physical threats/ demands; social threats/ demands)
- Repeated stressors (e.g., family violence, chronic illness, terminal illness)

References

Al-Hassan, M. & Sagr, L. (2002). Stress and stressors of myocardial infarction patients in the early period after discharge. *Journal of Advanced Nursing* **40**: 181–8.

Bay, E., Hagerty, B., Williams, R.A., & Kirsch, N. (2005). Chronic stress, salivary cortisol response, interpersonal relatedness, and depression among community-dwelling survivors of traumatic brain injury. *Journal of Neuroscience Nursing* **37**(1): 4–14.

Boardman, J.D. (2004). Stress and physical health: The role of neighborhoods as mediating and moderating mechanisms. *Social Science and Medicine* **58**: 2473–83.

Domain 9

Booth, K., Beaver, K., Kitchener, H., O'Neill, J., & Farrell, C. (2005). Women's experiences of information, psychological distress and worry after treatment for gynecological cancer. *Patient Education and Counseling* **56**: 225–32.

Carlson-Catalano, J. (1998). Nursing diagnoses and interventions for postacute phase battered women. *Nursing Diagnoses* **9**: 101–10.

Choenarom, C., Williams, R.A., & Hagerty, B.M. (2005). The role of sense of belonging and social support on stress and depression in individuals with depression. *Archives in Psychiatric Nursing* **19**(1): 18–29.

Cropley, M. & Steptoe, A. (2005). Social support, life events and physical symptoms: A prospective study of chronic and recent life stress in men and women. *Psychology, Health and Medicine* **10**: 317–25.

Davidson, M., Penney, E.D., Muller, B., & Grey, M. (2004). Stressors and self care challenges faced by adolescents living with type 1 diabetes. *Applied Nursing Research* **2**: 72–80.

Diong, S.M., Bishop, G.D., Enkelmann, H.C., et al. (2005). Anger, stress, coping, social support and health: Modelling the relationships. *Psychology and Health* **20**: 467–95.

Drew, D., Goodenough, B., Maurice, L., Foreman, T., & Willis, L. (2005). Parental grieving after a child dies from cancer: Is stress from stem cell transplant a factor? *International Journal of Palliative Nursing* **11**: 266–73.

Eby, K.K. (2004). Exploring the stressors of low-income women with abusive partners: Understanding their needs and developing effective community responses. *Journal of Family Violence* **19**: 251–32.

Golden-Kreutz, D.M., Thorton, L.M., Wells-Di Gregoria, S., et al. (2005). Traumatic stress, perceived global stress, and life events: Prospectively predicting quality of life in breast cancer patients. *Health Psychology* **24**: 288–96.

Hannigan, B., Edwards, D., & Burnard, P. (2004). Stress and stress management in clinical psychology: Findings from a systematic review. *Journal of Mental Health* **13**: 235–45.

Harwood, L., Locking-Cusolito, H., Spittal, J., Wilson, B., & White, S. (2005). Preparing for hemodialysis: Patients' stressors and responses. *Nephrology Nursing Journal* **32**: 295–303.

Holmes. T.H. & Rahe, R.H. (1967). The Social Readjustment Rating Scale. *Journal of Psychometric Research* **11**: 213–18.

Hung, C-H. (2005), Measuring postpartum stress. *Journal of Advanced nursing* **50**: 417–24.

Ilgen, M.A. & Hutchinson, K.E. (2005). A history of major depressive disorder and the response to stress. *Journal of Affective Disorders* **86**: 143–50.

Janz, N.K., Dodge, J.A., Janevic, M.R., Lin, X., Donaldson, A.E., & Clark, N.M. (2004). Understanding and reducing stress and psychological distress in older women with heart disease. *Journal of Women & Aging* **16** (3/4): 19–38.

Kanner, A.D., Coyne, J.C., Schaefer, C., & Lazarus, R.S. (1981). Comparison of two measures of stress measurement: Daily hassles and uplifts versus major life events. *Journal of Behavioral Medicine* **4**: 1–37.

Keil, R.M.K. (2004). Coping and stress: A conceptual analysis. *Journal of Advanced Nursing* **45**: 659–65.

Krause, N. (2004). Stressors arising in highly valued roles, meaning in life, and the physical health status of older adults. *Journal of Gerontology: Social Sciences* **59**b: S287–97.

Lazarus, R.S. & Folkman, S. (1984). *Stress, appraisal, and coping*. New York: Springer.

Lim, L., Williams, D., & Hagan, P. (2005). Validation of a five-point self rated stress score. *American Journal of Health Promotion* **19**: 438–41.

Lloyd, C., Smith, J., & Weinger, (K. 2005). Stress and diabetes: A review of the links. *Diabetes Spectrum* **18**: 121–7.

Lunney, M. & Myszak, C. (1997). Abstract: Stress overload: A new diagnosis. In: Rantz, M.J. & LeMone, P. (eds), *Classification of nursing diagnoses: Proceedings of the twelfth conference, North American Nursing Diagnosis Association*. Glendale, CA: CINAHL Information Systems, pp. 190–191.

Domain 9

Lustky, M.K., Widman, L., Paschane, A., & Ecker, E. (2004). Stress, Quality of life and physical activity in women with varying degrees of premenstrual symptomatology. *Women & Health* **39**(3): 35–44.

McNulty, P.A.F. (2005). Reported stressors and health care needs of active duty Navy personnel during three phases of deployment in support of the war in Iraq. *Military Medicine* **170**: 530–5.

Maller, M.H., Almeida, D.M., & Neupert, S.D. (2005). Women's daily physical health symptoms and stressful experiences across adulthood. *Psychology and Health* **20**: 389–403.

Mariano, C. (1993). Case study: The method. In: Munhall, P.L. & Oiler, C.O. (eds), *Nursing research: A qualitative perspective*, 2nd edn. New York: National League for Nursing, pp. 311–37.

Miles, M.B. & Huberman, A.M. (1984). *Qualitative data analysis: A sourcebook of new methods*. Newbury Park, CA: Sage.

Motzer, S.A. & Hertig, V. (2004). Stress, stress response and health. *Nursing Clinics of North America* **39**: 1–17.

Neilsen, N.R., Zuo-Fend, Z., Kristenses, T., Netterstrem, B., Schnohr, P., & Grebaek, M. (2005). Self reported stress and risk of breast cancer. *British Medical Journal* **331**: 548–50.

Pender, N.J., Murtaugh, C.L., & Parsons, M.A. (2006). *Health promotion in nursing practice*, 5th edn. Upper Saddle River, NJ: Prentice Hall.

Power, T.G. (2004). Stress and coping in childhood: The parents' role. *Parenting: Science and Practice* **4**: 271–317.

Ridner, S.H. (2004). Psychological distress: Concept analysis. *Journal of Advanced Nursing* **45**: 536–45.

Robinson, K.L., McBeth, J., & McFarlane, G.J. (2004). Psychological distress and premature mortality in the general population: A prospective study. *Annals of Epidemiology* **14**: 467–72.

Ryan, M. (2001). Biases that influence the diagnostic process. In: Lunney, M. (ed.), *Critical thinking and nursing diagnoses: Case studies and analyses*. Philadelphia: NANDA, pp. 8, 156–8.

Ryan-Wenger, N.A., Sharrer, V.W., & Campbell, K.K. (2005). Changes in children's stressors over the past 30 years. *Pediatric Nursing* **31**: 282–91.

Sarid, O., Anson, O., Yaari, A., & Margalith, M. (2004). Academic stress, immunological reaction, and academic performance among students of nursing and physiotherapy. *Research in Nursing & Health* **27**: 370–7.

Scollan-Koliopoulos, M. (2005). Managing stress response to control hypertension in type 2 diabetes. *The Nurse Practitioner* **30**(2): 46–9.

Selye, H. (1956). *The Stress of Life*. New York: McGraw Hill.

Selye, H. (1974). *Stress without Distress*. Philadelphia: J.B. Lippincott.

Selye, H. (1976). Further thoughts on "stress without distress." *Medical Times* **104**: 124–32.

Sepa, A., Wahlberg, J., Vaarsala, O., Frodi, A. & Ludvigsson, J. (2005). Psychological stress may induce diabetes-related autoimmunity in infancy. *Diabetes Care* **28**: 290–5.

So, H.M. & Chan, D.S.K. (2004). Perceptions of stressors by patients and nurses of critical care units in Hong Kong. *International Journal of Nursing Studies* **41**: 77–84.

Sternberg, E. (2001). *The balance within: The science of connecting health and emotions*. New York: W.H. Freeman.

Stewart, K.E., Cianfrani, L.R., & Walker, J.F. (2005). Stress, social support and housing are related to health status among HIV-positive persons in the Deep South of the United States. *AIDS Care* **17**: 350–8.

Taxis, J.C., Rew, L., Jackson, K., & Kouzekanani, K. (2004). Protective resources and perceptions of stress in a multi-ethnic sample of school-age children. *Pediatric Nursing* **30**: 477–87.

Vondras, D.D., Powless, M.R., Olson, A.K., Wheeler, D., & Snudden, A.L. (2005). Differential effects of everyday stress on the episodic memory test performances of young, mid-life, and older adults. *Aging & Mental Health* **9**(1): 60–70.

Domain 9

Autonomic Dysreflexia (00009)
(1988)

Domain 9: Coping/Stress Tolerance
Class 3: Neurobehavioral Stress

Definition Life-threatening, uninhibited sympathetic response of the nervous system to a noxious stimulus after a spinal cord injury at T7 or above

Defining Characteristics

- Blurred vision
- Bradycardia
- Chest pain
- Chilling
- Conjunctival congestion
- Diaphoresis (above the injury)
- Headache (a diffuse pain in different portions of the head and not confined to any nerve distribution area)
- Horner's syndrome
- Metallic taste in mouth
- Nasal congestion
- Pallor (below the injury)
- Paraesthesia
- Paroxysmal hypertension
- Pilomotor reflex
- Red splotches on skin (above the injury)
- Tachycardia

Related Factors

- Bladder distension
- Bowel distension
- Deficient caregiver knowledge
- Deficient patient knowledge
- Skin irritation

Risk for Autonomic Dysreflexia (00010)
(1998, 2000)

Domain 9: Coping/Stress Tolerance
Class 3: Neurobehavioral Stress

Definition At risk for life-threatening, uninhibited response of the sympathetic nervous system, post spinal shock, in an individual with spinal cord injury or lesion at T6 or above (has been demonstrated in patients with injuries at T7 and T8)

Risk Factors

An injury at T6 or above or a lesion at T6 or above AND at least one of the following noxious stimuli.

Cardiopulmonary Stimuli

- Deep vein thrombosis
- Pulmonary emboli

Gastrointestinal Stimuli

- Bowel distention
- Constipation
- Difficult passage of feces
- Digital stimulation
- Enemas
- Esophageal reflux
- Fecal impaction
- Gallstones
- Gastric ulcers
- Gastrointestinal system pathology
- Hemorrhoids
- Suppositories

Musculoskeletal–Integumentary Stimuli

- Cutaneous stimulation (e.g., pressure ulcer, ingrown toenail, dressings, burns, rash)
- Fractures
- Heterotopic bone
- Pressure over bony prominences
- Pressure over genitalia
- Range-of-motion exercises
- Spasm
- Sunburns
- Wounds

Neurological Stimuli

- Irritating stimuli below level of injury
- Painful stimuli below level of injury

Regulatory Stimuli

- Extreme environmental temperatures
- Temperature fluctuations

Reproductive Stimuli

- Ejaculation
- Labor and delivery
- Menstruation

- Ovarian cyst
- Pregnancy
- Sexual intercourse

Situational Stimuli

- Constrictive clothing (e.g., straps, stockings, shoes)
- Drug reactions (e.g., decongestants, sympathomimetics, vasoconstrictors)
- Narcotic/opiate withdrawal
- Positioning
- Surgical procedure

Urological Stimuli

- Bladder distension
- Bladder spasm
- Calculi
- Catheterization
- Cystitis
- Detrusor sphincter dyssynergia
- Epididymitis
- Instrumentation
- Surgery
- Urethritis
- Urinary tract infection

Domain 9

Domain 9: Coping/Stress Tolerance
Class 3: Neurobehavioral Stress

Definition Disintegrated physiological and neurobehavioral responses of infant to the environment

Defining Characteristics

Attention–Interaction System

- Abnormal response to sensory stimuli (e.g., difficult to soothe, inability to sustain alert status)

Motor System

- Altered primitive reflexes
- Changes to motor tone
- Finger splaying
- Fisting
- Hands to face
- Hyperextension of extremities
- Jittery
- Startles
- Tremors
- Twitches
- Uncoordinated movement

Physiological

- Arrhythmias

- Bradycardia
- Desaturation
- Feeding intolerances
- Skin color changes
- Tachycardia
- Time-out signals (e.g., gaze, grasp, hiccough, cough, sneeze, sigh, slack jaw, open mouth, tongue thrust)

Regulatory Problems

- Inability to inhibit startle
- Irritability

State–Organization System

- Active–awake (fussy, worried gaze)
- Diffuse sleep
- Irritable crying
- Quiet–awake (staring, gaze aversion)
- State–oscillation

Related Factors

Caregiver

- Cue knowledge deficit

- Cue misreading
- Environmental stimulation contribution

Domain 9

Environmental

- Lack of containment within environment
- Physical environment inappropriateness
- Sensory deprivation
- Sensory inappropriateness
- Sensory overstimulation

Individual

- Gestational age
- Illness
- Immature neurological system
- Postconceptual age

Postnatal

- Feeding intolerance
- Invasive procedures
- Malnutrition
- Motor problems
- Oral problems
- Pain
- Prematurity

Prenatal

- Congenital disorders
- Genetic disorders
- Teratogenic exposure

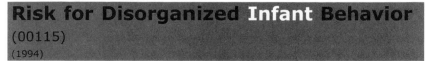

Risk for Disorganized Infant Behavior
(00115)
(1994)

Domain 9: Coping/Stress Tolerance
Class 3: Neurobehavioral Stress

Definition Risk for alteration in integrating and modulation of the physiological and behavioral systems of functioning (i.e., autonomic, motor, state–organization, self-regulatory, and attentional–interactional systems)

Risk Factors

- Environmental overstimulation
- Invasive procedures
- Lack of containment within environment
- Motor problems
- Oral problems
- Pain
- Painful procedures
- Prematurity

Readiness for Enhanced Organized Infant Behavior (00117)

(1994)

Domain 9: Coping/Stress Tolerance
Class 3: Neurobehavioral Stress

Definition A pattern of modulation of the physiologic and behavioral systems of functioning (i.e., autonomic, motor, state–organization, self-regulatory, and attentional–interactional systems) in an infant who is satisfactory but can be improved

Defining Characteristics

- Definite sleep–wake states
- Response to stimuli (e.g., visual, auditory)
- Stable physiologic measures
- Use of some self-regulatory behaviors

Decreased Intracranial Adaptive Capacity (00049)

(1994)

Domain 9: Coping/Stress Tolerance
Class 3: Neurobehavioral Stress

Definition Intracranial fluid dynamic mechanisms that normally compensate for increases in intracranial volumes are compromised, resulting in repeated disproportionate increases in intracranial pressure (ICP) in response to a variety of noxious and non-noxious stimuli

Defining Characteristics

- Baseline ICP ≥10 mmHg
- Disproportionate increase in ICP following stimulus
- Elevated P2 ICP waveform
- Repeated increases of >10 mmHg for more than 5 minutes following any of a variety of external stimuli
- Volume pressure response test variation (volume: pressure ratio 2, pressure volume index <10)
- Wide-amplitude ICP waveform

Related Factors

- Brain injuries
- Decreased cerebral perfusion ≤50–60 mmHg
- Sustained increase in ICP of 10–15 mmHg
- Systemic hypotension with intracranial hypertension

Domain 9

Domain 10
Life Principles

Readiness for Enhanced Hope (00185)

(2006, LOE 2.1)

Domain 10: Life Principles
Class 1: Values
Class 2: Beliefs
Domain 6: Self-Perception
Class 1: Self-Concept

Definition   A pattern of expectations and desires that is sufficient for mobilizing energy on one's own behalf and can be strengthened

Defining Characteristics

- Expresses desire to enhance ability to set achievable goals
- Expresses desire to enhance belief in possibilities
- Expresses desire to enhance congruency of expectations with desires
- Expresses desire to enhance hope

- Expresses desire to enhance interconnectedness with others
- Expresses desire to enhance problem-solving to meet goals
- Expresses desire to enhance sense of meaning to life
- Expresses desire to enhance spirituality

References

Benzein, E.G. (2005). The level of and relation between hope, hopelessness and fatigue in patients and family members in palliative care. *Palliative Medicine* **19**: 234–40.

Benzein, E. & Saveman, B-L. (1998). One step towards the understanding of hope: A concept analysis. *International Journal of Nursing Studies* **35**: 322–9.

Davis, B. (2005). Mediators of the relationship between hope and well-being in older adults. *Clinical Nursing Research* **14**: 253–72.

Domain 10

Domain 10: Life Principles
Class 2: Beliefs

Definition Ability to experience and integrate meaning and purpose in life through connectedness with self, others, art, music, literature, nature, and/or a power greater than oneself that can be strengthened

Defining Characteristics

Connections to Self

- Expresses desire for enhanced acceptance
- Expresses desire for enhanced coping
- Expresses desire for enhanced courage
- Expresses desire for enhanced forgiveness of self
- Expresses desire for enhanced hope
- Expresses desire for enhanced joy
- Expresses desire for enhanced love
- Expresses desire for enhanced meaning in life
- Expresses desire for enhanced purpose in life
- Expresses desire for enhanced satisfying philosophy of life
- Expresses desire for enhanced surrender
- Expresses desire for enhanced serenity (e.g., peace)
- Meditation

Connections with Others

- Provides service to others
- Requests interactions with significant others
- Requests interactions with spiritual leaders
- Requests forgiveness of others

Connections with Art, Music, Literature, Nature

- Displays creative energy (e.g., writing, poetry, singing)
- Listens to music
- Reads spiritual literature
- Spends time outdoors

Connections with Power Greater Than Self

- Expresses awe
- Expresses reverence
- Participates in religious activities
- Prays
- Reports mystical experiences

Decisional Conflict (00083)

(1988, 2006, LOE 2.1)

Domain 10: Life Principles
Class 3: Value/Belief/Action Congruence

Definition Uncertainty about course of action to be taken when choice among competing actions involves risk, loss, or challenge to values and beliefs

Defining Characteristics

- Delayed decision-making
- Physical signs of distress or tension (e.g., increased heart rate, increased muscle tension, restlessness)
- Questioning moral principles while attempting a decision
- Questioning moral rules while attempting a decision
- Questioning moral values while attempting a decision
- Questioning personal beliefs while attempting a decision
- Questioning personal values while attempting a decision
- Self-focusing
- Vacillation among alternative choices
- Verbalizes feeling of distress while attempting a decision
- Verbalizes uncertainty about choices
- Verbalizes undesired consequences of alternative actions being considered

Related Factors

- Divergent sources of information
- Interference with decision-making
- Lack of experience with decision-making
- Lack of relevant information
- Moral obligations require performing action
- Moral obligations require not performing action
- Moral principles support mutually inconsistent courses of action
- Moral rules support mutually inconsistent courses of action
- Moral values support mutually inconsistent courses of action
- Multiple sources of information
- Perceived threat to value system
- Support system deficit
- Unclear personal beliefs
- Unclear personal values

Domain 10

References

Audi, R. (1999). *The Cambridge dictionary of philosophy*, 2nd edn. New York: Cambridge University Press.

Beauchamp, T.L. & Childress, J.F. (2001). *Principles of biomedical ethics*, 5th edn. New York: Oxford University Press.

Canadian Nurses' Association (2002). *Code of ethics for registered nurses*. Ottawa, ON: Canadian Nurses' Association.

Fletcher, J.C., Lombardo, P.A., Marshall, M.F., & Miller, F.G. (1995). *Introduction to Clinical Ethics*, 2nd edn. Hagerston, HD: University Publishing.

Jameton, A. (1984). *Nursing practice: The ethical issues*. Englewood Cliffs, NJ: Prentice-Hall.

Kopala, B. & Burkhart, L. (2005). Ethical dilemma and moral distress: Proposed new NANDA diagnoses. *International Journal of Nursing Terminologies and Classifications* **16**(1): 3–13.

Redman, B.K. & Fry, S.T. (1998). Ethical conflicts reported by certified registered rehabilitation nurses. *Rehabilitation Nursing* **23**: 179–84.

Webster, G.C. & Baylis, F. (2000). Moral residue. In: Rubin, S.B. & Zoloth, L. (eds), *Margin of error. The ethics of mistakes in the practice of medicine*. Hagerstown, MD: University Publishing.

Domain 10

Domain 10: Life Principles
Class 3: Values/Belief/Action Congruence

Definition Response to the inability to carry out one's chosen ethical/moral decision/action

Defining Characteristics

■ Expresses anguish (e.g., powerlessness, guilt, frustration, anxiety, self- doubt, fear) over difficulty acting on one's moral choice

Related Factors

■ Conflict among decision-makers
■ Conflicting information guiding ethical decision-making
■ Conflicting information guiding moral decision-making

■ Cultural conflicts
■ End-of-life decisions
■ Loss of autonomy
■ Physical distance of decision-maker
■ Time constraints for decision-making
■ Treatment decisions

References

Audi, R. (1999). *The Cambridge dictionary of philosophy*, 2nd edn. New York: Cambridge University Press.

Beauchamp, T.L. & Childress, J.F. (2001). *Principles of biomedical ethics*, 5th edn. New York: Oxford University Press.

Berger, M.C., Seversen, A., & Chvatal, R. (1991). Ethical issues in nursing. *Western Journal of Nursing Research* **13**: 514–21.

Burkhardt, M.A. & Nathaniel, A.K. (2002). *Ethics & Issues in Contemporary Nursing*. Albany, NY: Delmar.

Canadian Nurses' Association (2002). *Code of ethics for registered nurses*. Ottawa, ON: Canadian Nurses' Association.

Corley, M.C, Elswick, RK, Gorman, M., Clor, & T. (2001). Development and evaluation of a moral distress scale. *Journal of Advanced Nursing* **33**: 250–6.

Ferrell, B.R. & Rivera, (L.M. 1995). Ethical decision making in oncology. *Cancer Practice* **3**: 94–9.

Fry, S.T. & Duffy, M.E. (2001). The development and psychometric evaluation of the ethical issues scale. *Image: Journal of Nursing Scholarship* **33**: 273–7.

Gwin, R.R. & Richters, J.E. (1998). Selected ethical issues in cancer care. In: Itano, J., & Taoka, K. (eds), *Core curriculum for oncology nurses*, 3rd edn. Philadelphia, PA: pp. 741–5.

Jameton, A. (1984). *Nursing Practice: The ethical issues*. Englewood Cliffs, NJ: Prentice-Hall.

Jameton, A. (1993). Dilemmas of moral distress: Moral responsibility and nursing practice. *AWHONN's Clinical Issues in Perinatal & Women's Health Nursing* 4: 542–51.

Kopala, B. & Burkhart, L. (2005). Ethical dilemma and moral distress: Proposed new NANDA diagnoses. *International Journal of Nursing Terminologies and Classifications* 16(1): 3–13.

McGee, G., Spanogle, J.P., Caplan, A.L., & Asch, D.A. (2001). A national study of ethics committees. *AJOB* 1(4): 60–4.

Moore, M.L. (2000). Ethical issues for nurses providing perinatal care in community settings. *Journal of Perinatal & Neonatal Nursing* 14(2): 25–35.

Omery, A., Henneman, E., Billet, B., Luna-Raines, M., & Brown-Saltzman, K. (1995). Ethical issues in hospital-based nursing practice. *Journal of Cardiovascular Nursing* 9: 43–53.

Pinch, W.J. & Spielman, M.L. (1993). Parental perceptions of ethical issues post-NICU discharge. *Western Journal of Nursing Research* 15: 422–40.

Redman, B.K. & Fry, S.T. (1998). Ethical conflicts reported by certified registered rehabilitation nurses. *Rehabilitation Nursing* 23: 179–84.

Redman, B.K. & S.T., Fry (1998). Ethical conflicts reported by registered nurse/certified diabetes educators: a replication. *Journal of Advanced Nursing* 28: 1320–5.

Rodney, P. & Starzomsky, R. (1993). Constraints on the moral agency of nurses. *Canadian Nurse* 89(9): 23–6.

Scanlon, C. (1994). Survey yields significant results. *American Nurses Association Center for Ethics and Human Rights Communique* 3(3).

Tiedje, L.B. (2000). Moral distress in perinatal nursing. *Journal of Perinatal and Neonatal Nursing* 14(2): 36–43.

Volbrecht, R.M. (2002). *Nursing ethics: Communities in dialogue*. Upper Saddle River, NJ: Prentice Hall.

Wilkinson, J.M. (1987/88). Moral distress in nursing practice: Experience and effect. *Nursing Forum* 23(1): 16–28.

Webster, G.C. & Baylis, F. (2000). Moral residue. In: Rubin, S.B. & Zoloth, L. (eds). *Margin of error: The ethics of mistakes in the practice of medicine*. Hagerstown, MD: University Publishing.

Noncompliance (00079)

(1973, 1996, 1998)

Domain 10: Life Principles
Class 3: Value/Belief/Action Congruence

Definition Behavior of person and/or caregiver that fails to coincide with a health-promoting or therapeutic plan agreed on by the person (and/or family and/or community) and healthcare professional. In the presence of an agreed-on, health promoting or therapeutic plan, person's or caregiver's behavior is fully or partially nonadherent and may lead to clinically ineffective or partially ineffective outcomes

Defining Characteristics

- Behavior indicative of failure to adhere
- Evidence of development of complications
- Evidence of exacerbation of symptoms
- Failure to keep appointments
- Failure to progress
- Objective tests (e.g., physiological measures, detection of physiologic markers)

Related Factors

Health System

- Access to care
- Client/provide relationships
- Communication skills of the provider
- Convenience of care
- Credibility of provider
- Individual health coverage
- Provider continuity
- Provider regular follow-up
- Provider reimbursement
- Satisfaction with care
- Teaching skills of the provider

Individual

- Cultural influences
- Developmental abilities
- Health beliefs
- Individual's value system
- Knowledge relevant to the regimen behavior
- Motivational forces
- Personal abilities
- Significant others
- Skill relevant to the regimen behavior
- Spiritual values

Healthcare Plan

- Complexity
- Cost
- Duration
- Financial flexibility of plan
- Intensity

Network

- Involvement of members in health plan
- Perceived beliefs of significant others
- Social value regarding plan

Domain 10

Impaired Religiosity (00169)

(2004, LOE 2.1)

Domain 10: Life Principles
Class 3: Value/Belief/Action Congruence

Definition Impaired ability to exercise reliance on beliefs and/or participate in rituals of a particular faith tradition

Defining Characteristics

- Difficulty adhering to prescribed religious beliefs
- Difficulty adhering to prescribed religious rituals (e.g., religious ceremonies, dietary regulations, clothing, prayer, worship/religious services, private religious behaviors/reading religious materials/media, holiday observances, meetings with religious leaders)
- Expresses emotional distress because of separation from faith community
- Expresses a need to reconnect with previous belief patterns
- Expresses a need to reconnect with previous customs
- Questions religious belief patterns
- Questions religious customs

Related Factors

Developmental and Situational

- Aging
- End-stage life crises
- Life transitions

Physical

- Illness
- Pain

Psychological

- Anxiety
- Fear of death
- Ineffective coping
- Ineffective support

- Lack of security
- Personal crisis
- Use of religion to manipulate

Sociocultural

- Cultural barriers to practicing religion
- Environmental barriers to practicing religion
- Lack of social integration
- Lack of sociocultural interaction

Spiritual

- Spiritual crises
- Suffering

Domain 10: Life Principles
Class 3: Value/Belief/Action Congruence

Definition Ability to increase reliance on religious beliefs and/or participate in rituals of a particular faith tradition

Defining Characteristics

- Expresses desire to strengthen religious belief patterns that have provided comfort in the past
- Expresses desire to strengthen religious belief patterns that have provided religion in the past
- Expresses desire to strengthen religious customs that have provided comfort in the past
- Expresses desire to strengthen religious customs that have provided comfort in the past
- Questions belief patterns that are harmful
- Questions customs that are harmful
- Rejects belief patterns that are harmful

- Rejects customs that are harmful
- Requests assistance expanding religious options
- Request for assistance to increase participation in prescribed religious beliefs (e.g., religious ceremonies, dietary regulations/rituals, clothing, prayer, worship/ religious services, private religious behaviors, reading religious materials/media, holiday observances)
- Requests forgiveness
- Requests meeting with religious leaders/facilitators
- Requests reconciliation
- Requests religious experiences
- Requests religious materials

Domain 10

Risk for Impaired Religiosity (00170)

(2004, LOE 2.1)

Domain 10: Life Principles
Class 3: Value/Belief/Action Congruence

Definition At risk for an impaired ability to exercise reliance on religious beliefs and/or participate in rituals of a particular faith tradition

Risk Factors

Developmental

- Life transitions

Environmental

- Barriers to practicing religion
- Lack of transportation

Physical

- Hospitalization
- Illness
- Pain

Psychological

- Depression

- Ineffective caregiving
- Ineffective coping
- Ineffective support
- Lack of security

Sociocultural

- Cultural barrier to practicing religion
- Lack of social interaction
- Social isolation

Spiritual

- Suffering

Spiritual Distress (00066)

(1978, 2002, LOE 2.1)

Domain 10: Life Principles
Class 3: Value/Belief/Action Congruence

Definition Impaired ability to experience and integrate meaning and purpose in life through connectedness with self, others, art, music, literature, nature, and/or a power greater than oneself

Defining Characteristics

Connections to Self

- Anger
- Expresses lack of acceptance
- Expresses lack of courage
- Expresses lack of self-forgiveness
- Expresses lack of hope
- Expresses lack of love
- Expresses lack of meaning in life
- Expresses lack of purpose in life
- Expresses lack of serenity (e.g., peace)
- Guilt
- Poor coping

Connections with Others

- Expresses alienation
- Refuses interactions with significant others
- Refuses interactions with spiritual leaders
- Verbalizes being separated from support system

Connections with Art, Music, Literature, Nature

- Disinterest in nature
- Disinterest in reading spiritual literature
- Inability to express previous state of creativity (e.g., singing/listening to music/writing)

Connections with Power Greater than Self

- Expresses being abandoned
- Expresses having anger toward God
- Expresses hopelessness
- Expresses suffering
- Inability to be introspective
- Inability to experience the transcendent
- Inability to participate in religious activities
- Inability to pray
- Requests to see a religious leader
- Sudden changes in spiritual practices

Domain 10

Related Factors

- Active dying
- Anxiety
- Chronic illness
- Death
- Life change
- Loneliness
- Pain
- Self-alienation
- Social alienation
- Sociocultural deprivation

Risk for Spiritual Distress (00067)

(1998, 2004, LOE 2.1)

Domain 10: Life Principles
Class 3: Value/Belief/Action Congruence

Definition At risk for an impaired ability to experience and integrate meaning and purpose in life through connectedness with self, others, art, music, literature, nature, and/or a power greater than oneself

Risk Factors

Developmental

■ Life changes

Environmental

■ Environmental changes
■ Natural disasters

Physical

■ Chronic illness
■ Physical illness
■ Substance abuse

Psychosocial

■ Anxiety
■ Blocks to experiencing love
■ Change in religious rituals
■ Change in spiritual practices
■ Cultural conflict
■ Depression
■ Inability to forgive
■ Loss
■ Low self-esteem
■ Poor relationships
■ Racial conflict
■ Separated support systems
■ Stress

Domain 10

Domain 11
Safety/Protection

Risk for Infection (00004)
(1986)

Domain 11: Safety/Protection
Class 1: Infection

Definition At increased risk for being invaded by pathogenic organisms

Risk Factors

- Chronic disease
- Inadequate acquired immunity
- Inadequate primary defenses (e.g., broken skin, traumatized tissue, decrease in ciliary action, stasis of body fluids, change in pH secretions, altered peristalsis)
- Inadequate secondary defenses (e.g., decreased hemoglobin, leukopenia, suppressed inflammatory response)
- Increased environmental exposure to pathogens
- Immunosuppression
- Invasive procedures
- Insufficient knowledge to avoid exposure to pathogens
- Malnutrition
- Pharmaceutical agents (e.g., immunosuppressants)
- Premature rupture of amniotic membranes
- Prolonged rupture of amniotic membranes
- Trauma
- Tissue destruction

Ineffective Airway Clearance (00031)

(1980, 1996, 1998)

Domain 11: Safety/Protection
Class 2: Physical Injury

Definition Inability to clear secretions or obstructions from the respiratory tract to maintain a clear airway

Defining Characteristics

- Absent cough
- Adventitious breath sounds
- Changes in respiratory rate
- Changes in respiratory rhythm
- Cyanosis
- Difficulty vocalizing
- Diminished breath sounds
- Dyspnea
- Excessive sputum
- Ineffective cough
- Orthopnea
- Restlessness
- Wide-eyed

Related Factors

Environmental

- Second-hand smoke
- Smoke inhalation
- Smoking

Obstructed Airway

- Airway spasm
- Excessive mucus
- Exudate in the alveoli
- Foreign body in airway
- Presence of artificial airway

- Retained secretions
- Secretions in the bronchi

Physiological

- Allergic airways
- Asthma
- Chronic obstructive pulmonary disease
- Hyperplasia of the bronchial walls
- Infection
- Neuromuscular dysfunction

Domain 11

Risk for Aspiration (00039)
(1988)

Domain 11: Safety/Protection
Class 2: Physical Injury

Definition At risk for entry of gastrointestinal secretions, oropharyngeal secretions, solids, or fluids into tracheobronchial passages

Risk Factors

- Decreased gastrointestinal motility
- Delayed gastric emptying
- Depressed cough
- Depressed gag reflex
- Facial surgery
- Facial trauma
- Gastrointestinal tubes
- Incompetent lower esophageal sphincter
- Increased gastric residual
- Increased intragastric pressure
- Impaired swallowing
- Medication administration
- Neck surgery
- Neck trauma
- Oral surgery
- Oral trauma
- Presence of endotracheal tube
- Presence of tracheostomy tube
- Reduced level of consciousness
- Situations hindering elevation of upper body
- Tube feedings
- Wired jaws

Risk for Sudden Infant Death Syndrome (00156)

(2002, LOE 3.3)

Domain 11: Safety/Protection
Class 2: Physical Injury

Definition Presence of risk factors for sudden death of an infant under 1 year of age

Risk Factors

Modifiable

- Delayed prenatal care
- Infant overheating
- Infant overwrapping
- Infants placed to sleep in the prone position
- Infants placed to sleep in the side-lying position
- Lack of prenatal care
- Postnatal infant smoke exposure
- Prenatal infant smoke exposure
- Soft underlayment (loose articles in the sleep environment)

Potentially Modifiable

- Low birth weight
- Prematurity
- Young maternal age

Nonmodifiable

- Ethnicity (e.g., African–American or Native American)
- Male gender
- Seasonality of sudden infant death syndrome (SIDS) deaths (e.g., winter and fall months)
- Infant age of 2–4 months

Impaired Dentition (00048)
(1998)

Domain 11: Safety/Protection
Class 2: Physical Injury

Definition Disruption in tooth development/eruption patterns or structural integrity of individual teeth

Defining Characteristics

- Abraded teeth
- Absence of teeth
- Asymmetrical facial expression
- Crown caries
- Erosion of enamel
- Excessive calculus
- Excessive plaque
- Halitosis
- Incomplete eruption for age (may be primary or permanent teeth)
- Loose teeth
- Malocclusion
- Missing teeth
- Premature loss of primary teeth
- Root caries
- Tooth enamel discoloration
- Tooth fracture(s)
- Tooth misalignment
- Toothache
- Worn down teeth

Related Factors

- Barriers to self-care
- Bruxism
- Chronic use of coffee
- Chronic use of tea
- Chronic use of red wine
- Chronic use of tobacco
- Chronic vomiting
- Deficient knowledge regarding dental health
- Dietary habits
- Economic barriers to professional care
- Excessive use of abrasive cleaning agents
- Excessive intake of fluorides
- Genetic predisposition
- Ineffective oral hygiene
- Lack of access to professional care
- Nutritional deficits
- Selected prescription medications
- Sensitivity to cold
- Sensitivity to heat

Risk for Falls (00155)
(2000)

Domain 11: Safety/Protection
Class 2: Physical Injury

Definition Increased susceptibility to falling that may cause physical harm

Risk Factors

Adults

- Age 65 or over
- History of falls
- Lives alone
- Lower limb prosthesis
- Use of assistive devices (e.g., walker, cane)
- Wheelchair use

Children

- <2 years of age
- Bed located near window
- Lack of automobile-restraints
- Lack of gate on stairs
- Lack of window guard
- Lack of parental supervision
- Male gender when <1 year of age
- Unattended infant on elevated surface (e.g., bed/changing table)

Cognitive

- Diminished mental status

Environment

- Cluttered environment
- Dimly lit room
- No antislip material in bath
- No antislip material in shower
- Restraints
- Throw rugs
- Unfamiliar room
- Weather conditions (e.g., wet floors, ice)

Medications

- Angiotensin-converting enzyme (ACE) inhibitors
- Alcohol use
- Antianxiety agents
- Antihypertensive agents
- Diuretics
- Hypnotics
- Narcotics/opiates
- Tranquilizers
- Tricyclic antidepressants

Physiological

- Anemias
- Arthritis
- Diarrhea
- Decreased lower extremity strength
- Difficulty with gait
- Faintness when extending neck
- Faintness when turning neck
- Foot problems
- Hearing difficulties
- Impaired balance

- Impaired physical mobility
- Incontinence
- Neoplasms (i.e., fatigue/limited mobility)
- Neuropathy
- Orthostatic hypotension
- Postoperative conditions
- Postprandial blood sugar changes
- Presence of acute illness
- Proprioceptive deficits
- Sleeplessness
- Urgency
- Vascular disease
- Visual difficulties

Risk for Injury (00035)
(1978)

Domain 11: Safety/Protection
Class 2: Physical Injury

Definition At risk of injury as a result of environmental
conditions interacting with the individual's adaptive and defensive
resources

Risk Factors

External

- Biological (e.g., immunization level of community, microorganism)
- Chemical (e.g., poisons, pollutants, drugs, pharmaceutical agents, alcohol, nicotine, preservatives, cosmetics, dyes)
- Human (e.g., nosocomial agents, staffing patterns, or cognitive, affective, psychomotor factors)
- Mode of transport
- Nutritional (e.g., vitamins, food types)
- Physical (e.g., design, structure, and arrangement of community, building, and/or equipment)

Internal

- Abnormal blood profile (e.g., leukocytosis/leukopenia, altered clotting factors, thrombocytopenia, sickle cell, thalassemia, decreased hemoglobin)
- Biochemical dysfunction
- Developmental age (physiological, psychosocial)
- Effector dysfunction
- Immune–autoimmune dysfunction
- Integrative dysfunction
- Malnutrition
- Physical (e.g., broken skin, altered mobility)
- Psychological (affective orientation)
- Sensory dysfunction
- Tissue hypoxia

Domain 11: Safety/Protection
Class 2: Physical Injury

Definition At risk for inadvertent anatomical and physical changes as a result of posture or equipment used during an invasive/surgical procedure

Risk Factors

- Disorientation
- Edema
- Emaciation
- Immobilization
- Muscle weakness
- Obesity
- Sensory/perceptual disturbances due to anesthesia

References

Ali, A.A., Breslin, D.S., Hardman, H.D. & Martin, G. (2003). Unusual presentation and complication of the prone position for spinal surgery. *Journal of Clinical Anesthesia* **15**: 471–3.

Blumenreich, G.A. (1998). Positioning, padding, documentation, and the CRNA. *AANA Journal* **66**: 435–8.

Fritzlen, T., Kremer, M., & Biddle, C. (2003). The AANA Foundation Closed Malpractice Claims Study on nerve injuries during anesthesia care. *AANA Journal* **71**: 347–52.

Li, W.W., Lee, T.W., & Yim, A.P. (2004). Shoulder function after thoracic surgery. *Thoracic Surgical Clinics* **14**: 331–43.

Litwiller, J.P., Wells, R.E., Halliwill, J.R., Carmichael, S.W., & Warner, M.A. (2004). Effect of lithotomy positions on strain of the obturator and lateral femoral cutaneous nerves. *Clinical Anatomy* **17**(1): 45–9.

McEwen, D.R. (1996 June). Intraoperative positioning of surgical patients. *AORN Journal* **63**: 1059–63, 1066–79; quiz 1080–6.

Murphy, E.K. (2004). Negligence cases concerning positioning injuries. *AORN Journal* **79**: 1017–18.

Impaired Oral Mucous Membrane
(00045)
(1982, 1998)

Domain 11: Safety/Protection
Class 2: Physical Injury

Definition   Disruption of the lips and/or soft tissue of the oral cavity

Defining Characteristics

- Bleeding
- Bluish masses (e.g., hemangiomas)
- Cheilitis
- Coated tongue
- Desquamation
- Difficult speech
- Difficulty eating
- Difficulty swallowing
- Diminished taste
- Edema
- Enlarged tonsils
- Fissures
- Geographic tongue
- Gingival hyperplasia
- Gingival pallor
- Gingival recession
- Halitosis
- Hyperemia
- Macroplasia
- Mucosal denudation
- Mucosal pallor
- Nodules
- Oral discomfort
- Oral lesions
- Oral pain
- Oral ulcers
- Papules
- Pocketing deeper than 4 mm
- Presence of pathogens
- Purulent drainage
- Purulent exudates
- Red masses (e.g., hemangiomas)
- Reports bad taste in mouth
- Smooth atrophic tongue
- Spongy patches
- Stomatitis
- Vesicles
- White, curd-like exudate
- White patches
- White plaques
- Xerostomia

Related Factors

- Barriers to oral self-care
- Barriers to professional care
- Chemotherapy
- Chemical irritants (e.g., alcohol, tobacco, acidic foods, drugs, regular use of inhalers or other noxious agents)
- Cleft lip
- Cleft palate
- Decreased platelets
- Decreased salivation
- Deficient knowledge of appropriate oral hygiene

- Dehydration
- Depression
- Diminished hormone levels (women)
- Ineffective oral hygiene
- Infection
- Immunocompromised
- Immunosuppressed
- Loss of supportive structures
- Malnutrition
- Mechanical factors (e.g., ill-fitting dentures, braces, tubes [endotracheal/nasogastric], surgery in oral cavity)
- Medication side effects
- Mouth breathing
- Nil by mouth (NPO) for more than 24 hours
- Radiation therapy
- Stress
- Trauma

Risk for Peripheral Neurovascular Dysfunction (00086)
(1992)

Domain 11: Safety/Protection
Class 2: Physical Injury

Definition At risk for disruption in circulation, sensation, or motion of an extremity

Risk Factors

- Burns
- Fractures
- Immobilization
- Mechanical compression (e.g., tourniquet, cane, cast, brace, dressing, restraint)

- Orthopedic surgery
- Trauma
- Vascular obstruction

Ineffective Protection (00043)
(1990)

Domain 11: Safety/Protection
Class 2: Physical Injury

Definition   Decrease in the ability to guard self from internal or external threats such as illness or injury

Defining Characteristics

- Altered clotting
- Anorexia
- Chilling
- Cough
- Deficient immunity
- Disorientation
- Dyspnea
- Fatigue
- Immobility
- Impaired healing
- Insomnia
- Itching
- Maladaptive stress response
- Neurosensory alteration
- Perspiring
- Pressure ulcers
- Restlessness
- Weakness

Related Factors

- Abnormal blood profiles (e.g., leukopenia, thrombocytopenia, anemia, coagulation)
- Alcohol abuse
- Cancer
- Drug therapies (e.g., antineoplastic, corticosteroid, immune, anticoagulant, thrombolytic)
- Extremes of age
- Immune disorders
- Inadequate nutrition
- Treatments (e.g., surgery, radiation)

Impaired Skin Integrity (00046)

(1975, 1998)

Domain 11: Safety/Protection
Class 2: Physical Injury

Definition   Altered epidermis and/or dermis

Defining Characteristics

- Destruction of skin layers
- Disruption of skin surface
- Invasion of body structures

Related Factors

External

- Chemical substance
- Extremes in age
- Humidity
- Hyperthermia
- Hypothermia
- Mechanical factors (e.g., shearing forces, pressure, restraint)
- Medications
- Moisture
- Physical immobilization
- Radiation

Internal

- Changes in fluid status
- Changes in pigmentation
- Changes in turgor
- Developmental factors
- Imbalanced nutritional state (e.g., obesity, emaciation)
- Immunological deficit
- Impaired circulation
- Impaired metabolic state
- Impaired sensation
- Skeletal prominence

Risk for Impaired Skin Integrity (00047)
(1975, 1998)

Domain 11: Safety/Protection
Class 2: Physical Injury

Definition At risk for skin being adversely altered

Risk Factors

External

- Chemical substance
- Excretions
- Extremes of age
- Hyperthermia
- Hypothermia
- Humidity
- Mechanical factors (e.g., shearing forces, pressure, restraint)
- Moisture
- Physical immobilization
- Radiation
- Secretions

Internal

- Changes in pigmentation
- Changes in skin turgor
- Developmental factors
- Imbalanced nutritional state (e.g., obesity, emaciation)
- Impaired circulation
- Impaired metabolic state
- Impaired sensation
- Immunologic factors
- Medications
- Psychogenetic factors
- Skeletal prominence

Note: risk should be determined by use of a standardized risk assessment tool.

Risk for Suffocation (00036)
(1980)

Domain 11: Safety/Protection
Class 2: Physical Injury

Definition Accentuated risk of accidental suffocation (inadequate air available for inhalation)

Risk Factors

External

- Discarding refrigerators without removed doors
- Eating large mouthfuls of food
- Hanging a pacifier around infant's neck
- Household gas leaks
- Inserting small objects into airway
- Leaving children unattended in water
- Low-strung clothesline
- Pillow placed in infant's crib
- Playing with plastic bags
- Propped bottle placed in infant's crib
- Smoking in bed
- Fuel-burning heaters not vented to outside
- Vehicle warming in closed garage

Internal

- Cognitive difficulties
- Disease process
- Emotional difficulties
- Injury process
- Lack of safety education
- Lack of safety precautions
- Reduced motor abilities
- Reduced olfactory sensation

Domain 11: Safety/Protection
Class 2: Physical Injury

Definition Damage to mucous membrane, corneal, integumentary, or subcutaneous tissues

Defining Characteristics

- Damaged tissue (e.g., cornea, mucous membrane, integumentary, subcutaneous)
- Destroyed tissue

Related Factors

- Altered circulation
- Chemical irritants
- Fluid deficit
- Fluid excess
- Impaired physical mobility
- Knowledge deficit
- Mechanical factors (e.g., pressure, shear, friction)
- Nutritional factors (e.g., deficit or excess)
- Radiation
- Temperature extremes

Risk for Trauma (00038)

(1980)

Domain 11: Safety/Protection
Class 2: Physical Injury

Definition Accentuated risk of accidental tissue injury (e.g., wound, burn, fracture)

Risk Factors

External

- Accessibility of guns
- Bathing in very hot water (e.g., unsupervised bathing of young children)
- Bathtub without antislip equipment
- Children playing with dangerous objects
- Children playing without gate at top of stairs
- Children riding in the front seat in car
- Contact with corrosives
- Contact with intense cold
- Contact with rapidly moving machinery
- Defective appliances
- Delayed lighting of gas appliances
- Driving a mechanically unsafe vehicle
- Driving at excessive speeds
- Driving while intoxicated
- Driving without necessary visual aids
- Entering unlighted rooms
- Experimenting with chemicals
- Exposure to dangerous machinery
- Faulty electrical plugs
- Flammable children's clothing
- Flammable children's toys
- Frayed wires
- Grease waste collected on stoves
- High beds
- High-crime neighborhood
- Inappropriate call-for-aid mechanisms for bedresting client
- Inadequate stair rails
- Inadequately stored combustibles (e.g., matches, oily rags)
- Inadequately stored corrosives (e.g., lye)
- Knives stored uncovered
- Lack of protection from heat source
- Large icicles hanging from the roof
- Misuse of necessary headgear
- Misuse of seat restraints
- Nonuse of seat restraints
- Obstructed passageways
- Overexposure to radiation
- Overloaded electrical outlets
- Overloaded fuse boxes
- Physical proximity to vehicle pathways (e.g., driveways, lanes, railroad tracks)
- Playing with explosives
- Pot handles facing toward front of stove
- Potential igniting of gas leaks

- Slippery floors (e.g., wet or highly waxed)
- Smoking in bed
- Smoking near oxygen
- Struggling with restraints
- Unanchored electric wires
- Unanchored rugs
- Unsafe road
- Unsafe walkways
- Unsafe window protection in homes with young children
- Use of cracked dishware
- Use of unsteady chairs
- Use of unsteady ladders
- Wearing flowing clothes around open flame

Internal

- Balancing difficulties
- Cognitive difficulties
- Emotional difficulties
- History of previous trauma
- Insufficient finances
- Lack of safety education
- Lack of safety precautions
- Poor vision
- Reduced hand–eye coordination
- Reduced muscle coordination
- Reduced sensation
- Weakness

Risk for Vascular Trauma (00213)

(2008, LOE 2.1)

Domain 11: Safety/Protection
Class 2: Physical Injury

Definition At risk for damage to a vein and its surrounding tissues related to the presence of a catheter and/or infused solutions

Risk Factors

- Catheter type
- Catheter width
- Impaired ability to visualize the insertion site
- Inadequate catheter fixation
- Infusion rate

- Insertion site
- Length of insertion time
- Nature of solution (e.g., concentration, chemical irritant, temperature, pH)

References

Adami N., Gutierrez M., Fonseca S. & Almeida, E. (2005). Risk management of extravasation of cytostatic drugs at the adult chemotherapy outpatient clinic of a university hospital. *Journal of Clinical Nursing* **14**: 876–82

Arreguy-Sena, C. & de Carvalho, E.C. (2003). Punção venosa periférica: análise dos critérios adotados por uma equipe de enfermagem para avaliar e remover um dispositivo endovenoso. *Escola Anna Nery Revista de Enfermagem*. Rio de Janeiro: EEAN-UFRJ **7**: 351–60.

Arreguy-Sena, C. (2002). *A trajetória de construção e validação dos diagnósticos de enfermagem: Trauma Vascular e Risco para Trauma Vascular*. [Tese] Ribeirão Preto: Escola de Enfermagem de Ribeirão Preto-USP, p. 280.

Phillips, L. (2005). *Manual of IV Therapeutics*, 4th edn. Philadelphia, PA: Davis.

Polimeno, N., Hara, M., Appezzato, L., Fernandes, V., Cintra, L., & Hara, C. (1995) Incidência e caracterização da tromboflebite superficial (TFS) pós-venóclise em Hospital Universitário. *Jornal Brasileiro de Medicina* **69**: 196–204.

Self-Mutilation (00151)
(2000)

Domain 11: Safety/Protection
Class 3: Violence

Definition Deliberate self-injurious behavior causing tissue damage with the intent of causing nonfatal injury to attain relief of tension

Defining Characteristics

- Abrading
- Biting
- Constricting a body part
- Cuts on body
- Hitting
- Ingestion of harmful substances
- Inhalation of harmful substances
- Insertion of object into body orifice
- Picking at wounds
- Scratches on body
- Self-inflicted burns
- Severing

Related Factors

- Adolescence
- Autistic individual
- Battered child
- Borderline personality disorder
- Character disorder
- Childhood illness
- Childhood sexual abuse
- Childhood surgery
- Depersonalization
- Developmentally delayed individual
- Dissociation
- Disturbed body image
- Disturbed interpersonal relationships
- Eating disorders
- Emotionally disturbed
- Family alcoholism
- Family divorce
- Family history of self-destructive behaviors
- Feels threatened with loss of significant relationship
- History of inability to plan solutions
- History of inability to see long-term consequences
- History of self-injurious behavior
- Impulsivity
- Inability to express tension verbally
- Incarceration
- Ineffective coping
- Irresistible urge to cut self
- Irresistible urge to damage self
- Isolation from peers
- Labile behavior
- Lack of family confidant
- Living in nontraditional setting (e.g., foster, group, or institutional care)

Domain 11

- Low self-esteem
- Mounting tension that is intolerable
- Needs quick reduction of stress
- Negative feelings (e.g., depression, rejection, self-hatred, separation anxiety, guilt, depersonalization)
- Peers who self-mutilate
- Perfectionism
- Poor communication between parent and adolescent
- Psychotic state (e.g., command hallucinations)
- Sexual identity crisis
- Substance abuse
- Unstable body image
- Unstable self-esteem
- Use of manipulation to obtain nurturing relationship with others
- Violence between parental figures

Risk for Self-Mutilation (00139)
(1992, 2000)

Domain 11: Safety/Protection
Class 3: Violence

Definition At risk for deliberate self-injurious behavior causing tissue damage with the intent of causing nonfatal injury to attain relief of tension

Risk Factors

- Adolescence
- Autistic individuals
- Battered child
- Borderline personality disorders
- Character disorders
- Childhood illness
- Childhood sexual abuse
- Childhood surgery
- Depersonalization
- Developmentally delayed individuals
- Dissociation
- Disturbed body image
- Disturbed interpersonal relationships
- Eating disorders
- Emotionally disturbed child
- Family alcoholism
- Family divorce
- Family history of self-destructive behaviors
- Feels threatened with loss of significant relationship
- History of inability to plan solutions
- History of inability to see long-term consequences
- History of self-injurious behavior
- Impulsivity
- Inability to express tension verbally
- Inadequate coping
- Incarceration
- Irresistible urge to damage self
- Isolation from peers
- Living in nontraditional setting (e.g., foster, group, or institutional care)
- Loss of control over problem-solving situations
- Loss of significant relationship(s)
- Low self-esteem
- Mounting tension that is intolerable
- Needs quick reduction of stress
- Negative feelings (e.g., depression, rejection, self-hatred, separation anxiety, guilt)
- Peers who self-mutilate
- Perfectionism
- Psychotic state (e.g., command hallucinations)
- Sexual identity crisis
- Substance abuse
- Unstable self-esteem
- Use of manipulation to obtain nurturing relationship with others
- Violence between parental figures

Domain 11

Risk for Suicide (00150)
(2000)

Domain 11: Safety/Protection
Class 3: Violence

Definition At risk for self-inflicted, life-threatening injury

Risk Factors

Behavioral

- Buying a gun
- Changing a will
- Giving away possessions
- History of prior suicide attempt
- Impulsiveness
- Making a will
- Marked changes in attitude
- Marked changes in behavior
- Marked changes in school performance
- Stockpiling medicines
- Sudden euphoric recovery from major depression

Demographic

- Age (e.g., elderly people, young adult males, adolescents)
- Divorced
- Male gender
- Race (e.g., white, Native American)
- Widowed

Physical

- Chronic pain
- Physical illness
- Terminal illness

Psychological

- Childhood abuse
- Family history of suicide
- Guilt
- Homosexual youth
- Psychiatric disorder
- Psychiatric illness
- Substance abuse

Situational

- Adolescents living in nontraditional settings (e.g., juvenile detention center, prison, half-way house, group home)
- Economic instability
- Institutionalization
- Living alone
- Loss of autonomy
- Loss of independence
- Presence of gun in home
- Relocation
- Retired

Social

- Cluster suicides
- Disrupted family life
- Disciplinary problems
- Grief
- Helplessness

- Hopelessness
- Legal problems
- Loneliness
- Loss of important relationship
- Poor support systems
- Social isolation

Verbal

- States desire to die
- Threats of killing oneself

Domain 11

Risk for Other-Directed Violence (00138)

(1980, 1996)

Domain 11: Safety/Protection
Class 3: Violence

Definition At risk for behaviors in which an individual demonstrates that he or she can be physically, emotionally, and/or sexually harmful to others

Risk Factors

- Availability of weapon(s)
- Body language (e.g., rigid posture, clenching of fists and jaw, hyperactivity, pacing, breathlessness, threatening stances)
- Cognitive impairment (e.g., learning disabilities, attention deficit disorder, decreased intellectual functioning)
- Cruelty to animals
- Firesetting
- History of childhood abuse
- History of indirect violence (e.g., tearing off clothes, ripping objects off walls, writing on walls, urinating on floor, defecating on floor, stamping feet, temper tantrum, running in corridors, yelling, throwing objects, breaking a window, slamming doors, sexual advances)
- History of substance abuse
- History of threats of violence (e.g., verbal threats against property, verbal threats against person, social threats, cursing, threatening notes/letters, threatening gestures, sexual threats)
- History of witnessing family violence
- History of violence against others (e.g., hitting someone, kicking someone, spitting at someone, scratching someone, throwing objects at someone, biting someone, attempted rape, rape, sexual molestation, urinating/defecating on a person)
- History of violent antisocial behavior (e.g., stealing, insistent borrowing, insistent demands for privileges, insistent interruption of meetings, refusal to eat, refusal to take medication, ignoring instructions)
- Impulsivity
- Motor vehicle offenses (e.g., frequent traffic violations, use of a motor vehicle to release anger)
- Neurological impairment (e.g., positive EEG, CT, MRI, neurological findings, head trauma, seizure disorders)
- Pathological intoxication
- Perinatal complications
- Prenatal complications
- Psychotic symptomatology (e.g., auditory, visual, command hallucinations; paranoid delusions; loose, rambling, or illogical thought processes)
- Suicidal behavior

Risk for Self-Directed Violence (00140)
(1994)

Domain 11: Safety/Protection
Class 3: Violence

Definition At risk for behaviors in which an individual demonstrates that he or she can be physically, emotionally and/or sexually harmful to self

Risk Factors

- Age 15–19
- Age >45
- Behavioral clues (e.g., writing forlorn love notes, directing angry messages at a significant other who has rejected the person, giving away personal items, taking out a large life insurance policy)
- Conflictual interpersonal relationships
- Emotional problems (e.g., hopelessness, despair, increased anxiety, panic, anger, hostility)
- Employment problems (e.g., unemployed, recent job loss/ failure)
- Engagement in autoerotic sexual acts
- Family background (e.g., chaotic or conflictual, history of suicide)
- History of multiple suicide attempts
- Lack of personal resources (e.g., poor achievement, poor insight, affect unavailable and poorly controlled)
- Lack of social resources (e.g., poor rapport, socially isolated, unresponsive family)
- Physical health problems (e.g., hypochondriasis, chronic or terminal illness)
- Marital status (single, widowed, divorced)
- Mental health problems (e.g., severe depression, psychosis, severe personality disorder, alcoholism or drug abuse)
- Occupation (executive, administrator/owner of business, professional, semiskilled worker)
- Sexual orientation (bisexual [active], homosexual [inactive])
- Suicidal ideation
- Suicidal plan
- Verbal clues (e.g., talking about death, "better off without me", asking questions about lethal dosages of drugs)

Contamination (00181)

(2006, LOE 2.1)

Domain 11: Safety/Protection
Class 4: Environmental Hazards

Definition Exposure to environmental contaminants in doses sufficient to cause adverse health effects

Defining Characteristics

(Defining characteristics are dependent on the causative agent. Agents cause a variety of individual organ responses as well as systemic responses.)

Pesticides

- Dermatological effects of pesticide exposure
- Gastrointestinal effects of pesticide exposure
- Neurological effects of pesticide exposure
- Pulmonary effects of pesticide exposure
- Renal effects of pesticide exposure
- Major categories of pesticides: insecticides, herbicides, fungicides, antimicrobials, rodenticides
- Major pesticides: organophosphates, carbamates, organochlorines, pyrethrum, arsenic, glycophosphates, bipyridyls, chlorophenoxy

Chemicals

- Dermatological effects of chemical exposure
- Gastrointestinal effects of chemical exposure
- Immunologic effects of chemical exposure
- Neurological effects of chemical exposure
- Pulmonary effects of chemical exposure
- Renal effects of chemical exposure
- Major chemical agents: petroleum-based agents, anticholinesterases type I agents act on proximal tracheobronchial portion of the respiratory tract, type II agents act on alveoli; type III agents produce systemic effects

Biologics

- Dermatological effects of exposure to biologics
- Gastrointestinal effects of exposure to biologics
- Pulmonary effects of exposure to biologics
- Neurological effects of exposure to biologics
- Renal effects of exposure to biologics (toxins from living

organisms [bacteria, viruses, fungi])

Pollution

- Neurological effects of pollution exposure
- Pulmonary effects of pollution exposure (major locations: air, water, soil; major agents: asbestos, radon, tobacco, heavy metal, lead, noise, exhaust)

Waste

- Dermatological effects of waste exposure
- Gastrointestinal effects of waste exposure

- Hepatic effects of waste exposure
- Pulmonary effects of waste exposure (categories of waste: trash, raw sewage, industrial waste)

Radiation

- External exposure through direct contact with radioactive material
- Genetic effects of radiation exposure
- Immunologic effects of radiation exposure
- Neurological effects of radiation exposure
- Oncological effects of radiation exposure

Related Factors

External

- Chemical contamination of food
- Chemical contamination of water
- Exposure to bioterrorism
- Exposure to disaster (natural or man-made)
- Exposure to radiation (occupation in radiology, employment in nuclear industries and electrical generating plants, living near nuclear industries and/or electrical generating plants)
- Exposure through ingestion of radioactive material (e.g., food/water contamination)
- Flaking, peeling paint in presence of young children

- Flaking, peeling plaster in presence of young children
- Flooring surface (carpeted surfaces hold contaminant residue more than hard floor surfaces)
- Geographic area (living in area where high level of contaminants exist)
- Household hygiene practices
- Inadequate municipal services (trash removal, sewage treatment facilities)
- Inappropriate use of protective clothing
- Lack of breakdown of contaminants once indoors (breakdown is inhibited without sun and rain exposure)

- Lack of protective clothing
- Lacquer in poorly ventilated areas
- Lacquer without effective protection
- Living in poverty (increases potential for multiple exposure, lack of access to health care, poor diet)
- Paint in poorly ventilated areas
- Paint without effective protection
- Personal hygiene practices
- Playing in outdoor areas where environmental contaminants are used
- Presence of atmospheric pollutants
- Use of environmental contaminants in the home (e.g., pesticides, chemicals, environmental tobacco smoke)

- Unprotected contact with chemicals (e.g., arsenic)
- Unprotected contact with heavy metals (e.g., chromium, lead)

Internal

- Age (children <5 years, older adults)
- Concomitant exposures
- Developmental characteristics of children
- Female gender
- Gestational age during exposure
- Nutritional factors (e.g., obesity, vitamin and mineral deficiencies)
- Pre-existing disease states
- Pregnancy
- Previous exposures
- Smoking

References

Baker, J. E. (1992). Primary, secondary, and tertiary prevention in reducing pesticide related illness in farmers. *Journal of Community Health Nursing* **9**: 245–53.

Berkowitz, G. S., Obel, J., Deych, E., Lapinski, R., Godbold, J., & Liu, Z. (2003). Exposure to indoor pesticides during pregnancy in a multiethnic, urban cohort. *Environmental Health Perspectives* **111**(1): 79–84.

Brender, J., Suarez, L., Hendricks, K., Baetz, R.A., & Larsen, R. (2002). Parental occupation and neural tube defect-affected pregnancies among Mexican Americans. *Journal of Occupational and Environmental Medicine* **44**: 650–6.

Butterfield, P.G. (2002). Upstream reflections on environmental health: An abbreviated history and framework for action. *Advances in Nursing Science* **25**(1): 32–49.

Center for Disease Control and Prevention (2005). Third national report on human exposure to environmental chemicals: Executive summary. Atlanta, GA: Center for Disease Control and Prevention. NCEH Pub # 05-0725.

Center for Disease Control and Prevention (2004). Agency for Toxic Substances and Disease Registry. Available at: www.atsdr.cdc.gov (accessed May 23, 2008).

Chalupka, S.M. (2001). Essentials of environmental health. Enhancing your occupational health nursing practice. (Part I). *American Association of Occupational Health Nurses or Nursing* **49**: 137–54.

Chalupka, S.M. (2001). Essentials of environmental health. Enhancing your occupational health nursing practice. (Part II). *American Association of Occupational Health Nurses or Nursing* **49**(4), 194–213.

Children's Environmental Health Network. (2004). Resource guide on children's environmental health. Available at: www.cehn.org.

Children's Environmental Health Network. (2005). Training manual on pediatric environmental health: Putting it into practice. Available at: www.cehn.org.

Diaz, J. & Lopez, M.A. (1999). Voluntary ingestion of organophosphate insecticide by a young farmer. *Journal of Emergency Nursing* **25**: 266–8.

Dixon, J.K. & Dixon, J.P. (2002). An integrative model for environmental health research. *Advances in Nursing Science* **24**: 43–57.

Environmental Protection Agency (2004). Understanding radiation health effects. EPA. Available at www.epa.gov (accessed May 23, 2008).

Gerrard, C.E. (1998). Farmer's occupational health: Cause for concern, cause for action. *Journal of Advanced Nursing* **28** :155–63.

Goldman, L.R., Shannon, M.W., & the Committee on Environmental Health. (2001). Technical report: Mercury in the environment: Implications for physicians. *Pediatrics* **108**: 197–205.

King, C. & Harber, (P. 1998). Community environmental health concerns and the nursing process. *American Association of Occupational Health Nursing Journal* **46**: 20–7.

Larsson, L.S. & Butterfield, P. (2002). Mapping the future of environmental health and nursing: Strategies for integrating national competencies into nursing practice. *Public Health Nursing* **19**: 301–8.

Massey-Stokes, M. & Lanning, B. (2002). Childhood cancer and environmental toxins: The debate continues. *Family and Community Health* **24**(4): 27–38.

McCauley, L.A., Michaels, S., Rothlein, J., Muniz, J., Lasarev, M., & Ebbert, C. (2003). Pesticide exposure and self-reported home hygiene. *American Association of Occupational Health Nurses or Nursing* **51**: 113–19.

Meeker, B.J., Curruth, A., & Holland, C.B. (2002). Health hazards and preventive measures of farm women. *AAOHN* **50**: 307–14.

Melum, M.F. (2001). Organophosphate toxicity. *American Journal of Nursing* **101**(5): 57–8.

Schneider, D. & Freeman, N. (2001). Children's environmental health risks: A state of the art conference. *Archives of Environmental Health* **56**(2): 103–110.

Silbergeld, E.K. & Flaws, J.A. (2002). Environmental exposures and women's health. *Clinical Obstetrics and Gynecology* **45**: 1119–28.

Thornton, J.W., McCally, M., & Houlihan, J. (2002). Biomonitoring of industrial pollutants: Health and policy implications of the chemical body burden. *Public Health Reports* **117**: 315–23.

Domain 11: Safety/Protection
Class 4: Environmental Hazards

Definition Accentuated risk of exposure to environmental contaminants in doses sufficient to cause adverse health effects

Risk Factors

External

- Chemical contamination of food
- Chemical contamination of water
- Exposure to bioterrorism
- Exposure to disaster (natural or man-made)
- Exposure to radiation (occupation in radiography, employment in nuclear industries and electrical generating plants, living near nuclear industries and/or electrical generating plants)
- Flaking, peeling paint in presence of young children
- Flaking, peeling plaster in presence of young children
- Flooring surface (carpeted surfaces hold contaminant residue more than hard floor surfaces)
- Geographic area (living in area where high level of contaminants exist)
- Household hygiene practices
- Inadequate municipal services (e.g., trash removal, sewage treatment facilities)
- Inappropriate use of protective clothing

- Lack of breakdown of contaminants once indoors (breakdown is inhibited without sun and rain exposure)
- Lack of protective clothing
- Lacquer in poorly ventilated areas
- Lacquer without effective protection
- Living in poverty (increases potential for multiple exposure, lack of access to health care, poor diet)
- Paint, lacquer, etc. in poorly ventilated areas
- Paint, lacquer, etc. without effective protection
- Personal hygiene practices
- Playing in outdoor areas where environmental contaminants are used
- Presence of atmospheric pollutants
- Use of environmental contaminants in the home (e.g., pesticides, chemicals, environmental tobacco smoke
- Unprotected contact with chemicals (e.g., arsenic)
- Unprotected contact with heavy metals (e.g., chromium, lead)

Internal

- Age (children <5 years, older adults)
- Concomitant exposures
- Developmental characteristics of children
- Female gender
- Gestational age during exposure
- Nutritional factors (e.g., obesity, vitamin and mineral deficiencies)
- Pre-existing disease states
- Pregnancy
- Previous exposures
- Smoking

References

Baker, J. E. (1992). Primary, secondary, and tertiary prevention in reducing pesticide related illness in farmers. *Journal of Community Health Nursing* 9: 245–53.

Berkowitz, G. S., Obel, J., Deych, E., Lapinski, R., Godbold, J., & Liu, Z. (2003). Exposure to indoor pesticides during pregnancy in a multiethnic, urban cohort. *Environmental Health Perspectives* 111(1): 79–84.

Brender, J., Suarez, L., Hendricks, K., Baetz, R.A., & Larsen, R. (2002). Parental occupation and neural tube defect-affected pregnancies among Mexican Americans. *Journal of Occupational and Environmental Medicine* 44: 650–6.

Butterfield, P.G. (2002). Upstream reflections on environmental health: An abbreviated history and framework for action. *Advances in Nursing Science* 25(1): 32–49.

Center for Disease Control and Prevention (2004). Agency for Toxic Substances and Disease Registry. Available at: www.atsdr.cdc.gov (accessed May 23, 2008).

Center for Disease Control and Prevention (2005). *Third national report on human exposure to environmental chemicals: Executive summary.* Atlanta, GA: Center for Disease Control and Prevention. NCEH Pub # 05–0725.

Chalupka, S.M. (2001). Essentials of environmental health. Enhancing your occupational health nursing practice. (Part I). *American Association of Occupational Health Nurses or Nursing* 49: 137–54.

Chalupka, S.M. (2001). Essentials of environmental health. Enhancing your occupational health nursing practice. (Part II). *American Association of Occupational Health Nurses or Nursing* 49(4): 194–213.

Children's Environmental Health Network (2004). Resource guide on children's environmental health. Available at: www.cehn.org.

Children's Environmental Health Network (2005). Training manual on pediatric environmental health: Putting it into practice. Available at: www.cehn.org.

Diaz, J. & Lopez, M.A. (1999). Voluntary ingestion of organophosphate insecticide by a young farmer. *Journal of Emergency Nursing* 25: 266–8.

Dixon, J.K. & Dixon, J.P. (2002). An integrative model for environmental health research. *Advances in Nursing Science* 24: 43–57.

Environmental Protection Agency (2004). Understanding radiation health effects. Available at www.epa.gov (accessed May 23, 2008).

Gerrard, C.E. (1998). Farmer's occupational health: Cause for concern, cause for action. *Journal of Advanced Nursing* 28: 155–63.

Goldman, L.R., Shannon, M.W., & the Committee on Environmental Health. (2001). Technical report: Mercury in the environment: Implications for physicians. *Pediatrics* 108: 197–205.

King, C. & Harber, (P. 1998). Community environmental health concerns and the nursing process. *American Association of Occupational Health Nursing Journal* 46: 20–7.

Domain 11

Larsson, L.S. & Butterfield, P. (2002). Mapping the future of environmental health and nursing: Strategies for integrating national competencies into nursing practice. *Public Health Nursing* **19**: 301–8.

McCauley, L.A., Michaels, S., Rothlein, J., Muniz, J., Lasarev, M., & Ebbert, C. (2003). Pesticide exposure and self-reported home hygiene. *American Association of Occupational Health Nurses or Nursing* **51**: 113–19.

Massey-Stokes, M. & Lanning, B. (2002). Childhood cancer and environmental toxins: The debate continues. *Family and Community Health* **24**(4): 27–38.

Meeker, B.J., Curruth, A., & Holland, C.B. (2002). Health hazards and preventive measures of farm women. *AAOHN* **50**: 307–14.

Melum, M.F. (2001). Organophosphate toxicity. *American Journal of Nursing* **101**(5): 57–8.

Schneider, D. & Freeman, N. (2001). Children's environmental health risks: A state of the art conference. *Archives of Environmental Health* **56**(2): 103–110.

Silbergeld, E.K. & Flaws, J.A. (2002). Environmental exposures and women's health. *Clinical Obstetrics and Gynecology* **45**: 1119–28.

Thornton, J.W., McCally, M., & Houlihan, J. (2002). Biomonitoring of industrial pollutants: Health and policy implications of the chemical body burden. *Public Health Reports* **117**: 315–23.

Domain 11

Risk for Poisoning (00037)

(1980, 2006, LOE 2.1)

Domain 11: Safety/Protection
Class 4: Environmental Hazards

Definition Accentuated risk of accidental exposure to, or ingestion of, drugs or dangerous products in doses sufficient to cause poisoning

Risk Factors

External

- Availability of illicit drugs potentially contaminated by poisonous additives
- Dangerous products placed within reach of children
- Dangerous products placed within reach of confused individuals
- Large supplies of drugs in house
- Medicines stored in unlocked cabinets accessible to children
- Medicines stored in unlocked cabinets accessible to confused individuals

Internal

- Cognitive difficulties
- Emotional difficulties
- Lack of drug education
- Lack of proper precaution
- Lack of safety education
- Reduced vision
- Verbalization that occupational setting is without adequate safeguards

Reference

Center for Disease Control and Prevention (2005). *Third national report on human exposure to environmental chemicals: Executive summary.* Atlanta, GA: Center for Disease Control and Prevention. NCEH Pub # 05–0725.

Latex Allergy Response (00041)

(1998, 2006, LOE 2.1)

Domain 11: Safety/Protection
Class 5: Defensive Processes

Definition A hypersensitive reaction to natural latex rubber products

Defining Characteristics

Life-threatening Reactions occurring <1 Hour after Exposure to Latex Protein

- Bronchospasm
- Cardiac arrest
- Contact urticaria progressing to generalized symptoms
- Dyspnea
- Edema of the lips
- Edema of the throat
- Edema of the tongue
- Edema of the uvula
- Hypotension
- Respiratory arrest
- Syncope
- Tightness in chest
- Wheezing

Orofacial Characteristics

- Edema of eyelids
- Edema of sclera
- Erythema of the eyes
- Facial erythema
- Facial itching
- Itching of the eyes
- Oral itching
- Nasal congestion
- Nasal erythema
- Nasal itching
- Rhinorrhea
- Tearing of the eyes

Gastrointestinal Characteristics

- Abdominal pain
- Nausea

Generalized Characteristics

- Flushing
- Generalized discomfort
- Generalized edema
- Increasing complaint of total body warmth
- Restlessness

Type IV Reactions occurring >1 Hour after Exposure to Latex Protein

- Discomfort reaction to additives such as thiurams and carbamates
- Eczema
- Irritation
- Redness

Related Factors

- Hypersensitivity to natural latex rubber protein

References

American Society of Anesthesiologists (2005). *Natural rubber latex allergy: Considerations for anesthesiologists* (a practice guideline). Park Ridge, IL: American Society of Anesthesiologists.

AORN (2004). AORN latex guideline. In *AORN standards, recommended practices and guidelines* (pp. 103.118). Denver, CO: AORN.

Kelly, K.J. (2000). Latex allergy: Where do we go from here? *Canadian Journal of Allergy and Clinical Immunology* **5**: 337–40.

Sussman, G.L. (2000) Latex allergy: An overview. *Canadian Journal of Allergy and Clinical Immunology* **5**: 317–21.

Swanson, M.C. & Olson, D.Q. (2000). Latex allergen affinity for starch powders applied to natural rubber gloves and released as an aerosol. *Canadian Journal of Allergy and Clinical Immunology* **5**: 328–36.

Domain 11

Risk for Latex Allergy Response (00042)
(1998, 2006, LOE 2.1)

Domain 11: Safety/Protection
Class 5: Defensive Processes

Definition Risk of hypersensitivity to natural latex rubber products

Risk Factors

- Allergies to avocados
- Allergies to bananas
- Allergies to chestnuts
- Allergies to kiwis
- Allergies to poinsettia plants
- Allergies to tropical fruits
- History of allergies
- History of asthma
- History of reactions to latex
- Multiple surgical procedures, especially from infancy
- Professions with daily exposure to latex

References

American Society of Anesthesiologists (2005). *Natural rubber latex allergy: Considerations for anesthesiologists* (a practice guideline). Park Ridge, IL: American Society of Anesthesiologists.

AORN (2004). AORN latex guideline. In *AORN standards, recommended practices and guidelines* (pp. 103.118). Denver, CO: AORN.

Kelly, K.J. (2000). Latex allergy: Where do we go from here? *Canadian Journal of Allergy and Clinical Immunology* **5**: 337–40.

Sussman, G.L. (2000) Latex allergy: An overview. *Canadian Journal of Allergy and Clinical Immunology* **5**: 317–21.

Swanson, M.C. & Olson, D.Q. (2000). Latex allergen affinity for starch powders applied to natural rubber gloves and released as an aerosol. *Canadian Journal of Allergy and Clinical Immunology* **5**: 328–36.

Risk for Imbalanced Body Temperature (00005)

(1986, 2000)

Domain 11: Safety/Protection
Class 6: Thermoregulation

Definition At risk for failure to maintain body temperature within normal range

Risk Factors

- Altered metabolic rate
- Dehydration
- Exposure to extremes of environmental temperature
- Extremes of age
- Extremes of weight
- Illness affecting temperature regulation
- Inactivity
- Inappropriate clothing for environmental temperature
- Medications causing vasoconstriction
- Medications causing vasodilation
- Sedation
- Trauma affecting temperature regulation
- Vigorous activity

Hyperthermia (00007)
(1986)

Domain 11: Safety/Protection
Class 6: Thermoregulation

Definition Body temperature elevated above normal range

Defining Characteristics

- Convulsions
- Flushed skin
- Increase in body temperature above normal range
- Seizures
- Tachycardia
- Tachypnea
- Warm to touch

Related Factors

- Anesthesia
- Decreased perspiration
- Dehydration
- Exposure to hot environment
- Inappropriate clothing
- Increased metabolic rate
- Illness
- Medications
- Trauma
- Vigorous activity

Hypothermia (00006)
(1986, 1988)

Domain 11: Safety/Protection
Class 6: Thermoregulation

Definition Body temperature below normal range

Defining Characteristics

- Body temperature below
  normal range
- Cool skin
- Cyanotic nail beds
- Hypertension

- Pallor
- Piloerection
- Shivering
- Slow capillary refill
- Tachycardia

Related Factors

- Aging
- Consumption of alcohol
- Damage to hypothalamus
- Decreased ability to shiver
- Decreased metabolic rate
- Evaporation from skin in cool
  environment

- Exposure to cool environment
- Illness
- Inactivity
- Inadequate clothing
- Malnutrition
- Medications
- Trauma

Ineffective Thermoregulation (00008)
(1986)

Domain 11: Safety/Protection
Class 6: Thermoregulation

Definition Temperature fluctuation between hypothermia and hyperthermia

Defining Characteristics

- Cool skin
- Cyanotic nail beds
- Fluctuations in body temperature above and below the normal range
- Flushed skin
- Hypertension
- Increased respiratory rate
- Increase in body temperature above normal range
- Mild shivering
- Moderate pallor
- Piloerection
- Reduction in body temperature below normal range
- Seizures
- Slow capillary refill
- Tachycardia
- Warm to touch

Related Factors

- Aging
- Fluctuating environmental temperature
- Illness
- Immaturity
- Trauma

Domain 11

Domain 12
Comfort

Readiness for Enhanced Comfort (00183)
(2006, LOE 2.1)

Domain 12: Comfort
Class 1: Physical Comfort
Class 2: Environmental Comfort

Definition
A pattern of ease, relief, and transcendence in physical, psychospiritual, environmental, and/or social dimensions that can be strengthened

Defining Characteristics

- Expresses desire to enhance comfort
- Expresses desire to enhance feeling of contentment
- Expresses desire to enhance relaxation
- Expresses desire to enhance resolution of complaints

References

Arruda, E., Larson, P., & Meleis, A. (1992). Immigrant Hispanic cancer patients' views. *Cancer Nursing* **15**: 387–95.

Cameron, B.L. (1993). The nature of comfort to hospitalized medical surgical patients. *Journal of Advanced Nursing* **18**: 424–36.

Duggleby, W. & Berry, P. (2005). Transitions in shifting goals of care for palliative patients and their families. *Clinical Journal of Oncology Nursing* **9**: 425–8.

Gropper, E.I. (1992). Promoting health by promoting comfort. *Nursing Forum* **27**(2): 5–8.

Jenny, J. & Logan, J. (1996). Caring and comfort metaphors used by patients in critical care. *Image: Journal of Nursing Scholarship* **28**: 349–52.

Kolcaba, K. (1991). A taxonomic structure for the concept comfort. *Image: Journal of Nursing Scholarship* **23**: 237–40.

Kolcaba, K. (1992). Holistic comfort: Operationalizing the construct as a nurse-sensitive outcome. *Advances in Nursing Science* **15**: 1–10.

Kolcaba, K. (1994). A theory of holistic comfort for nursing. *Journal of Advanced Nursing* **19**: 1178–84.

Kolcaba, K. & Kolcaba, R. (1991). An analysis of the concept of comfort. *Journal of Advanced Nursing* **16**: 1301–10.

Malinowski, A. & Stamler, L.L. (2002). Comfort: Exploration of the concept in nursing. *Journal of Advanced Nursing* **39**: 599–606.

Morse, J.M. (2000). On comfort and comforting. *American Journal of Nursing* **100**(9): 34–8.

Morse, J.M., Bottoroff, J.L., & Hutchinson, S. (1994). The phenomenology of comfort. *Journal of Advanced Nursing* **20**: 189–95.

Mitchell, G.J. & Pilkington, F.B. (2000). Comfort-discomfort with ambiguity: Flight and freedom in nursing practice. *Nursing Science Quarterly* **13**(1): 31–6.

Domain 12

Impaired Comfort (00214)

(2008, LOE 2.1)

Domain 12: Comfort
Class 1: Physical Comfort
Class 2: Environmental Comfort
Class 3: Social Comfort

Definition
Perceived lack of ease, relief and transcendence in physical, psychospiritual, environmental and social dimensions

Defining Characteristics

- Anxiety
- Crying
- Disturbed sleep pattern
- Fear
- Illness-related symptoms
- Inability to relax
- Insufficient resources (e.g., financial, social support)
- Irritability
- Lack of environmental control
- Lack of privacy
- Lack of situational control
- Moaning
- Noxious environmental stimuli
- Reports being uncomfortable
- Reports being cold
- Reports being hot
- Reports distressing symptoms
- Reports hunger
- Reports itching
- Reports lack of contentment in situation
- Reports lack of ease in situation
- Restlessness
- Treatment-related side effects (e.g., medication, radiation)

Reference

Kolcaba, K. (2003). *Comfort theory and practice: A vision for holistic health care and research.* New York: Springer Publishing Co.

Nausea (00134)

(1998, 2002, LOE 2.1)

Domain 12: Comfort
Class 1: Physical Comfort

Definition A subjective unpleasant, wave-like sensation in the back of the throat, epigastrium, or abdomen that may lead to the urge or need to vomit

Defining Characteristics

- Aversion toward food
- Gagging sensation
- Increased salivation
- Increased swallowing
- Report of nausea
- Sour taste in mouth

Related Factors

Biophysical

- Biochemical disorders (e.g., uremia, diabetic ketoacidosis)
- Esophageal disease
- Gastric distension
- Gastric irritation
- Increased intracranial pressure
- Intra-abdominal tumors
- Labyrinthitis
- Liver capsule stretch
- Localized tumors (e.g., acoustic neuroma, primary or secondary brain tumors, bone metastases at base of skull)
- Meningitis
- Menière's disease
- Motion sickness
- Pain
- Pancreatic disease
- Pregnancy
- Splenetic capsule stretch
- Toxins (e.g., tumor-produced peptides, abnormal metabolites due to cancer)

Situational

- Anxiety
- Fear
- Noxious odors
- Noxious taste
- Pain
- Psychological factors
- Unpleasant visual stimulation

Treatment

- Gastric distension
- Gastric irritation
- Pharmaceuticals

Domain 12

Acute Pain (00132)
(1996)

Domain 12: Comfort
Class 1: Physical Comfort

Definition Unpleasant sensory and emotional experience arising from actual or potential tissue damage or described in terms of such damage (International Association for the Study of Pain); sudden or slow onset of any intensity from mild to severe with an anticipated or predictable end and a duration of <6 months

Defining Characteristics

- Changes in appetite
- Changes in blood pressure
- Changes in heart rate
- Changes in respiratory rate
- Coded report
- Diaphoresis
- Distraction behavior (e.g., pacing, seeking out other people and/or activities, repetitive activities)
- Expressive behavior (e.g., restlessness, moaning, crying, vigilance, irritability, sighing)
- Facial mask (e.g., eyes lack luster, beaten look, fixed or scattered movement, grimace)
- Guarding behavior
- Narrowed focus (e.g., altered time perception, impaired thought processes, reduced interaction with people and environment)
- Observed evidence of pain
- Positioning to avoid pain
- Protective gestures
- Pupillary dilation
- Self-focus
- Sleep disturbance
- Verbal report of pain

Related Factors

- Injury agents (e.g., biological, chemical, physical, psychological)

Chronic Pain (00133)
(1986, 1996)

Domain 12: Comfort
Class 1: Physical Comfort

Definition Unpleasant sensory and emotional experience arising from actual or potential tissue damage or described in terms of such damage (International Association for the Study of Pain); sudden or slow onset of any intensity from mild to severe, constant or recurring without an anticipated or predictable end and a duration of >6 months

Defining Characteristics

- Altered ability to continue previous activities
- Anorexia
- Atrophy of involved muscle group
- Changes in sleep pattern
- Coded report
- Depression
- Facial mask (e.g. eyes lack luster, beaten look, fixed or scattered movement, grimace)
- Fatigue
- Fear of reinjury
- Guarding behavior
- Irritability
- Observed protective behavior
- Reduced interaction with people
- Restlessness
- Self-focusing
- Sympathetic mediated responses (e.g., temperature, cold, changes of body position, hypersensitivity)
- Verbal report of pain

Related Factors

- Chronic physical disability
- Chronic psychosocial disability

Social Isolation (00053)

(1982)

Domain 12: Comfort
Class 3: Social Comfort

Definition Aloneness experienced by the individual and perceived as imposed by others and as a negative or threatening state

Defining Characteristics

Objective

- Absence of supportive significant other(s)
- Developmentally inappropriate behaviors
- Dull affect
- Evidence of handicap (e.g., physical, mental)
- Exists in a subculture
- Illness
- Meaningless actions
- No eye contact
- Preoccupation with own thoughts
- Projects hostility
- Repetitive actions
- Sad affect
- Seeks to be alone
- Shows behavior unaccepted by dominant cultural group
- Uncommunicative
- Withdrawn

Subjective

- Expresses feelings of aloneness imposed by others
- Expresses feelings of rejection
- Developmentally inappropriate interests
- Inadequate purpose in life
- Inability to meet expectations of others
- Expresses values unacceptable to the dominant cultural group
- Experiences feelings of differences from others
- Insecurity in public

Related Factors

- Alterations in mental status
- Alterations in physical appearance
- Altered state of wellness
- Factors contributing to the absence of satisfying personal relationships (e.g., delay in accomplishing developmental tasks)
- Immature interests
- Inability to engage in satisfying personal relationships
- Inadequate personal resources
- Unaccepted social behavior
- Unaccepted social values

Domain 13
Growth/Development

Domain 13: Growth/Development
Class 1: Growth

Definition Progressive functional deterioration of a physical and cognitive nature. The individual's ability to live with multisystem diseases, cope with ensuing problems, and manage his or her care is remarkably diminished.

Defining Characteristics

- Altered mood state
- Anorexia
- Apathy
- Cognitive decline
  - Demonstrated difficulty responding to environmental stimuli
  - Demonstrated difficulty in concentration
  - Demonstrated difficulty in decision-making
  - Demonstrated difficulty in judgment
  - Demonstrated difficulty in memory
  - Demonstrated difficulty in reasoning
  - Decreased perception
- Consumption of minimal to no food at most meals (e.g., consumes <75% of normal requirements)
- Decreased participation in activities of daily living
- Decreased social skills
- Expresses loss of interest in pleasurable outlets
- Frequent exacerbations of chronic health problems
- Inadequate nutritional intake
- Neglect of home environment
- Neglect of financial responsibilities
- Physical decline (e.g., fatigue, dehydration, incontinence of bowel and bladder)
- Self-care deficit
- Social withdrawal
- Unintentional weight loss (e.g., 5% in 1 month, 10% in 6 months)
- Verbalizes desire for death

Related Factors

- Depression

Domain 13

Delayed Growth and Development
(00111)
(1986)

Domain 13: Growth/Development
Class 1: Growth
Class 2: Development

Definition Deviations from age-group norms

Defining Characteristics

- Altered physical growth
- Decreased response time
- Delay in performing skills typical of age group
- Difficulty in performing skills typical of age group
- Inability to perform self care activities appropriate for age
- Inability to perform self-control activities appropriate for age
- Flat affect
- Listlessness

Related Factors

- Effects of physical disability
- Environmental deficiencies
- Inadequate caretaking
- Inconsistent responsiveness
- Indifference
- Multiple caretakers
- Prescribed dependence
- Separation from significant others
- Stimulation deficiencies

Risk for Disproportionate Growth

(00113)

(1998)

Domain 13: Growth/Development
Class 1: Growth

Definition At risk for growth above the 97th percentile or below the 3rd percentile for age, crossing two percentile channels

Risk Factors

Caregiver

- Abuse
- Learning difficulties (mental handicap)
- Mental illness
- Severe learning disability

Environmental

- Deprivation
- Lead poisoning
- Natural disasters
- Poverty
- Teratogen
- Violence

Individual

- Anorexia

- Caregiver's maladaptive feeding behaviors
- Chronic illness
- Individual maladaptive feeding behaviors
- Infection
- Insatiable appetite
- Prematurity
- Malnutrition
- Substance abuse

Prenatal

- Congenital disorders
- Genetic disorders
- Maternal infection
- Maternal nutrition
- Multiple gestation
- Teratogen exposure
- Substance abuse
- Substance use

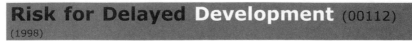

Risk for Delayed Development (00112)
(1998)

Domain 13: Growth/Development
Class 2: Development

Definition At risk for delay of 25% or more in one or more of the areas of social or self-regulatory behavior, or in cognitive, language, gross or fine motor skills

Risk Factors

Prenatal

- Endocrine disorders
- Genetic disorders
- Illiteracy
- Inadequate nutrition
- Infections
- Lack of prenatal care
- Late prenatal care
- Maternal age <15 years
- Maternal age >35 years
- Inadequate prenatal care
- Poverty
- Substance abuse
- Unplanned pregnancy
- Unwanted pregnancy

Individual

- Adopted child
- Behavior disorders
- Brain damage (e.g., hemorrhage in postnatal period, shaken baby, abuse, accident)
- Chemotherapy
- Chronic illness
- Congenital disorders

- Failure to thrive
- Foster child
- Frequent otitis media
- Genetic disorders
- Hearing impairment
- Inadequate nutrition
- Lead poisoning
- Natural disasters
- Positive drug screen(s)
- Prematurity
- Radiation therapy
- Seizures
- Substance abuse
- Technology dependent
- Vision impairment

Environmental

- Poverty
- Violence

Caregiver

- Abuse
- Learning disabilities
- Mental illness
- Severe learning disability

Part 3
Taxonomy II
2009–2011

Part 3 describes the historical development and structure of Taxonomy II. It includes a discussion of the multiaxial structure of Taxonomy II with its three levels, Domains, Classes, and Nursing Diagnoses; the mapping of the nursing diagnoses in the NANDA-I, NIC, and NOC (NNN) Common Structure; and the NNN Taxonomy of Nursing Practice).

History of the Development of Taxonomy II

Following the biennial conference in April 1994, the Taxonomy Committee met to place newly submitted diagnoses into the Taxonomy I revised structure. The committee had considerable difficulty, however, categorizing some of these diagnoses. Given this difficulty and the expanding number of submissions at level 1.4 and higher, the committee felt that a new taxonomic structure was necessary. This possibility gave rise to considerable discussion as to how this might be accomplished.

To start, the committee agreed to determine whether there were categories that arose naturally from the data, i.e., from accepted diagnoses. Round 1 of a naturalistic Q-sort was completed at the eleventh biennial conference in 1994 in Nashville, Tennessee (USA). Round 2 was completed and the analysis presented at the twelfth biennial conference in 1996 in Pittsburgh, Pennsylvania (USA). That Q-sort yielded 21 categories-far too many to be useful or practical.

In 1998, the Taxonomy Committee sent four Q-sorts using four different frameworks to the NANDA Board of Directors. Framework 1, reported in 1996, was in the naturalistic style. Framework 2 used Jenny's (1994) ideas. Framework 3 used the Nursing Outcomes Classifications (NOC) (Johnson & Maas, 1997), and Framework 4 used Gordon's (1998) Functional Health Patterns. None of these frameworks was entirely satisfactory, although Gordon's was the best fit. With Gordon's permission, the Taxonomy Committee modified this framework to create Framework 5, which was presented to the membership in April 1998 at the thirteenth biennial conference in St Louis, Missouri (USA). At that conference, the Taxonomy Committee invited the members to sort the diagnoses according to the domains that had been selected. By the end of the conference, 40 usable sets of data were available for analysis. During the data collection phase at the conference, members of the Taxonomy Committee took careful notes of the questions asked, the confusion expressed by members, and the suggestions for improvements.

Based on the analysis of the data and the field notes, additional modifications were made to the framework. One domain of the original framework was divided into two to reduce the number of classes and diagnoses falling within it. A separate domain was added for growth and development because the original framework did not contain that domain. Several other domains were renamed to better reflect the content of the diagnoses within them. The final taxonomic structure is much less like Gordon's original, but has reduced misclassification errors and redundancies to near zero, which is a much-desired state in a taxonomic structure.

Finally, definitions were developed for all the domains and classes within the structure. The definition of each diagnosis was then compared with that of the class and the domain in which it was placed. Revisions and modifications in the diagnosis placements were made to ensure maximum match among domain, class, and diagnosis.

In 2002, following the NANDA, NIC, and NOC (NNN) Conference in Chicago, the approved nursing diagnoses were placed in Taxonomy II. These included 11 health-promotion nursing diagnoses as well as the revised and newly approved nursing diagnoses. In the future, as new nursing diagnoses were developed and approved, they will be added to the taxonomic structure in the appropriate locations. In January 2003, the Taxonomy Committee met in Chicago (USA) and made further refinements to the terminology in Taxonomy II. Following the 2004 NNN Conference in Chicago, the Taxonomy Committee placed the newly approved nursing diagnoses in their appropriate categories. The Taxonomy Committee, to foster its international focus, reviewed the axes in Taxonomy II and compared them with the International Standards Organization (ISO) Reference Terminology Model for a Nursing Diagnosis.

For this edition, the nursing diagnoses and supporting materials that were approved by the Diagnostic Development Committee were made available for voting to members on the NANDA-I website. This was the first time that this method of approval was used for the ongoing expansion and revision of Taxonomy II. Following approval by the membership of the nursing diagnoses, they were placed in both the NANDA-I Taxonomy II and the NNN Taxonomy of Nursing Practice.

Structure of Taxonomy II

Clinicians are primarily concerned with the diagnoses within the taxonomy and rarely need to use the taxonomic structure itself. Familiarity with how a diagnosis is structured will, however, aid the clinician who needs to find information quickly and those who wish to submit new diagnoses. A brief explanation of how the taxonomy is designed is therefore included here.

Taxonomy II has three levels: domains, classes, and nursing diagnoses. Figure 3.1 (see pp. 368–369) depicts the organization of domains and classes in Taxonomy II. Some nursing diagnoses lend themselves to placement in more than one domain and class. This occurs because the nursing diagnosis label, definition, defining characteristics or related factors in the instance of "risk for", lend themselves to appropriate location in more than one domain and class.

Table 3.1 (page 370–380) shows Taxonomy II with 13 domains, 47 classes, and numbers of diagnoses. A domain is a sphere of activity, study or interest (Roget, 1980, p. 287). A class is "a subdivision of a larger group; a division of persons or things by quality, rank, or grade" (Roget, p. 157). "A nursing diagnosis is a clinical judgment about an individual, family or community response to actual or potential health problems/life processes which provides the basis for definitive therapy toward achievement of outcomes for which a nurse is accountable" (see p. 364).

The Taxonomy II code structure is a 32-bit integer (or if the user's database uses another notation, the code structure is a five-digit code). This structure provides for the growth and development of the classification structure without having to change codes when new diagnoses, refinements, and revisions are added. New codes are assigned to the nursing diagnoses when they are approved by the Board of Directors upon the recommendation of the Diagnosis Development Committee and approval by the NANDA-I membership.

Taxonomy II has a code structure that is compliant with recommendations from the National Library of Medicine (NLM) concerning healthcare terminology codes. The NLM recommends that codes do not contain information about the classified concept, as did the Taxonomy I code structure, which included information about the location and the level of the diagnosis.

The NANDA-I Taxonomy II is a recognized nursing language that meets the criteria established by the Committee for Nursing Practice Information Infrastructure (CNPII) of the American Nurses Association (ANA) (Coenen et al., 2001). The benefit of being included as a recognized nursing language indicates that the classification system is accepted as supporting nursing practice by providing clinically useful terminology. The ANA recognition facilitates the inclusion of NANDA-I in the ANA Nursing Information and Data Set Evaluation Center (NIDSEC) criteria for clinical information systems (nursingworld.org/nidsec/index.htm) and the National Library of Medicine's (NLM's) Unified Medical Language System (UMLS) (www.nlm.nih.gov/research/umls/umlsmain.html).

The taxonomy is registered with Health Level Seven (HL7), a healthcare informatics standard, as a terminology to be used in identifying nursing diagnoses in electronic messages among clinical information systems (www.HL7.org). NANDA-I diagnoses have been modeled into SNOMED CT, which has been accepted as a terminology standard for the US Department of Health and Human Services, the US Consolidated Health Information Initiative, and the United Kingdom's National Health Service. A map of this modeling effort is available from SNOMED International (www.snomed.org).

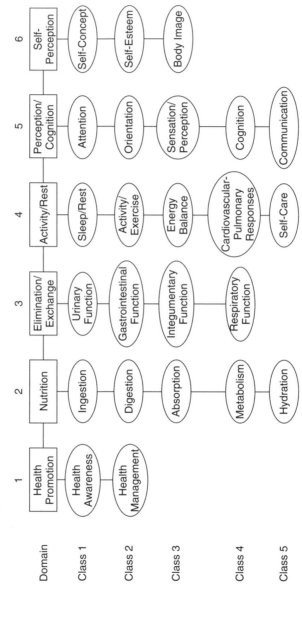

Figure 3.1 *Taxonomy II domains and classes*

Figure 3.1 *Continued*

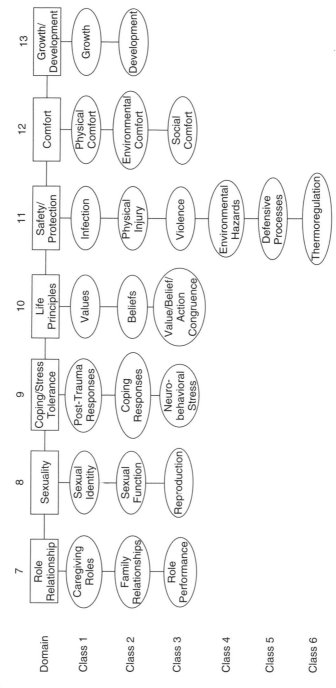

Table 3.1 *Taxonomy II: domains, classes, and diagnoses*

DOMAIN 1 HEALTH PROMOTION
The awareness of wellbeing or normality of function and the strategies used to maintain control of and enhance that wellbeing or normality of function

Class 1 Health Awareness Recognition of normal function and wellbeing

Approved Diagnoses
None at present time

Class 2 Health Management Identifying, controlling, performing, and integrating activities to maintain health and wellbeing

Approved Diagnoses
00078 Ineffective self health management
00080 Ineffective family therapeutic regimen management
00099 Ineffective health maintenance
00098 Impaired home maintenance
00162 Readiness for enhanced self health management
00163 Readiness for enhanced nutrition
00186 Readiness for enhanced immunization status
00193 Self neglect

DOMAIN 2 NUTRITION
The activities of taking in, assimilating, and using nutrients for the purposes of tissue maintenance, tissue repair, and the production of energy

Class 1 Ingestion Taking food or nutrients into the body

Approved Diagnoses
00107 Ineffective infant feeding pattern
00103 Impaired swallowing
00002 Imbalanced nutrition: less than body requirements
00001 Imbalanced nutrition: more than body requirements
00003 Risk for imbalanced nutrition: More than body requirements

Class 2 Digestion The physical and chemical activities that convert foodstuffs into substances suitable for absorption and assimilation

Approved Diagnoses
None at present time

Table 3.1 *Continued*

Class 3 Absorption The act of taking up nutrients through body tissues

Approved Diagnoses
None at present time

Class 4 Metabolism The chemical and physical processes occurring in living organisms and cells for the development and use of protoplasm, production of waste and energy, with the release of energy for all vital processes

Approved Diagnoses
00178 Risk for impaired liver function
00179 Risk for unstable blood glucose level
00194 Neonatal jaundice

Class 5 Hydration The taking in and absorption of fluids and electrolytes

Approved Diagnoses
00027 Deficient fluid volume
00028 Risk for deficient fluid volume
00026 Excess fluid volume
00160 Readiness for enhanced fluid balance
00195 Risk for electrolyte imbalance
00025 Risk for imbalanced fluid volume

DOMAIN 3 ELIMINATION AND EXCHANGE
Secretion and excretion of waste products from the body

Class 1 Urinary Function The process of secretion, reabsorption, and excretion of urine

Approved Diagnoses
00016 Impaired urinary elimination
00023 Urinary retention
00020 Functional urinary incontinence
00017 Stress urinary incontinence
00019 Urge urinary incontinence
00018 Reflex urinary incontinence
00022 Risk for urge urinary incontinence
00166 Readiness for enhanced urinary elimination
00176 Overflow urinary incontinence

Class 2 Gastrointestinal Function The process of absorption and excretion of the end products of digestion

Approved Diagnoses
00014 Bowel incontinence

Continued

Table 3.1 *Continued*

00013 *Diarrhea*
00011 *Constipation*
00015 *Risk for constipation*
00012 *Perceived constipation*
00196 *Dysfunctional gastrointestinal motility*
00197 *Risk for dysfunctional gastrointestinal motility*

Class 3 Integumentary Function The process of secretion and excretion through the skin

Approved Diagnoses
None at present time

Class 4 Respiratory Function The process of exchange of gases and removal of the end-products of metabolism

Approved Diagnoses
00030 *Impaired gas exchange*
00031 *Ineffective airway clearance*
00032 *Impaired spontaneous ventilation*

DOMAIN 4 ACTIVITY/REST
The production, conservation, expenditure, or balance of energy resources

Class 1 Sleep/Rest Slumber, repose, ease, relaxation, or inactivity

Approved Diagnoses
00096 *Sleep deprivation*
00165 *Readiness for enhanced sleep*
00095 *Insomnia*
00198 *Disturbed sleep pattern*

Class 2 Activity/Exercise Moving parts of the body (mobility), doing work, or performing actions often (but not always) against resistance

Approved Diagnoses
00040 *Risk for disuse syndrome*
00085 *Impaired physical mobility*
00091 *Impaired bed mobility*
00089 *Impaired wheelchair mobility*
00090 *Impaired transfer ability*
00088 *Impaired walking*
00097 *Deficient diversional activity*
00100 *Delayed surgical recovery*
00168 *Sedentary lifestyle*

Table 3.1 *Continued*

Class 3 Energy Balance A dynamic state of harmony between intake and expenditure of resources

Approved Diagnoses
00050 Disturbed energy field
00093 Fatigue

Class 4 Cardiovascular/Pulmonary Responses
Cardiopulmonary mechanisms that support activity/rest

Approved Diagnoses
00029 Decreased cardiac output
00033 Impaired spontaneous ventilation
00032 Ineffective breathing pattern
00092 Activity intolerance
00094 Risk for activity intolerance
00034 Dysfunctional ventilatory weaning response
00200 Risk for decreased cardiac tissue perfusion
00201 Risk for ineffective cerebral tissue perfusion
00202 Risk for ineffective gastrointestinal perfusion
00203 Risk for tissue perfusion
00204 Ineffective peripheral tissue perfusion
00205 Risk for shock
00206 Risk for bleeding

Class 5 Self-Care Ability to perform activities to care for one's body and bodily functions

Approved Diagnoses
00109 Dressing self-care deficit
00108 Bathing self-care deficit
00102 Feeding self-care deficit
00110 Toileting self-care deficit
00182 Readiness for enhanced self-care

DOMAIN 5 PERCEPTION/COGNITION
The human information processing system including attention, orientation, sensation, perception, cognition, and communication

Class 1 Attention Mental readiness to notice or observe

Approved Diagnoses
00123 Unilateral neglect

Class 2 Orientation Awareness of time, place, and person

Approved Diagnoses
00127 Impaired environmental interpretation syndrome
00154 Wandering

Continued

Table 3.1 *Continued*

Class 3   Sensation/Perception Receiving information through the senses of touch, taste, smell, vision, hearing, and kinesthesia and the comprehension of sense data resulting in naming, associating, and/or pattern recognition

Approved Diagnoses

00122   Disturbed sensory perception (specify: visual, auditory, kinesthetic, gustatory, tactile)

Class 4   Cognition Use of memory, learning, thinking, problem-solving, abstraction, judgment, insight, intellectual capacity, calculation, and language

Approved Diagnoses

00126   Deficient knowledge
00161   Readiness for enhanced knowledge
00128   Acute confusion
00129   Chronic confusion
00131   Impaired memory
00130   Disturbed thought processes
00184   Readiness for enhanced decision making
00173   Risk for acute confusion
00199   Ineffective activity planning

Class 5   Communication Sending and receiving verbal and nonverbal information

Approved Diagnoses

00051   Impaired verbal communication
00157   Readiness for enhanced communication

DOMAIN 6   SELF-PERCEPTION
Awareness about the self

Class 1   Self-Concept The perception(s) about the total self

Approved Diagnoses

00121   Disturbed personal identity
00125   Powerlessness
00152   Risk for powerlessness
00124   Hopelessness
00054   Risk for loneliness
00167   Readiness for enhanced self-concept
00187   Readiness for enhanced power
00174   Risk for compromised human dignity
00185   Readiness for enhanced hope

Table 3.1 *Continued*

Class 2 *Self-Esteem* Assessment of one's own worth, capability, significance, and success

Approved Diagnoses
00119 Chronic low self-esteem
00120 Situational low self-esteem
00153 Risk for situational low self-esteem

Class 3 *Body Image* A mental image of one's own body

Approved Diagnoses
00118 Disturbed body image

DOMAIN 7 ROLE RELATIONSHIPS
The positive and negative connections or associations between people or groups of people and the means by which those connections are demonstrated

Class 1 *Caregiving Roles* Socially expected behavior patterns by people providing care who are not healthcare professionals

Approved Diagnoses
00061 Caregiver role strain
00062 Risk for caregiver role strain
00056 Impaired parenting
00057 Risk for impaired parenting
00164 Readiness for enhanced parenting

Class 2 *Family Relationships* Associations of people who are biologically related or related by choice

Approved Diagnoses
00060 Interrupted family processes
00159 Readiness for enhanced family processes
00063 Dysfunctional family processes
00058 Risk for impaired attachment

Class 3 *Role Performance* Quality of functioning in socially expected behavior patterns

Approved Diagnoses
00106 Effective breastfeeding
00104 Ineffective breastfeeding
00105 Interrupted breastfeeding
00055 Ineffective role performance
00064 Parental role conflict
00052 Impaired social interaction
00207 Readiness for enhanced relationship

Continued

Table 3.1 *Continued*

DOMAIN 8 SEXUALITY
Sexual identity, sexual function, and reproduction

Class 1 Sexual Identity The state of being a specific person in regard to sexuality and/or gender

Approved Diagnoses
None at present time

Class 2 Sexual Function The capacity or ability to participate in sexual activities

Approved Diagnoses
00059 Sexual dysfunction
00065 Ineffective sexuality pattern

Class 3 Reproduction Any process by which human beings are produced

Approved Diagnoses
00208 Readiness for enhanced childbearing process
00209 Risk for disturbed maternal/fetal dyad

DOMAIN 9 COPING/STRESS TOLERANCE
Contending with life events/life processes

Class 1 Post-Trauma Responses Reactions occurring after physical or psychological trauma

Approved Diagnoses
00114 Relocation stress syndrome
00149 Risk for relocation stress syndrome
00142 Rape-trauma syndrome
00141 Post-trauma syndrome
00145 Risk for post-trauma syndrome

Class 2 Coping Responses The process of managing environmental stress

Approved Diagnoses
00148 Fear
00146 Anxiety
00147 Death anxiety
00137 Chronic sorrow
00072 Ineffective denial
00069 Ineffective coping
00073 Disabled family coping
00074 Compromised family coping
00071 Defensive coping

Table 3.1 *Continued*

00077 *Ineffective community coping*
00158 *Readiness for enhanced coping (individual)*
00075 *Readiness for enhanced family coping*
00076 *Readiness for enhanced community coping*
00172 *Risk for complicated grieving*
00177 *Stress overload*
00188 *Risk-prone health behavior*
00136 *Grieving*
00135 *Complicated grieving*
00210 *Impaired individual resilience*
00211 *Risk for compromised resilience*
00212 *Readiness for enhanced resilience*

Class 3 Neurobehavioral Stress Behavioral responses reflecting nerve and brain function

Approved Diagnoses
00009 *Autonomic dysreflexia*
00010 *Risk for autonomic dysreflexia*
00116 *Disorganized infant behavior*
00115 *Risk for disorganized infant behavior*
00117 *Readiness for enhanced organized infant behavior*
00049 *Decreased intracranial adaptive capacity*

DOMAIN 10 LIFE PRINCIPLES
Principles underlying conduct, thought, and behavior about acts, customs, or institutions viewed as being true or having intrinsic worth

Class 1 Values The identification and ranking of preferred modes of conduct or end states

Approved Diagnoses
00185 *Readiness for enhanced hope*

Class 2 Beliefs Opinions, expectations, or judgments about acts, customs, or institutions viewed as being true or having intrinsic worth

Approved Diagnoses
00068 *Readiness for enhanced spiritual wellbeing*
00185 *Readiness for enhanced hope*

Class 3 Value/Belief/Action Congruence The correspondence or balance achieved among values, beliefs, and actions

Approved Diagnoses
00066 *Spiritual distress*
00067 *Risk for spiritual distress*

Continued

Table 3.1 *Continued*

00083   *Decisional conflict (specify)*
00079   *Noncompliance (specify)*
00170   *Risk for impaired religiosity*
00169   *Impaired religiosity*
00171   *Readiness for enhanced religiosity*
00175   *Moral distress*
00184   *Readiness for enhanced decision making*

DOMAIN 11   SAFETY/PROTECTION

Freedom from danger, physical injury, or immune system damage; preservation from loss; and protection of safety and security

*Class 1   **Infection*** Host responses following pathogenic invasion

Approved Diagnoses

00004   *Risk for infection*
00186   *Readiness for enhanced immunization status*

*Class 2   **Physical Injury*** Bodily harm or hurt

Approved Diagnoses

00045   *Impaired oral mucous membrane*
00035   *Risk for injury*
00087   *Risk for perioperative positioning injury*
00155   *Risk for falls*
00038   *Risk for trauma*
00046   *Impaired skin integrity*
00047   *Risk for impaired skin integrity*
00044   *Impaired tissue integrity*
00048   *Impaired dentition*
00036   *Risk for suffocation*
00039   *Risk for aspiration*
00031   *Ineffective airway clearance*
00086   *Risk for peripheral neurovascular dysfunction*
00043   *Ineffective protection*
00156   *Risk for sudden infant death syndrome*
00213   *Risk for vascular trauma*

*Class 3   **Violence*** The exertion of excessive force or power so as to cause injury or abuse

Approved Diagnoses

00139   *Risk for self-mutilation*
00151   *Self-mutilation*
00138   *Risk for other-directed violence*
00140   *Risk for self-directed violence*
00150   *Risk for suicide*

Table 3.1 *Continued*

Class 4   Environmental Hazards Sources of danger in the surroundings

Approved Diagnoses
00037   Risk for poisoning
00180   Risk for contamination
00181   Contamination

Class 5   Defensive Processes The processes by which the self protects itself from the nonself

Approved Diagnoses
00041   Latex allergy response
00042   Risk for latex allergy response
00186   Readiness for enhanced immunization status

Class 6   Thermoregulation The physiologic process of regulating heat and energy within the body for purposes of protecting the organism

Approved Diagnoses
00005   Risk for imbalanced body temperature
00008   Ineffective thermoregulation
00006   Hypothermia
00007   Hyperthermia

DOMAIN 12   COMFORT
Sense of mental, physical, or social wellbeing or ease

Class 1   Physical Comfort Sense of wellbeing or ease and/or freedom from pain

Approved Diagnoses
00132   Acute pain
00133   Chronic pain
00134   Nausea
00183   Readiness for enhanced comfort
00214   Impaired comfort

Class 2   Environmental Comfort Sense of wellbeing or ease in/ with one's environment

Approved Diagnoses
00183   Readiness for enhanced comfort
00214   Impaired comfort

Continued

Table 3.1 *Continued*

Class 3 Social Comfort Sense of wellbeing or ease with one's social situations

Approved Diagnoses
00053 Social isolation
00214 Impaired comfort

DOMAIN 13 GROWTH/DEVELOPMENT
Age-appropriate increases in physical dimensions, maturation of organ systems, and/or progression through the developmental milestone

Class 1 Growth Increases in physical dimensions or maturity of organ systems

Approved Diagnoses
00111 Delayed growth and development
00113 Risk for disproportionate growth
00101 Adult failure to thrive

Class 2 Development Progression or regression through a sequence of recognized milestones in life

Approved Diagnoses
00111 Delayed growth and development
00112 Risk for delayed development

The NANDA-I Taxonomy II nursing diagnoses also comply with the International Standards Organization (ISO) terminology model for a nursing diagnosis (Figure 3.2, page 381).

The Multiaxial System

Taxonomy II is multiaxial in form. This format substantially improves the flexibility of the nomenclature and allows for easy additions and modifications.

An axis, for the purpose of the NANDA-I Taxonomy II, is operationally defined as a dimension of the human response that is considered in the diagnostic process.

There are seven axes. The NANDA-I Model of a Nursing Diagnosis displays the seven axes and their relationship to each other (Figure 3.3, page 381). The ordering and some of the labels and definitions have been changed since the 2005–2006 edition of this book in order to parallel the International Standards Reference Model for a Nursing Diagnosis.

Figure 3.2 *The ISO reference terminology model for a nursing diagnosis*

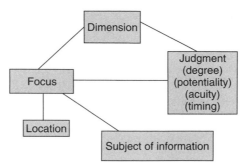

Figure 3.3 *The NANDA-I model of a nursing diagnosis*

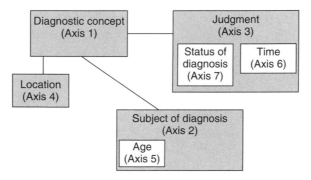

- Axis 1: the diagnostic concept
- Axis 2: subject of the diagnosis (individual, family, group, community)
- Axis 3: judgment (e.g., impaired, ineffective)
- Axis 4: location (e.g., bladder, auditory, cerebral)
- Axis 5: age (e.g., infant, child, adult)
- Axis 6: time (chronic, acute, intermittent)
- Axis 7: status of the diagnosis (actual, risk, wellness, health promotion).

The axes are represented in the named/coded nursing diagnoses through their values. In some cases, they are named explicitly, e.g., *Ineffective Community Coping* and *Compromised Family Coping*, in which the subject of the diagnosis (in the first instance "community" and in the second instance "family") is named using the two values "community" and "family" taken from Axis 2 (subject of the diagnosis). "Ineffective" and "compromised" are two of the values contained in Axis 3 (judgment).

In some cases, the axis is implicit, e.g., *Activity intolerance*, in which the subject of the diagnosis (Axis 2) is always the individual. In some instances an axis may not be pertinent to a particular diagnosis and therefore is not part of the nursing diagnostic label or code. For example, the time axis may not be relevant to every diagnosis.

Axis 1 (the diagnostic concept) and Axis 3 (judgment) are essential components of a nursing diagnosis. In some cases, however, the diagnostic concept contains the judgment (e.g., *Nausea*); in these cases the judgment is not explicitly separated out in the diagnostic label. Axis 2 (subject of the diagnosis) is also essential, although, as described above, it may be implied and therefore not included in the label. The Diagnostic Development Committee requires these axes for submission; the other axes may be used where relevant for clarity.

Definitions of the Axes

Axis 1 The Diagnostic Concept

The diagnostic concept is the principal element or the fundamental and essential part, the root, of the diagnostic statement. It describes the "human response" that is the core of the diagnosis.

The diagnostic concept may consist of one or more nouns. When more than one noun is used (e.g., *Activity intolerance*), each one contributes a unique meaning to the concept, as if the two were a single noun; the meaning of the combined term, however, is different from when the nouns are stated separately. Frequently, an adjective (e.g., *Spiritual*) may be used with a noun (e.g., *Distress*) to denote the diagnostic concept *Spiritual Distress*.

In some cases, the diagnostic concept and the diagnosis are one and the same, e.g., *Nausea*. This occurs when the nursing diagnosis is stated at its most clinically useful level and the separation of the diagnostic concept adds no meaningful level of abstraction.

The diagnostic concepts in Taxonomy II are:

- Activity tolerance
- Adaptive capacity
- Airway clearance
- Anxiety
- Aspiration
- Attachment
- Autonomic dysreflexia
- Bathing self-care
- Bed mobility
- Behavior
- Bleeding
- Blood glucose level
- Body image
- Body temperature
- Breastfeeding
- Breathing pattern
- Cardiac output
- Caregiver role strain
- Childbearing process
- Communication

- Comfort
- Confusion
- Constipation
- Comfort
- Electrolyte imbalance
- Elimination
- Energy field
- Environmental interpretation
- Falls
- Family processes
- Fatigue
- Fear
- Feeding self-care
- Feeding pattern
- Fluid balance
- Fluid volume
- Functional incontinence
- Gas exchange
- Grieving
- Growth
- Health maintenance
- Health behavior
- Home maintenance
- Hope
- Hopelessness
- Human dignity
- Hyperthermia
- Hypothermia
- Identity
- Immunization status
- Incontinence
- Infection
- Injury
- Insomnia
- Intracranial adaptive behavior
- Jaundice
- Knowledge
- Latex allergy response
- Liver function
- Loneliness
- Maternal / fetal dyad
- Memory
- Mobility
- Moral distress
- Motility
- Mucous membrane
- Nausea
- Neurovascular function
- Noncompliance
- Nutrition
- Pain
- Parental role conflict
- Parenting
- Perfusion
- Perioperative positioning injury
- Peripheral neurovascular dysfunction
- Personal identity
- Physical mobility
- Planning
- Poisoning
- Post-trauma response
- Power
- Powerlessness
- Protection
- Rape-trauma syndrome
- Reflex incontinence
- Religiosity
- Relationship
- Relocation stress syndrome
- Resilience
- Retention
- Role conflict
- Role performance
- Sedentary lifestyle
- Self-care
- Self-concept
- Self-esteem
- Self health management
- Self-mutilation
- Self-neglect
- Sensory perception
- Sexual dysfunction
- Sexual function
- Sexuality patterns
- Shock

- Skin integrity
- Sleep
- Sleep deprivation
- Sleep pattern
- Social interaction
- Social isolation
- Sorrow
- Spiritual distress
- Spiritual wellbeing
- Spontaneous ventilation
- Stress incontinence
- Stress overload
- Sudden infant death syndrome
- Suicide
- Suffocation
- Surgical recovery

- Swallowing
- Therapeutic regimen management
- Thermoregulation
- Thought process
- Tissue integrity
- Tissue perfusion
- Toileting self-care
- Transfer ability
- Unilateral neglect
- Urge incontinence
- Ventilatory weaning response
- Violence
- Walking
- Wandering
- Wheelchair mobility

Axis 2 Subject of the Diagnosis

The subject of the diagnosis is defined as the person(s) for whom a nursing diagnosis is determined. The values in Axis 2 are individual, family, group, and community:

- *Individual:* a single human being distinct from others, a person.
- *Family:* two or more people having continuous or sustained relationships, perceiving reciprocal obligations, sensing common meaning, and sharing certain obligations toward others; related by blood and/or choice.
- *Group:* a number of people with shared characteristics
- *Community:* a group of people living in the same locale under the same governance. Examples include neighborhoods and cities.

When the subject of the diagnosis is not explicitly stated, it becomes the individual by default.

Axis 3 Judgment

A judgment is a descriptor or modifier that limits or specifies the meaning of the diagnostic concept. The diagnostic concept together with the nurse's judgment about it forms the diagnosis. The values in Axis 3 are:

Value	Definition
Compromised	Damaged, made vulnerable
Complicated	Intricately involved, complex
Decreased	Lessened (in size, amount, or degree)
Defensive	Used or intended to defend or protect
Deficient	Insufficient, inadequate
Delayed	Late, slow, or postponed
Disabled	Limited, handicapped
Disorganized	Not properly arranged or controlled
Disproportionate	Too large or too small in comparison with norm
Disturbed	Agitated, interrupted, interfered with
Dysfunctional	Not operating normally
Effective	Producing the intended or desired effect
Enhanced	Improved in quality, value, or extent
Excessive	Greater than necessary or desirable
Imbalanced	Out of proportion or balance
Impaired	Damaged, weakened
Ineffective	Not producing the intended or desired effect
Interrupted	Having its continuity broken
Low	Below the norm
Organized	Properly arranged or controlled
Perceived	Observed through the senses
Readiness for	In a suitable state for an activity or situation
Situational	Related to a particular circumstance

Axis 4 Location

Location describes the parts/regions of the body and/or their related functions – all tissues, organs, anatomical sites, or structures. The values in Axis 4 are:

- Auditory
- Bladder
- Bowel
- Cardiac
- Cardiopulmonary
- Cerebral
- Gastrointestinal
- Gustatory
- Intracranial
- Kinesthetic
- Mucous membranes
- Oral
- Olfactory
- Peripheral

- Neurovascular
- Peripheral vascular
- Renal
- Skin
- Tactile
- Tissue
- Vascular
- Verbal
- Visual
- Urinary.

Axis 5 Age

Age refers to the age of the person who is the subject of the diagnosis (Axis 2). The values in Axis 5 are:

- Fetus
- Neonate
- Infant
- Toddler
- Preschool child
- School-age child
- Adolescent
- Adult
- Older adult.

Axis 6 Time

Time describes the duration of the diagnostic concept (Axis 1). The values in Axis 6 are:

- *Acute:* lasting <6 months
- *Chronic:* lasting >6 months
- *Intermittent:* stopping or starting again at intervals, periodic, cyclic
- *Continuous:* uninterrupted, going on without stop.

Axis 7 Status of the Diagnosis

Status of the diagnosis refers to the actuality or potentiality of the problem or to the categorization of the diagnosis as a wellness/health promotion diagnosis. The values in Axis 7 are:

- *Actual:* existing in fact or reality, existing at the present time

- *Health Promotion:* behavior motivated by the desire to increase well-being and actualize human health potential (Pender, Murduagh, & Parsons, 2006)
- *Risk:* vulnerability, especially as a result of exposure to factors that increase the chance of injury or loss
- *Wellness:* the quality or state of being healthy. May be stated as:
  - actual (although it is understood to exist if not specifically stated).

Construction of a Nursing Diagnostic Statement

A nursing diagnosis is constructed by combining the values from Axis 1 (the diagnostic concept), Axis 2 (subject of the diagnosis), and Axis 3 (judgment) where needed, and adding values from the other axes for relevant clarity. Thus you start with the diagnostic concept (Axis 1) and add the judgment (Axis 3) about it. Remember that these two axes are sometimes combined into a single diagnostic concept, e.g., *Pain*. Next, you specify the subject of the diagnosis (Axis 2). If the subject is an "individual," you need not make it explicit (Figure 3.4 below). You can then use the remaining axes, if they are appropriate, to add more detail. Figures 3.5 and 3.6 illustrate other examples, using the risk diagnoses (Figure 3.5, page 388) and readiness for enhanced diagnoses (Figure 3.6, page 388).

Please see Part 1, The Process for Development of an Approved NANDA-I Nursing Diagnosis, on preparing a nursing diagnosis for acceptance into the NANDA-I taxonomy, page 41, for a detailed explanation on the diagnosis submission process for new and revised diagnoses.

Figure 3.4 *A NANDA-I nursing diagnosis model: (Individual) Ineffective Coping*

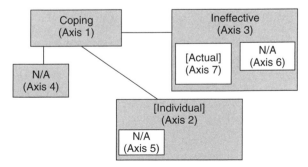

Figure 3.5 *A NANDA-I nursing diagnosis model: Risk for Disorganized Infant Behaviour*

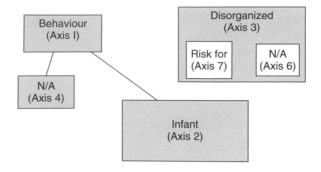

Figure 3.6 *A NANDA-I nursing diagnosis model: Readiness for Enhanced Family Coping*

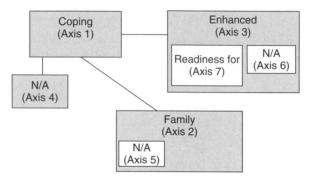

The NNN Taxonomy of Nursing Practice

The NANDA-I Taxonomy II appeared for the first time in *NANDA Nursing Diagnoses: Definitions & Classification 2001–2002*. During this period, NANDA-I began to negotiate an alliance with the Classification Center at the College of Nursing, University of Iowa, Iowa City, Iowa (USA). As a part of that alliance, the possibility of developing a common taxonomic structure was explored. The purposes of a common structure are to make relationships among the three classifications – nursing diagnoses, nursing interventions, and nursing outcomes – visible and to facilitate the linkage of the three systems. The possibilities were discussed among members of the NANDA-I Board of Directors and the leadership of the Classification Center.

Dr Dorothy Jones, representing NANDA-I, and Dr Joanne McCloskey, representing the Classification Center, developed a proposal to convene an invitational conference. The proposal was funded by the National Library of Medicine, and a 3-day meeting was held August 2001 at the Starved Rock Conference Center in Utica, Illinois. It was attended by 24 experts in standardized nursing language development, testing, and refinement. The goal was to develop a common taxonomic structure for nursing practice, including NANDA-I (nursing diagnoses), NIC (nursing interventions), and NOC (nursing outcomes), with the possibility of including other languages. A detailed account of the conference, as well as the history and development, can be found in *Unifying nursing languages: The harmonization of NANDA, NIC, and NOC* (Dochterman & Jones, 2003).

The NANDA Taxonomy Committee met in January 2003 to place the nursing diagnoses from the *NANDA-I Nursing Diagnoses: Definitions and Classifications 2003–2004* into the NNN Taxonomy of Nursing Practice. The committee established rules governing the placement of the nursing diagnoses:

1. The nursing diagnosis definition, defining characteristics or risk factors guide the placement of the nursing diagnosis.
2. When a nursing diagnosis bridges two or more domains, the Taxonomy Committee reviews the nursing diagnosis definition, defining characteristics or risk factors, and places it in the domain clinically consistent with that information.
3. Upon review of the definition, defining characteristics or risk factors of a nursing diagnosis; if it is clinically consistent with two or more domains, the nursing diagnosis is placed where the practicing nurse would expect to find it.
4. Some nursing diagnoses cannot be placed because there is no consensus among the members of the Taxonomy Committee. For example, *Deficient Diversional Activity* and *Delayed Surgical Recovery* were not placed because they could fall in several domains and classes.
5. "Risk for" or "Readiness for Enhanced" nursing diagnoses are placed in the same domain and class as the actual nursing diagnosis, when one exists.

Table 3.2 (page 390) shows the placement of the 206 current nursing diagnosis approved by NANDA-I in the NNN Taxonomy of Nursing Practice.

Further Development of the NANDA-I Taxonomy

A multiaxial framework allows clinicians to see where there are gaps and/or potentially useful new diagnoses. If you construct a new diagnosis or a set of diagnoses that is useful to your practice, please submit it (them) to NANDA-I so that others can share in the discovery. Submission guidelines are on page 412. Submission forms can also be found on the NANDA-I website (www.nanda.org) and on the NLINKS (Network for Language In Nursing Knowledge Systems) website (www.nlinks.org). The Diagnostic Development Committee (DDC)

Table 3.2 NNN Taxonomy of Nursing Practice: Placement of Nursing Diagnoses[1]

Domains	Classes	Diagnoses, Outcomes and Interventions	NANDA-I Nursing Diagnoses
I. Functional Includes diagnoses, outcomes, and interventions to promote basic needs	**Activity/Exercise**	Physical activity, including energy conservation and expenditure	*Activity intolerance* *Risk for activity intolerance* *Risk for disuse syndrome* *Risk for falls* *Fatigue* *Impaired bed mobility* *Impaired physical mobility* *Impaired wheelchair mobility* *Impaired transfer ability* *Impaired walking* *Sedentary lifestyle*
	Comfort	A sense of emotional, physical, and spiritual well being and relative freedom from distress	*Nausea* *Acute pain* *Chronic pain* *Disturbed energy field* *Readiness for enhanced comfort* *Impaired comfort*
	Growth and Development	Physical, emotional, and social growth and development milestones	*Risk for delayed development* *Adult failure to thrive* *Delayed growth and development* *Risk for disproportionate growth* *Disorganized infant behavior* *Risk for disorganized infant behavior* *Readiness for enhanced organized infant behavior* *Readiness for enhanced childbearing process*

Nutrition	Processes related to taking in, assimilating, and using nutrients	*Effective breastfeeding* *Ineffective breastfeeding* *Interrupted breastfeeding* *Ineffective infant feeding pattern* *Imbalanced nutrition: less than body requirements* *Imbalanced nutrition: more than body requirements* *Risk for imbalanced nutrition: more than body requirements* *Readiness for enhanced nutrition* *Impaired swallowing*
Self-Care	Ability to accomplish basic and instrumental activities of daily living	*Bathing self-care deficit* *Dressing self-care deficit* *Feeding self-care deficit* *Toileting self-care deficit* *Readiness for enhanced self-care* *Self neglect*
Sexuality	Maintenance or modification of sexual identity and patterns	*Sexual dysfunction* *Ineffective sexuality patterns*
Sleep/Rest	The quantity and quality of sleep, rest and relaxation patterns	*Sleep deprivation* *Insomnia* *Readiness for enhanced sleep* *Disturbed sleep pattern*
Values/Beliefs	Ideas, goals, perceptions, spiritual and other beliefs that influence choices or decisions	*Spiritual distress* *Risk for spiritual distress* *Readiness for enhanced spiritual wellbeing* *Impaired religiosity* *Risk for impaired religiosity* *Readiness for enhanced religiosity* *Moral distress*

Continued

Table 3.2 *Continued*

Domains	*Classes*	*Diagnoses, Outcomes and Interventions*	*NANDA-I Nursing Diagnoses*
II. Physiological Includes diagnoses, outcomes, and interventions to promote optimal biophysical health	**Cardiac Function**	Cardiac mechanisms used to maintain tissue perfusion	*Decreased cardiac output* *Ineffective tissue perfusion* *Risk for decreased cardiac tissue perfusion* *Risk for ineffective cerebral tissue perfusion* *Risk for ineffective gastrointestinal perfusion* *Risk for ineffective renal perfusion* *Ineffective peripheral tissue perfusion* *Risk for shock*
	Elimination	Processes related to secretion and excretion of body wastes	*Bowel incontinence* *Constipation* *Perceived constipation* *Risk for constipation* *Diarrhea* *Functional urinary incontinence* *Reflex urinary incontinence* *Stress urinary incontinence* *Urge urinary incontinence* *Risk for urge urinary incontinence* *Impaired urinary elimination* *Urinary retention* *Readiness for enhanced urinary elimination* *Overflow incontinence* *Neonatal jaundice* *Dysfunctional gastrointestinal motility* *Risk for dysfunctional gastrointestinal motility*

Fluid & Electrolyte	Regulation of fluids/ electrolytes and acid–base balance	Deficient fluid volume Excess fluid volume Risk for deficient fluid volume Readiness for enhanced fluid balance Risk for bleeding Risk for electrolyte imbalance
Neurocognition	Mechanisms related to the nervous system and neurocognitive functioning, including memory, thinking, and judgment	Autonomic dysreflexia Risk for autonomic dysreflexia Acute confusion Ineffective activity planning Chronic confusion Risk for acute confusion Impaired environmental interpretation syndrome Decreased intracranial adaptive capacity Impaired memory Unilateral neglect Disturbed thought processes Wandering
Pharmacological Function	Effects (therapeutic and adverse) of medications or drugs and other pharmacologically active products	

Continued

Table 3.2 *Continued*

Domains	Classes	Diagnoses, Outcomes and Interventions	NANDA-I Nursing Diagnoses
II. Physiological *(Continued)*	Physical Regulation	Body temperature, endocrine, and immune system responses to regulate cellular processes	Latex allergy response Risk for latex allergy response Risk for imbalanced body temperature Hyperthermia Hypothermia Ineffective thermoregulation Risk for infection Risk for peripheral neurovascular dysfunction Ineffective protection Risk for unstable blood glucose level Risk for impaired liver function
	Reproduction	Processes related to human procreation and birth	Risk for disturbed maternal/fetal dyad
	Respiratory Function	Ventilation adequate to maintain arterial blood gases within normal limits	Ineffective airway clearance Risk for aspiration Ineffective breathing pattern Impaired gas exchange Risk for suffocation Impaired spontaneous ventilation Dysfunctional ventilatory weaning response

Sensation/ Perception	Intake and interpretation of information through the senses, including seeing, hearing, touching, tasting, smelling	*Disturbed sensory perception*
Tissue Integrity	Skin and mucous membrane protection to support secretion, excretion, and healing	*Impaired dentition* *Impaired oral mucous membrane* *Impaired skin integrity* *Risk for impaired skin integrity* *Impaired tissue integrity*
Behavior	Actions that promote, maintain, or restore health	*Ineffective health maintenance* *Health-seeking behaviors* *Noncompliance* *Ineffective family therapeutic regimen management* *Readiness for enhanced self-health management* *Ineffective self-health management* *Self-neglect*
Communication	Receiving, interpreting, and expressing spoken, written, and nonverbal messages	*Impaired verbal communication* *Readiness for enhanced communication*

III. Psychosocial
Includes diagnoses, outcomes, and interventions to promote optimal mental and emotional health and social functioning

Continued

Table 3.2 *Continued*

Domains	Classes	Diagnoses, Outcomes and Interventions	NANDA-I Nursing Diagnoses
III. **Psychosocial** *(Continued)*	**Coping**	Adjusting or adapting to stressful events	Risk-prone health behavior
			Decisional conflict
			Ineffective coping
			Ineffective community coping
			Readiness for enhanced community coping
			Defensive coping
			Compromised family coping
			Disabled family coping
			Readiness for enhanced family coping
			Ineffective denial
			Grieving
			Complicated grieving
			Risk for complicated grieving
			Post-trauma syndrome
			Risk for post-trauma syndrome
			Rape-trauma syndrome
			Relocation stress syndrome
			Risk for relocation stress syndrome
			Self-mutilation
			Risk for self-mutilation
			Risk for suicide
			Risk for self-directed violence
			Readiness for enhanced coping
			Stress overload
			Readiness for enhanced decision-making
			Impaired individual resilience
			Risk for compromised resilience
			Readiness for enhanced resilience

Emotional	A mental state or feeling that may influence perceptions of the world	Anxiety Death anxiety Fear Hopelessness Chronic sorrow Readiness for enhanced hope
Knowledge	Understanding and skill in applying information to promote, maintain, and restore health	Deficient knowledge Readiness for enhanced knowledge
Roles/ Relationships	Maintenance and/or modification of expected social behaviors and emotional connectedness with others	Risk for impaired attachment Caregiver role strain Risk for caregiver role strain Parental role conflict Dysfunctional family processes Interrupted family processes Impaired parenting Risk for impaired parenting Ineffective role performance Impaired social interaction Social isolation Risk for other-directed violence Readiness for enhanced family processes Readiness for enhanced parenting Readiness for enhanced relationship

Continued

Table 3.2 *Continued*

Domains	Classes	Diagnoses, Outcomes and Interventions	NANDA-I Nursing Diagnoses
III. Psychosocial *(Continued)*	**Self-Perception**	Awareness of one's body and personal identity	Disturbed body image Disturbed personal identity Risk for loneliness Powerlessness Risk for powerlessness Chronic low self-esteem Situational low self-esteem Risk for situational low self-esteem Readiness for enhanced self-concept Readiness for enhanced power Risk for compromised human dignity
IV. Environmental Includes diagnoses, outcomes, and interventions to promote and protect the environmental health and safety of individuals, systems, and communities	**Healthcare System**	Social, political, and economic structures and processes for the delivery of healthcare services	

| **Populations** | Aggregates of individuals or communities having characteristics in common | |
| **Risk Management** | Avoidance of identifiable health threats | *Impaired home maintenance*
Risk for injury
Risk for perioperative positioning injury
Risk for poisoning
Risk for trauma
Risk for sudden infant death syndrome
Readiness for enhanced immunization
Contamination
Risk for contamination
Risk for vascular trauma |

[1] The taxonomy shown in columns 1 to 3 is in the public domain and can be freely used without permission: neither this taxonomy nor a modification can be copyrighted by any person, group or organization: any use of the taxonomy should acknowledge the source.
Taxonomy from: Dochterman J & Jones D (eds) (2003) Unifying nursing languages: the harmonization of NANDA NIC and NOC. Washington DC: American nurses publishing.

will be glad to help you prepare the submission. For assistance and/or questions, contact the DDC committee chair through the NANDA-I website.

References

Coenen, A., McNeil, B., Bakken, S., Bickford, C., & Warren, J. (2001). Toward comparable nursing data: American Nurses Association criteria for data sets, classification systems, and nomenclatures. *Computers in Nursing* **19**: 240–8.

Dochterman, J.M. & Jones, D. (eds) (2003). *Unifying nursing languages: The harmonization of NANDA, NIC, and NOC.* Washington DC: American Nurses Association.

Gordon. M. (1998). *Manual of nursing diagnosis.* St Louis: Mosby.

Jenny, J. (1994). Advancing the science of nursing with nursing diagnosis. In: Rantz, M. & LeMone, P. (eds), *Classification of nursing diagnoses: Proceedings of the eleventh conference.* Glendale, CA: CINAHL, pp. 73–81.

Johnson, M. & Maas, M. (1997). *Nursing outcomes classification (NOC).* St Louis: Mosby.

NANDA (2001). *NANDA-I nursing diagnoses: Definitions and classifications 2001–2002.* Philadelphia: NANDA.

Pender, N.J., Murdaugh, C.L., & Parsons, M.A. (2006). *Health promotion in nursing practice,* 5th edn. Upper Saddle River, NJ: Pearson Prentice-Hall.

Roget's II: The new thesaurus (1980). Boston: Houghton Mifflin.

Part 4
Nursing Diagnoses Retired from the NANDA-I Taxonomy 2009–2011

Total Urinary Incontinence

Definition Continuous and unpredictable loss of urine

Defining Characteristics

- Constant flow of urine at unpredictable times without uninhibited bladder contractions/spasm or distension
- Lack of bladder filling
- Lack of perineal filling
- Nocturia
- Unawareness of incontinence
- Unsuccessful incontinence refractory treatments

Related Factors

- Anatomic (fistula)
- Disease affecting spinal cord nerves
- Independent contraction of detrusor reflex
- Neurological dysfunction
- Neuropathy preventing transmission of reflex indicating bladder fullness
- Trauma affecting spinal cord nerves

Note: this diagnosis has been removed from the NANDA-I Taxonomy, and will not appear in the Definitions & Classification text, 2012–2014 edition, unless significant work is done to bring this diagnosis up to a LOE 2.1. Any work completed on this diagnosis will need to be submitted to the Diagnosis Development Committee as a new diagnosis.

Rape-Trauma Syndrome: Compound Reaction
(1980)

Definition Forced violent sexual penetration against the victim's will and consent. The trauma syndrome that develops from this attack or attempted attack includes an acute phase of disorganization of the victim's lifestyle and a long-term process of reorganization of lifestyle

Defining Characteristics

- Change in lifestyle (e.g., changes in residence, dealing with repetitive nightmares and phobias, seeking family support, seeking social network support in long-term phase)
- Emotional reaction (e.g., anger, embarrassment, fear of physical violence and death, humiliation, revenge, self-blame in acute phase)
- Multiple physical symptoms (e.g., gastrointestinal irritability, genitourinary discomfort, muscle tension, sleep pattern disturbance in acute phase)
- Reactivated symptoms of previous conditions (e.g., physical illness, psychiatric illness in acute phase)
- Substance abuse (acute phase)

Related Factors

To be developed

Note: this diagnosis has been removed from the NANDA-I Taxonomy, and will not appear in the Definitions & Classification text, 2012–2014 edition, unless significant work is done to bring this diagnosis up to a LOE 2.1. Any work completed on this diagnosis will need to be submitted to the Diagnosis Development Committee as a new diagnosis.

Rape-Trauma Syndrome: Silent Reaction

(1980)

Definition Forced violent sexual penetration against the victim's will and consent. The trauma syndrome that develops from this attack or attempted attack includes an acute phase of disorganization of the victim's lifestyle and a long-term process of reorganization of lifestyle

Defining Characteristics

- Abrupt changes in relationships with men
- Increase in nightmares
- Increased anxiety during interview (e.g., blocking of associations, long periods of silence, minor stuttering, physical distress)
- No verbalization of the occurrence of rape
- Pronounced changes in sexual behavior
- Sudden onset of phobic reactions

Related Factors

To be developed

Note: this diagnosis has been removed from the NANDA-I Taxonomy, and will not appear in the Definitions & Classification text, 2012–2014 edition, unless significant work is done to bring this diagnosis up to a LOE 2.1. Any work completed on this diagnosis will need to be submitted to the Diagnosis Development Committee as a new diagnosis.

Definition Pattern of regulating and integrating into daily living a program for treatment of illness and its sequelae that are satisfactory for meeting specific health goals

Defining Characteristics

- Appropriate choices of daily activities for meeting the goals of a prevention program
- Appropriate choices of daily activities for meeting the goals of a treatment program
- Illness symptoms within a normal range of expectation
- Verbalizes desire to manage the treatment of illness
- Verbalizes desire to manage prevention of sequelae
- Verbalizes intent to reduce risk factors for progression of illness and sequelae

Related Factors

To be developed

Note: this diagnosis will be removed from the NANDA-I Taxonomy, and will not appear in the Definitions & Classification text, 2012–2014 edition, unless significant work is done to bring this diagnosis up to a LOE 2.1. Any work completed on this diagnosis will need to be submitted to the Diagnosis Development Committee as a new diagnosis.

Ineffective Community Therapeutic Regimen Management

(1994)

Definition Pattern of regulating and integrating into community processes programs for treatment of illness and the sequelae of illness that are unsatisfactory for meeting health-related goals

Defining Characteristics

- Deficits in advocates for aggregates
- Deficits in community activities for prevention
- Illness symptoms above the norm expected for the population
- Insufficient healthcare resources (e.g., people, programs)
- Unavailable healthcare resources for illness care
- Unexpected acceleration of illness

Related Factors

To be developed

Note: this diagnosis will be removed from the NANDA-I Taxonomy, and will not appear in the Definitions & Classification text, 2012–2014 edition, unless significant work is done to bring this diagnosis up to a LOE 2.1. Any work completed on this diagnosis will need to be submitted to the Diagnosis Development Committee as a new diagnosis.

Disturbed Thought Processes
(1973, 1996)

Definition Disruption in cognitive operations and activities

Defining Characteristics

- Cognitive dissonance
- Distractibility
- Egocentricity
- Hypervigilance
- Hypovigilance

- Inaccurate interpretation of environment
- Inappropriate thinking
- Memory deficit

Related Factors

To be developed

Note: this diagnosis will be removed from the NANDA-I Taxonomy, and will not appear in the Definitions & Classification text, 2012–2014 edition, unless significant work is done to bring this diagnosis up to a LOE 2.1. Any work completed on this diagnosis will need to be submitted to the Diagnosis Development Committee as a new diagnosis. Note: work is already underway on resubmitting this diagnosis into the NANDA-I Taxonomy.

Part 5
NANDA International
2009–2011

Proposed diagnoses and revisions of diagnoses undergo a systematic review to determine consistency with the established criteria for a nursing diagnosis. All submissions are subsequently staged according to evidence supporting either the level of development or validation.

Diagnoses may be submitted at various levels of development (e.g., label and definition; label, definition, defining characteristics, or risk factors; label, definition, defining characteristics, and related factors). All submissions must include supporting references. Articles used for the submission are to be catalogued in the reference section of the submission form using APA format.

NANDA-I diagnosis submission guidelines are available on the NANDA-I website (www.nanda.org) and the NLINKS website (www.nlinks.org; click on "diagnostic review"). Diagnoses may be submitted electronically using the form available on the NANDA-I website. Diagnoses not submitted electronically should be sent as an e-mail attachment to the DDC chair, using the form provided on the NANDA-I website.

On receipt, the diagnosis will be assigned to a primary reviewer from the Diagnosis Development Committee (DDC). This person will work with the submitter as the DDC reviews for submission.

Full Review Process

New diagnoses go through a *full review process*, which includes the following steps:

1. Review of submission by the primary reviewer.
2. Primary reviewer works with submitter to address changes that need to be made
3. Submission is forwarded to full DDC for review.
4. DDC recommends one of the following:
   (a) Approve with no recommendations
   (b) Approve pending follow-up with recommendations (most frequent DDC decision)
   (c) Disapprove.
5. The primary reviewer forwards the DDC recommendations to the submitter and works with the submitter to make the recommended changes.
6. Submissions approved by the DDC are presented to the NANDA-I membership electronically for review and vote. Recommended changes from the membership must be supported by the literature.
7. Once revisions recommended by the membership have been addressed, the submission is then forwarded to the NANDA International Board of Directors for final approval. Diagnoses accepted at the 2.1 level of evidence will be incorporated into both the

NANDA-I Taxonomy and the NNN Taxonomy of Nursing Practice, and will be published in the next edition of *NANDA-I Nursing Diagnoses: Definitions and Classification*.

Expedited Review Process

An expedited review process (ERP) is appropriate only for proposed revisions of current diagnoses. The ERP is a streamlined process to facilitate rapid review of proposed revisions of diagnoses, when those revisions are determined by the DDC to be minor in nature and when they do not alter the original intent of the diagnoses. Examples of such revisions may include:

- editing and clarification of definition
- limited addition or deletion of defining characteristics, risk factors or related factors.

An ERP includes the following steps:

1. Review of submission by the primary DDC reviewer.
2. Primary reviewer works with submitter to address any needed revisions that may need to be made to enable acceptance of the revised diagnosis.
3. Submission is forwarded to the DDC for review.
4. DDC recommends one of the following:
   (a) Approve with no recommendations
   (b) Approve pending follow-up with recommendations (most frequent DDC decision)
   (c) Disapprove.
5. The primary reviewer forwards the DDC recommendations to the submitter and works with the submitter to make the recommended changes.
6. Submissions approved by the DDC are presented to the NANDA International Board of Directors for final approval. Approval of the proposed revisions is posted on the NANDA-I website.

Submission Process for New Diagnoses

To submit a new diagnosis for consideration by the DDC, follow these steps:

1. Review this edition of *NANDA-I Nursing Diagnoses: Definitions and Classification* and review any potentially related diagnoses in the book. Refer to the NANDA-I Diagnosis Submission Guidelines on the NANDA-I website (www.nanda.org) and/or the NLINKS website (www.nlinks.org; click on "diagnostic review"). Follow the guidelines on the NANDA-I website in case they have been updated since publication of this edition of the NANDA-I book.

2. Contact the Chair of the DDC for more specific instructions, guidelines regarding format, criteria for assigning level of evidence, and protocol for submission.
3. Review "Glossary of Terms" in this edition of *NANDA-I Nursing Diagnoses: Definitions and Classification*.
4. Decide whether your diagnosis is an actual diagnosis, risk diagnosis, wellness diagnosis, or a health-promotion diagnosis.
5. Provide a label for the diagnosis, supported by references. Identify the references.
6. Provide a definition for the diagnosis that is supported by references. Identify the references.
7. Identify the defining characteristics or risk factors for the diagnosis. Actual, wellness, and health-promotion diagnoses have defining characteristics; risk diagnoses have risk factors. To facilitate coding, each defining characteristic and risk factor must contain a single concept rather than multiple concepts. For example, "nausea and vomiting" cannot be listed as a single concept, but rather as two separate concepts (e.g., "nausea" and "vomiting"). References from articles related to the concept (*not from textbooks*) should be used to back up each defining characteristic and risk factor. The references should be research based, if at all possible. If no research-based or nursing references are available, indicate this in your submission.
8. Identify related factors for the actual diagnosis. To facilitate coding, each related factor must contain a single concept rather than multiple concepts. Risk, wellness, and health promotion diagnoses do not have related factors. References are required for each related factor and must be identified (see point 7 above).
9. Develop a bibliography, including all the articles referenced. **The reference list must be in APA format**. Number each reference and link the reference to the component(s) of your submission that the reference supports (e.g., definition, defining characteristic, risk factor, or related factor).
10. Provide up to three examples of appropriate nursing outcomes and nursing interventions from one of the standardized nursing terminologies (e.g., NOC, NIC) for the diagnosis. Although not components of a diagnosis, interventions and outcomes are requested to delineate the role of nursing in treating the diagnosis and the accountability of nursing related to the proposed diagnosis.
11. Use the electronic submission process available on the NANDA-I website.
12. You will be notified when your work is received and will be given an estimate of the time that it will take before you can expect to receive a response from the DDC. Most submissions require some refinement before acceptance into the NANDA-I Taxonomy. You

will be assigned a mentor from the DDC to assist you through the process.

Submission Process for Revising a Current Nursing Diagnosis

To submit a revision of a current diagnosis for consideration by the DDC, follow these steps:

1. Review this edition of *NANDA-I Nursing Diagnoses: Definitions and Classification* and review any potentially related diagnoses in the book. Refer to the NANDA-I Diagnosis Submission Guidelines on the NANDA-I website (www.nanda.org) and/or the NLINKS website (www.nlinks.org; click on "diagnostic review"). Follow the guidelines on the NANDA-I website in case they have been updated since publication of this edition of the NANDA-I book.
2. Contact the Chair of the DDC for more specific instructions, guidelines regarding format, criteria for assigning level of evidence, and protocol for submission.
3. Review "Glossary of Terms" in this edition of *NANDA-I Nursing Diagnoses: Definitions and Classification*.
4. Identify whether the label of the diagnosis requires revision; revise as appropriate. The revision must be supported by references and the references must be identified.
5. Review the definition of the diagnosis to determine if revision is necessary; revise as appropriate. The revision must be supported by references and the references must be identified.
6. Review the defining characteristics or risk factors for the diagnosis. Actual, wellness, and health-promotion diagnoses have defining characteristics; risk diagnoses have risk factors. To facilitate coding, each defining characteristic and risk factor must contain a single concept rather than multiple concepts. For example, "nausea and vomiting" cannot be listed as a single concept, but rather as two separate concepts (e.g., "nausea" and "vomiting"). References from articles related to the concept (*not from text books*) should be used to back up each defining characteristic and risk factor, and must be identified. The references should be research based, if at all possible. If no research-based or nursing references are available, indicate this in your submission.
7. Review the related factors for the actual diagnosis. To facilitate coding, each related factor must contain a single concept rather than multiple concepts. Risk, wellness, and health promotion diagnoses do not have related factors. References are required for each related factor and must be identified (see point 7 above).

8. Develop a bibliography, including all the articles referenced. **The reference list must be in APA format**. Number each reference and link the reference to the component(s) of your submission that the reference supports (e.g., definition, defining characteristic, risk factor or related factor).
9. Use the electronic submission process available on the NANDA-I website.
10. You will be notified when your work is received and will be given an estimate of the time that it will take before you can expect to receive a response from the DDC. Revised diagnoses may undergo a full review process or an expedited review process, depending on the extent of the revisions being proposed. The DDC will make this decision and inform you which process will be followed. Most submissions require some refinement before acceptance into the NANDA-I Taxonomy. You will be assigned a mentor from the DDC to assist you through the process.

Procedure to Appeal a DDC Decision on Diagnosis Review

If a new or revised diagnosis is reviewed by the DDC and returned to the submitter(s) either for revision or because it is judged not to meet one or more criteria for staging a diagnosis, the submitter(s) may appeal the decision.

If the DDC chooses not to accept a new or revised diagnosis, notification of the lack of approval will be given to the submitter(s) with detailed rationale. One or more of the following reasons will be explained:

1. Reject diagnosis (e.g., does not meet criteria for the definition of a nursing diagnosis or does not meet level of evidence criteria)
2. Return – requires substantial revision (e.g., need to make major content changes)
3. Insufficient/old literature support (e.g., failure to reference meta-analyses, concept papers, current research or lack of research articles with reliance on textbooks only)
4. Return with editorial changes (e.g., solicit submitter response to DDC rationale and/or revision to submission).

If the submitter(s) choose(s) to appeal the DDC decision, the proposed new or revised diagnosis will be placed on the NANDA-I website (www.nanda.org) and the appeal will be announced in the journal. A period of 90 days after the distribution of the journal will be provided for members to submit evidence supporting, modifying, or rejecting the submission. After the close of 90 days, the DDC will review feedback and submit a second decision to the submitter(s).

If the DDC chooses not to accept a diagnosis after this second review, the submitter(s) will have an opportunity at the biennial conference to present the submission and the rationale for the disagreement with the DDC decision. The presentation will occur in an open session and require evidence-based argument from the submitter(s) and the DDC about the decision. Conference attendees will also have the opportunity to present evidence-based argument supporting, modifying, or rejecting the submission. Following this presentation, the DDC will review all information and forward a decision to the submitter(s) and the NANDA-I Board of Directors.

The NANDA-I Board of Directors will have an opportunity to provide evidence-based argument supporting, modifying or rejecting submission at two points:

1. During the open forum at the biennial conference
2. After the conference in its final review of the DDC recommendations for approval. A decision by the Board to modify or reject the DDC's recommendation must be evidence based and at the same LOE or higher as the evidence presented by the submitter(s) and/or by the DDC.

NANDA-I Diagnosis Submission: Level of Evidence Criteria

1. Received for Development (Consultation from DDC)

1.1 Label Only

This level is intended primarily for submission by organized groups rather than individuals. The label is clear, stated at a basic level, and is supported by literature references, and these are identified. The DDC will consult with the submitter and provide education related to diagnostic development through printed guidelines and workshops. At this stage the label is categorized as "Received for Development" and identified as such on the NANDA-I website.

1.2 Label and Definition

The label is clear and stated at a basic level. The definition is consistent with the label. The label and definition are distinct from other NANDA-I diagnoses and definitions. The definition differs from the defining characteristics and label, and these components are not included in the definition. At this stage, the diagnosis must be consistent with the current NANDA-I definition of nursing diagnosis (page 417). The label and definition is supported by literature references and these are identified.

2. Accepted for Publication and Inclusion in the NANDA-I Taxonomy

2.1 Label, Definition, Defining Characteristics or Risk Factors, Related Factors, and References

References are cited for the definition, each defining characteristic or risk factor, and each related factor. In addition, it is required that nursing outcomes and nursing interventions from a standardized nursing terminology (e.g., NOC, NIC) be provided for each diagnosis. If approved, the diagnosis will be forwarded to the Taxonomy Committee for classification within the NANDA-I taxonomy.

2.2 Concept Analysis

The criteria in 2.1 are met. In addition, a narrative review of relevant literature, culminating in a written concept analysis, is required to demonstrate the existence of a substantive body of knowledge underlying the diagnosis. The literature review/concept analysis supports the label and definition, and includes discussion and support of the defining characteristics, risk factors (for risk diagnoses), or related factors (for actual diagnoses).

2.3 Consensus Studies Related to Diagnosis Using Experts

The criteria in 2.1 are met. Studies include those soliciting expert opinion, Delphi, and similar studies of diagnostic components in which nurses are subjects.

3. Clinically Supported (Validation and Testing)

3.1 Literature Synthesis

The criteria in 2.2 are met. The synthesis is in the form of an integrated review of the literature. Search terms/MESH terms used in the review are provided to assist future researchers.

3.2 Clinical Studies Related to Diagnosis, but Not Generalizable to the Population

The criteria in 2.2 are met. The narrative includes a description of studies related to the diagnosis, which includes defining characteristics or risk factors, and related factors. Studies may be qualitative in nature, or quantitative studies using nonrandom samples in which patients are subjects.

3.3 Well-designed Clinical Studies with Small Sample Sizes

The criteria in 2.2 are met. The narrative includes a description of studies related to the diagnosis, which includes defining characteristics or risk factors, and related factors. Random sampling is used in these studies, but the sample size is limited.

3.4 Well-designed Clinical Studies with Random Sample of Sufficient Size to Allow for Generalizability to the Overall Population

The criteria in 2.2 are met. The narrative includes a description of studies related to the diagnosis, which includes defining characteristics or risk factors, and related factors. Random sampling is used in these studies and the sample size is sufficient to allow for generalizability of results to the overall population.

Glossary of Terms

Nursing Diagnoses

Nursing Diagnosis

A clinical judgment about individual, family, or community responses to actual or potential health problems/life processes. A nursing diagnosis provides the basis for selection of nursing interventions to achieve outcomes for which the nurse is accountable (approved at the ninth NANDA Conference, 1990).

Actual Nursing Diagnosis

Describes human responses to health conditions/life processes that exist in an individual, family, or community. It is supported by defining characteristics (manifestations, signs, and symptoms) that cluster in patterns of related cues or inferences.

Health-promotion Nursing Diagnosis

Clinical judgment of a person's, family's, or community's motivation and desire to increase wellbeing and actualize human health potential as expressed in the readiness to enhance specific health behaviors, such as nutrition and exercise. Health-promotion diagnoses can be used in any health state and do not require current levels of wellness. This readiness is supported by defining characteristics. Interventions are selected in concert with the individual/family/community to best ensure the ability to reach the stated outcomes.

Risk Nursing Diagnosis

Describes human responses to health conditions/life processes that may develop in a vulnerable individual, family, or community. It is supported by risk factors that contribute to increased vulnerability.

Syndrome

A cluster or group of signs and symptoms that almost always occur together. Together, these clusters represent a distinct clinical picture. (McCourt, 1991, p. 79)

Wellness Nursing Diagnosis

Describes human responses to levels of wellness in an individual, family, or community. It is supported by defining characteristics (manifestations, signs, and symptoms) that cluster in patterns of related cues or inferences.

Components of a Nursing Diagnosis
Diagnosis Label

Provides a name for a diagnosis. It is a concise term or phrase that represents a pattern of related cues. It may include modifiers.

Definition

Provides a clear, precise description; delineates its meaning and helps differentiate it from similar diagnoses.

Defining Characteristics

Observable cues/inferences that cluster as manifestations of an actual, wellness or health promotion diagnosis.

Risk Factors

Environmental factors and physiological, psychological, genetic, or chemical elements that increase the vulnerability of an individual, family, group or community to an unhealthy event.

Related Factors

Factors that appear to show some type of patterned relationship with the nursing diagnosis. Such factors may be described as antecedent to, associated with, related to, contributing to, or abetting. Only actual nursing diagnoses have related factors.

Definitions for Classification of Nursing Diagnoses
Classification

Systematic arrangement of related phenomena in groups or classes based on characteristics that objects have in common

Level of Abstraction

Describes the concreteness/abstractness of a concept:

- Very abstract concepts are theoretical, may not be directly measurable, defined by concrete concepts, inclusive of concrete concepts, disassociated from any specific instance, independent of time and space, have more general descriptors, and may not be clinically useful for planning treatment.
- Concrete concepts are observable and measurable, limited by time and space, constitute a specific category, more exclusive, name a real thing or class of things, restricted by nature, may be clinically useful for planning treatment.

Nomenclature

A system of designations (terms) elaborated according to pre-established rules (American Nurses Association, 1999)

Taxonomy

Classification according to presumed natural relationships among types and their subtypes (American Nurses Association, 1999)

References

American Nurses' Association (1999). *ANA CNP II Recognition Criteria and Definitions*. Washington DC: ANA.
McCourt, A. (1991). In: Carroll-Johnson, R.M. (ed.), *Classification of Nursing Diagnoses: Proceedings of the ninth conference*. Philadelphia, PA: Lippincott, p. 79.

NANDA International 2006–2008

NANDA International Board of Directors

President   T. Heather Herdman, RN, PhD
President-Elect   Dickon Weir-Hughes, RN, EdD, FRSH
Treasurer   Anne Perry, RN, EdD, FAAN
Directors   Jane Brokel, RN, PhD
                   Dame June Clark, RN, PhD, RHV, FRNC, DBE
                   Leann Scroggins, RN, MS, CRRN-A, APRN BC
                   Gunn Von Krogh, RN, MNSc

NANDA International Diagnosis Development Committee

Co-Chairs   Leann Scroggins, RN, MS, CRRN-A, APRN BC
                   Geralyn Meyer, RN, PhD
Members   Dorothy Jones, RN, EdD, FAAN
                   Shigemi Kamitsuru, RN, PhD
                   Marlene Lindeman, RN, MSN, CS
                   Meridean Maas, RN, PhD, FAAN
                   Lina Rahal, RN, Med

NANDA International Taxonomy Committee

Chair   Barbara Vassallo, RN, EdD, CS, ANPC
Members   Sally Decker, RN, PhD
                   Carme Espinosa, RN
                   J. Adolf Guirao Goris, RN
                   Marion Johnson, RN, PhD
                   Mikyoung Lee, RN, PhD
                   Carol Soares O'Hearn, RN, PhD, CPRQ
                   Elizabeth Rose, RN, PhD

An Invitation to Join
NANDA International

Words are powerful. They allow us to communicate ideas and experience to others so that they may share our understanding. Nursing diagnoses are an example of a powerful and precise terminology that highlights and renders visible the unique contribution of nursing to global health. Nursing diagnoses communicate the professional judgments that nurses make everyday to our patients, our colleagues, members of other disciplines, and the public. They are our words.

NANDA International's Commitment

NANDA International is a member-driven, grassroots organization committed to the development of nursing diagnostic terminology. The desired outcome of the Association's work is to provide nurses at all levels and in all areas of practice with a standardized nursing terminology with which to:

- name client responses to actual or potential health problems, life processes, and wellness
- document care for reimbursement of nursing services
- contribute to the development of informatics and information standards, ensuring the inclusion of nursing terminology in electronic healthcare records
- facilitate study of the phenomena of concern to nurses for the purpose of improving patient care.

Nursing terminology is the key to defining the future of nursing practice and NANDA International is in the forefront. Join us and become a part of this exciting process!

Involvement Opportunities

The participation of NANDA International members is critical to the growth and development of nursing terminology. Many opportunities exist for participation on committees, in the development, use, and refinement of diagnoses, and in research. Opportunities also exist for international liaison work and networking with nursing leaders.

Benefits of Membership

1. Subscription to the *International Journal of Nursing Terminologies and Classifications*
2. Reduced fee at the NANDA-I conference

3. Participation in debate and decisions about new and revised diagnoses
4. State-of-the-art information on development of nursing terminology systems, which enable nurses to communicate with each other around the world
5. Reduced rate on in-house publications, such as *Nursing Diagnoses: Definitions and Classification*
6. Resources for networking and research data
7. Access to the NANDA International web page – www.nanda.org – with links to minutes of Board meetings and all current decisions and initiatives
8. Access to NLINKS – www.nlinks.org – an online opportunity to participate in nursing diagnosis research

NANDA International:
A Member-driven Organization

Our Vision

NANDA International will be a global force for the development and use of nursing's standardized terminology to improve the healthcare of all people.

Our Mission

To facilitate the development, refinement, dissemination and use of standardized nursing diagnostic terminology.

- We provide the world's leading evidence-based nursing diagnoses for use in practice and to determine interventions and outcomes.
- We fund research through the NANDA-I Foundation.
- We are a supportive and energetic global network of nurses who are committed to improving the quality of nursing care through evidence-based practice.

Our Purpose

Implementation of nursing diagnosis enhances every aspect of nursing practice, from garnering professional respect to assuring accurate documentation for reimbursement.

NANDA International exists to develop, refine, and promote terminology that accurately reflects nurses' clinical judgments. This unique, evidence-based perspective includes social, psychological. and spiritual dimensions of care.

Our History

NANDA (North American Nursing Diagnosis Association), which was founded in 1982, grew out of the National Conference Group, a task force established at the First National Conference on the Classification of Nursing Diagnoses, held in St Louis, Missouri, USA in 1973.This conference and the ensuing task force ignited interest in the concept of standardizing nursing terminology. In 2002 NANDA was re-launched as NANDA International to reflect increasing worldwide interest in the field of nursing terminology development.

NANDA International has approved more than 200 diagnoses for clinical use, testing, and refinement. A dynamic, international process of diagnosis review and classification approves and updates terms and definitions for identified human responses. In collaboration with the Nursing Classification Center at the University of Iowa, USA, NANDA International has developed a nursing practice taxonomy and class structure. This system allows for the placement of NANDA International diagnoses in an organizing framework that accommodates interventions and outcomes from the Nursing Interventions Classification (NIC) and the Nursing Outcomes Classification (NOC), thus creating a comprehensive language system capable of documenting nursing care in a standardized manner.

NANDA International has international networks in Brazil, Argentina, Columbia, Peru, and Venezuela; other countries and/or language groups interested in forming a NANDA International Network should contact the President of NANDA International at president@nanda. org. NANDA-I also has collaborative links with nursing terminology societies around the world such as the Japanese Society of Nursing Diagnoses (JSND), the Association for Common European Nursing Diagnoses, Interventions and Outcomes (ACENDIO), the Asociacíon Española de Nomenclatura, Taxonomia y Diagnóstico de Enfermeria (AENTDE) and the Association Francophone Européenne des Diagnostics Interventions Résuitats Infirmiers (AFEDI). Joint membership is available with some of these organizations; contact us to see if a joint membership is available with other organizations related to standardized nursing language to which you belong.

NANDA International Taxonomy

- International Standards Organization (ISO) compatible
- Health Level 7 (HL7) registered
- SNOMED-CT available
- Unified Medical Language System (UMLS) compatible
- American Nurses' Association (ANA) recongnized terminology

The NANDA International taxonomy is available in: Chinese, Dutch, English (US and British), French, German, Icelandic, Italian, Japanese, Norwegian, Portuguese and Spanish.

For more information, and to apply for membership online, please visit www.nanda.org.

Our Services Include:

- Professional Networking
- Consulting Services
- International Conferences
- Member Discounts
- Reference Publications:
  - *Journal*
  - *Taxonomy*
  - *Books*
  - *Website*
- . . . and more!

Apply for membership online at: www.nanda.org

Or call: (+1) (920) 344-8670

Do You Have a Nursing Diagnosis to Contribute?

Nursing diagnostic terminology is a living, breathing creation. You are invited to submit your diagnoses or diagnostic refinements to our Diagnosis Development Committee. Contact the NANDA International Office for submission forms and guidelines or find them online at:
www.nanda.org or
www.nlinks.org

Your input matters!

NANDA International

P.O. Box 157
Kaukauna, WI 54130-0157

TEL (+1) (920) 344-8670

www.nanda.org

☐ YES! I WANT TO SUPPORT THE NURSING TERMINOLOGY MOVEMENT. PLEASE ACCEPT MY APPLICATION FOR NANDA INTERNATIONAL MEMBERSHIP:

☐ Regular Membership (RN's only).. USD $105*
☐ Retired Membership .... USD $65*
☐ Associate Membership (non RN's welcome)... USD $105*
☐ Student Membership.. USD $35*

(Open to matriculating undergraduate students. Proof of enrollment required; limited to three years.) Institutional membership is also available. Contact our office for details.

☐ Send _____ copy(ies) of Nursing Diagnoses
  at special member's price: @ USD $29.99/ea. $_____

☐ Send _____ copy(ies) of Critical Thinking & Nursing
  Diagnoses at special member's price: @ USD $19.95/ea. $_____

☐ I am also enclosing my tax deductible donation
  to the NANDA-I Foundation: $_____

TOTAL ENCLOSED $_____
NANDA-I's Federal Tax Identification Number is 41-1363777.

☐ Check enclosed   ☐ Money Order enclosed
(Payable to NANDA-I. NANDA-I can only accept checks in US dollars.)

☐ Charge my credit card: ☐ Amex   ☐ MC   ☐ Visa

CARD #_____
Signature_____   Exp. Date_____/_____

* USD $29 of this amount is for your one-year subscription to
The International Journal of Nursing Terminologies and Classifications.

PLEASE PRINT

_____
FIRST NAME   M.I.

_____
LAST NAME AND CREDENTIALS

_____
CURRENT LICENSE NUMBER

_____
POSITION / TITLE(S)

_____
COMPANY / INSTITUTION

_____
DEPARTMENT

_____
MAILING ADDRESS   ☐ HOME   ☐ BUSINESS

_____

_____
CITY

_____
STATE / PROVINCE   ZIP /POSTAL CODE

_____
COUNTRY

_____
TELEPHONE   FAX

_____
E-MAIL ADDRESS

Who referred you to NANDA International? _____

US-Registered RN's only: Are you an ANA Member?   ☐Yes   ☐No

What is your clinical specialty? _____

Please contact the NANDA-I office to see if a joint membership is available with other organizations that you belong to.

☐ Please remove my name for rented mail lists.

Index

Page numbers in *italics* refer to figures; those in **bold** to tables.

The Official Journal of NANDA International

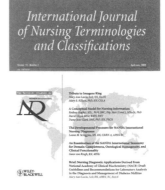

It's time to take a closer look at the *International Journal of Nursing Terminologies and Classifications* (IJNTC) – the official journal of NANDA International. *IJNTC* edited by Georgia Griffith Whitley, RN, EdD, is *the* nursing journal that documents the science behind the diagnoses and their applications for nurses, educators, and administrators. Each quarterly issue will help you stay current on global efforts to include critical nursing terminology in health databases. You'll want to read the journal articles for:

- Scientific documentation of the validity of individual diagnoses and the concepts underlying them
- Methodologies for development, testing, and classification of diagnoses
- Computer applications of standardized nursing language
- Linguistic dilemmas involved in translating diagnoses across different languages
- Educational ramifications of teaching and measuring critical thinking processes in students
- Expanded uses for standardized nursing languages across treatment settings and specialty areas
- NANDA International Society news

Plus, all issues are available online back to Volume 1! That means, through a member, individual, or library subscription, readers can conduct research on articles published dating back to 1990.

Subscriptions are available to individuals, and institutions and at a reduced rate to members of NANDA-International. To recommend a subscription to your library contact http://www.blackwellpublishing.com/librarians/librecfm.asp

For information on becoming a member (including institutional, student and retired memberships) of NANDA International or for details on your member access, please see http://www.nanda.org/html/membership.html

For individual subscriptions visit http://www.blackwellpublishing.com/ijnt